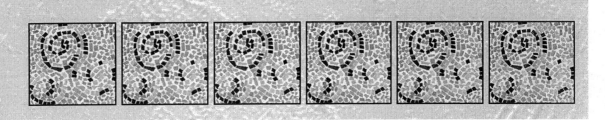

Study Guide for
Monahan and Neighbors

Medical-Surgical Nursing

*Foundations
for Clinical Practice*

2nd Edition

Karen L. Burger, PhD, RN, MSN

Professor
Department of Nursing
Columbus State Community College
Columbus, Ohio

W.B. SAUNDERS COMPANY

A Division of Harcourt Brace & Company

Philadelphia   London   Toronto   Montreal   Sydney   Tokyo

W.B. SAUNDERS COMPANY

A Division of Harcourt Brace & Company

The Curtis Center
Independence Square West
Philadelphia, Pennsylvania 19106

Study Guide for Monahan and Neighbors
MEDICAL-SURGICAL NURSING:
Foundations for Clinical Practice, Second Edition

ISBN 0-7216-7553-0

Printed in the United States of America.

Last digit is the print number: 9   8   7   6   5   4   3   2   1

PREFACE

This Study Guide was developed to accompany *Medical-Surgical Nursing: Foundations for Clinical Practice*, 2/e, by Frances Donovan Monahan and Marianne Neighbors. Its goal is to assist you in comprehending and applying basic information, concepts, disease processes, and nursing interventions as presented in the text.

While this guide is primarily intended for self-directed learning, it should also prove to be a valuable tool to use to review classroom material and to prepare for examinations, including the NCLEX exam.

The Study Guide follows the corresponding chapters in the text. Each Study Guide chapter begins with the learning objectives. Within each chapter are a variety of learning experiences that may include short answers, true/false questions, identification exercises, matching exercises, and multiple choice questions.

While some of the learning opportunities are a reflection of basic knowledge, others will require you to apply that knowledge in a variety of practice arenas. You will develop nursing care plans and use critical thinking skills as you answer the case studies that are included with each chapter.

Applying basic knowledge and using the nursing process to make appropriate nursing decisions are important nursing skills. This Study Guide should assist you in these endeavors. As always, this Study Guide was written with my students in mind. I hope it will be a useful tool.

CONTENTS

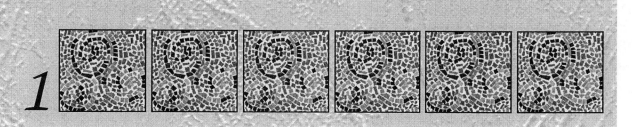

Introduction to the Practice of Medical-Surgical Nursing

Objectives

1.0 Demonstrate an understanding of the professional aspects of nursing.
    1.1 List five areas of practice for nurses.
    1.2 List two specialized roles for nurses.
    1.3 Define the practice of nursing.
    1.4 Define standards of practice.

2.0 Examine trends in nursing.
    2.1 Describe changes in society that will impact nursing.
    2.2 Describe ways that nurses can influence the changes in health care.
    2.3 Identify national policies that affect the nursing care of adults.

3.0 Demonstrate an understanding of the nursing process.
    3.1 List the five phases of the nursing process.
    3.2 Describe the nursing diagnosis statement.
    3.3 Explain the planning phase of the nursing process.
    3.4 Identify reasons for using the nursing process.

4.0 Demonstrate an understanding of clinical pathways.
    4.1 List the components of a clinical pathway.
    4.2 Identify reasons for using clinical pathways in medical-surgical practice.

Learning Activities

Short Answers

1. Probably one of the most compelling reasons for current changes in health care is a desire to _____ cost.

2. Changes in health care have resulted in _____ hospital stays.

3. A _____ _____ is a guideline for patient care.

4. Nurses today must recognize the needs of a _____ and _____ society.

5. The health profile of American adults is often determined by the analysis of _____.

Knowledge Base

6. List five areas of employment for nurses today.

7. List two of the specialized roles available in nursing.

8. Describe what you believe to be the nature of nursing practice today.

9. Define the term *standards of practice* and explain why it is important.

10. What organization was responsible for the development of the *Standards of Medical/Surgical Nursing Practice*?

11. List several changes in society that you believe will influence the future practice of nursing.

12. Based on the changes you have identified, describe how nurses can influence the future practice of nursing.

13. List several ways that the medical-surgical nurse can become more sensitive to the cultural norms and values of the patient.

14. Three broad goals for the United States that are published in *Healthy People 2000* are

    1.

    2.

    3.

15. What group was responsible for developing a system for nursing diagnoses?

16. List the five phases of the nursing process.

    1.

    2.

    3.

    4.

    5.

17. Define the term *nursing diagnosis*.

18. List and define the three components of the nursing diagnosis.
    1.

    2.

    3.

19. List the four steps of the planning phase of the nursing process.
    1.

    2.

    3.

    4.

20. How can the nurse determine if the patient outcome has been achieved?

21. How would the nurse determine which problem has the highest priority?

22. If, after the nursing care plan is implemented, the patient outcome is not achieved, what questions should the nurse ask?

True/False

23. _____ The nursing process can be described as the essence of nursing.

24. _____ The nursing process allows nursing care to be individualized.

25. _____ The nursing process only includes the patient in the nurse's care.

26. _____ The nursing diagnosis promotes continuity of care.

27. _____ Each nursing diagnosis can have only one patient outcome.

*L*earner Self-Evaluation

Do I fully understand the content? If no, then the areas I need to review are:

I need more information from my instructor on:

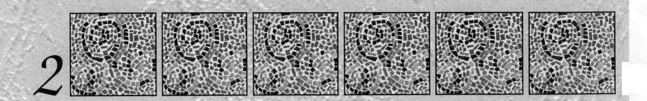

2

Medical-Surgical Nursing in Multiple Settings

*O*bjectives

1.0 Demonstrate an understanding of the changes in health care and society that affect nursing.

    1.1 Identify factors responsible for the shift in health care from the hospital to the community.

    1.2 Identify vulnerable populations in the U.S.

    1.3 Identify nonhospital settings where nurses work.

    1.4 Describe the role of the nurse in discharge planning.

    1.5 Identify future nursing roles.

2.0 Demonstrate an understanding of managed care and case management.

    2.1 Identify the members of the health-care team.

    2.2 Identify skills performed by different members of the health-care team.

    2.3 Examine the changing roles of nurses working in home care.

*L*earning Activities

Short Answers

1. List three factors that have contributed to the shift in patient care from the hospital to community-based services.

    1.

    2.

    3.

2. List four ways that patients cover health-care costs.

    1.

    2.

    3.

    4.

3. The U.S. Commerce Department's Census Bureau has reported that _____ million people were living below the poverty level in 1995.

4. Approximately _____ % of the nation's population does not have health insurance.

5. A significant change in society is the increased prevalence of _____ violence.

6. It has been estimated that before 2010, _____ percent of insured patients will receive care through a managed system.

7. In a nursing-managed care center, _____ and _____ are paramount.

8. _____ is a palliative system of health care that provides services to the terminally ill.

9. For a nurse working in a nonhospital practice setting, care is based on _____.

10. List several nonhospital settings in which nurses work.

True/False

11. _____ Health-care costs in the U.S. have risen faster and higher than in any other industrialized nation.

12. _____ Providing health care in community-based settings is one way to reduce health-care costs.

13. _____ There is no correlation between poverty and health status.

14. _____ Managed care organizations arrange for health care at predetermined rates.

15. _____ Many ambulatory care centers provide inpatient services.

16. _____ Nurses who work in the community are often part of a multidisciplinary health-care team.

17. _____ Nurse practitioners can engage in independent or collaborative nursing practice.

Knowledge Application

18. Health-care expenditures are measured as a percentage of the U.S. gross national product (GNP). How much of the GNP does the U.S. currently allocate for health care?
    A. 10%
    B. 16%
    C. 22%
    D. 33%

19. Which of the following statements about the population over age 65 in the U.S. is NOT true?
    A. Most older people have at least one chronic illness.
    B. Almost 25% of those living in the community need help with activities of daily living.
    C. Elderly patients will need community services and institutional based services.
    D. Since 1900, the percentage of U.S. citizens over 65 has doubled.

20. If a worker is part of a health maintenance organization (HMO), this means
    A. the health plan contracts with medical groups to provide a full range of services
    B. the patient can choose any physician within his or her county
    C. the plan reduces costs by establishing a network of preferred providers
    D. all costs are fully covered

21. In a case management system, the nurse
    A. helps determine costs
    B. coordinates health care of enrolled patients
    C. determines who is eligible
    D. provides direct patient care

22. The primary care providers in nurse-managed care centers are usually
    A. physicians
    B. licensed practical nurses
    C. associate degree nurses
    D. nurse practitioners

23. Facilities that have been established to care for frail, older patients during daytime hours are called
    A. outpatient care centers
    B. extended care facilities
    C. nursing clinics
    D. adult day health centers

24. In order for Medicare patients to be eligible for home-based care, they must meet which of the following criteria? (Check all that apply.)
    A. _____ They must be over age 65.
    B. _____ They must be homebound.
    C. _____ They must have a chronic illness.
    D. _____ They need intermittent skilled nursing care.
    E. _____ They need complete physical care.

25. The focus of care in a hospice is to
    A. prolong life
    B. improve the quality of life
    C. continue to seek curative treatment
    D. provide active treatment for the illness

26. Which of the following statements best defines unlicensed assistive personnel? They
    A. help the nurse with direct patient care
    B. can do anything the nurse delegates
    C. perform without direct supervision
    D. are trained and certified but not licensed to perform nursing tasks

27. To be sure that all patients receive continuity of health care, an agency will often employ a
    A. physician planner
    B. social worker
    C. discharge planner
    D. home care nurse

28. The roles of the home health nurse are diverse. Which of the following services would the home health nurse provide? (Check all that apply.)
    A. _____ Do patient evaluations.
    B. _____ Develop a plan of care.
    C. _____ Provide skilled nursing care.
    D. _____ Serve as case manager.
    E. _____ Make referrals.

Food for Thought

Who will care for the aging population in the U.S. if the current Medicare/Medicaid system fails?

Is access to health care related to the ability to pay?

Do you believe that the use of unlicensed assistive personnel changes the quality of health care?

How do you think the delivery of health care may change by the next century?

*L*earner Self-Evaluation

Do I fully understand the content? If no, then the
areas I need to review are:

I need more information from my instructor on:

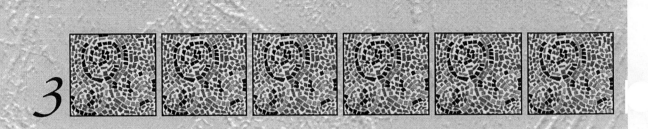

3

Death, Dying, and Bereavement

*O*bjectives

1.0 Demonstrate an understanding of death as a developmental stage of life.
    1.1 List the five stages of death and dying.
    1.2 List several of the final tasks to be completed if one is to achieve acceptance of death.
    1.3 Develop a nursing care plan that reflects the psychosocial care of the dying patient.
    1.4 Demonstrate an understanding of the nurse's role in working with individuals who are dying.

2.0 Demonstrate an understanding of the bereavement process.
    2.1 Apply the nursing process to the person suffering bereavement.
    2.2 Demonstrate application of the nursing process to the care of the person with dysfunctional grieving.

3.0 Demonstrate an understanding of how religious beliefs and practices relate to death and bereavement.
    3.1 Identify characteristics of several religious beliefs.
    3.2 Demonstrate application of the nursing process to the care of the dying patient in spiritual distress.

4.0 Review other aspects of death and dying.
    4.1 List the characteristics found in an ideal hospice .
    4.2 List several of the core experiences of a near-death experience.
    4.3 List the legal criteria for death.
    4.4 Demonstrate an understanding of do not resuscitate (DNR) orders.
    4.5 Examine your personal beliefs about death and dying.

*L*earning Activities

Short Answers

1. _____ is a natural part of life.

2. Kubler-Ross called death the final state of ___ _____ .

3. When the reality of death registers, individuals often exhibit signs of _____ .

4. _____ is the antidote for fear and despair.

5. A basic human drive that motivates all of us is a desire for _____.

6. _____ of death is not fully experienced by many.

7. After the death of a child, parents are often overwhelmed by feelings of _____.

8. Dying is the final _____ stage of life.

9. List the five stages of grief and dying as identified by Elisabeth Kubler-Ross.
    1.

    2.

    3.

    4.

    5.

10. List four of the final tasks that the dying person must accomplish to reach the final stage of acceptance of death.
    1.

    2.

    3.

    4.

11. List several of the characteristics found in an ideal hospice.

12. List some of the common characteristics of the phenomenon of near-death experience.

13. List four of the six criteria for the definition of brain death that is commonly used today.
    1.

    2.

    3.

    4.

Knowledge Application

14. It is essential that nurses provide hope because it is the antidote to
    A. depression
    B. grief
    C. fear
    D. anger

15. The stage of death and dying in which the individual promises to do a particular thing in exchange for a longer life is
    A. anger
    B. depression
    C. decision-making
    D. bargaining

16. One way that the nurse can help a patient with a terminal illness cope with death would be to encourage the patient to
    A. review his or her life
    B. make up a living will
    C. seek spiritual guidance
    D. focus on recovering

17. The first emotion felt by the bereaved individual after the death of a loved one is usually
    A. anger
    B. shock
    C. depression
    D. disbelief

18. During a conversation with the nurse, a patient says, "Why bother getting dressed or eating, it won't make any difference." This indicates the stage of

    A. depression

    B. grief

    C. indifference

    D. melancholy

19. As a health-care professional, the nurse is aware that the grieving process can last as long as

    A. 3–6 months

    B. 6–12 months

    C. 1–2 years

    D. 2–4 years

20. Which of the individuals listed would be most at risk for developing dysfunctional grieving?

    A. a parent who has lost a young child in an accident

    B. a daughter who has emotional problems and fought frequently with her mother who has died

    C. a wife who lost her husband to cancer after two years

    D. a son who loses his father from a stroke at age 64

21. After an unexpected death, survivors often show signs of emotional stress. This is often due to the fact that

    A. the survivor feels guilty

    B. opportunities for closure are denied

    C. the survivor wishes they had died instead

    D. death is always stressful

22. Mourning is a process of "letting go." Which of the following tasks would NOT be considered part of this process?

    A. accepting the reality of the loss

    B. emotionally withdrawing energy from the deceased

    C. focusing on an environment that includes the deceased

    D. working through the pain of grief

23. In which of the following religions would the nurse recognize that after death only family and close friends may touch the body?

    A. Hinduism

    B. Christianity

    C. Judaism

    D. Islam

24. For members of which major religious group would it be inappropriate to ask permission for organ donation?

    A. Buddhism

    B. Hinduism

    C. Judaism

    D. Islam

True/False

25. _____ All dying patients will experience all the stages of grief and dying.

26. _____ The stages of death and dying follow the same sequence for all patients.

27. _____ Nurses should examine their own philosophies about death to be better equipped to care for dying patients.

28. _____ Spiritual needs do not have a significant effect during a time of illness.

29. _____ To meet the spiritual needs of patients, nurses must be very religious themselves.

30. _____ The living will is a legally binding document.

Nursing Care Plans

31. Write a nursing care plan that addresses the needs of Ms. H., who is dying from lung cancer, using the following nursing diagnosis.

    Nursing diagnosis: Anticipatory grieving related to impending death.

    Patient outcome:

    Interventions:

32. Write a nursing care plan for Mrs. N., who is exhibiting signs of spiritual distress following the death of her spouse of 50 years. Use the following nursing diagnosis.

    Nursing diagnosis: Spiritual distress related to inability to engage in usual religious practices.

    Patient outcome:

    Interventions:

33. As an office nurse you receive a call from 21-year-old Ms. D., who has symptoms of dysfunctional grieving following the death of her father. Use the following nursing diagnosis

    Nursing diagnosis: Dysfunctional grieving related to ambivalent feelings resulting from unresolved conflict with the deceased.

    Patient outcome:

    Interventions:

Food for Thought

Examine your personal beliefs about death and dying. Have any of your beliefs changed since studying nursing? Can you successfully interact with a dying patient?

Case Study

Mrs. F. is 78 years old and has terminal cancer. Currently she is hospitalized for dehydration. She is expected to live less than two weeks. She is very weak and in constant pain. She lives alone and has no family.

34. If Mrs. F. should suddenly stop breathing, what would be an appropriate intervention by the nurse?

    A. Start CPR.

    B. Call the physician.

    C. Do nothing.

    D. Get the chart.

35. Mrs. F. has made out a living will. This means

    A. if sudden death occurs you would do nothing

    B. it is an expression of her wishes only, but not legally binding in all states

    C. it means you must follow her wishes or risk prosecution

    D. it is meaningless; you would still resuscitate her

36. Mrs. F. says, "I was very angry when I first found out I had cancer, but now I just don't care about anything at all." What stage is she in?

    A. bargaining

    B. denial

    C. depression

    D. acceptance

37. In order for this patient to reach the final stage of acceptance, what should the patient do?

    A. develop awareness of impending death

    B. balance hope and fear

    C. detach herself from former experiences

    D. all of the above

38. The nurse notices a Bible and a crucifix at the bedside. What would be an appropriate question to determine if the patient is in need of spiritual comfort?

    A. "Would you like to tell me about your spiritual beliefs?"

    B. "What can I do to help you spiritually?"

    C. "Would you like to see a spiritual advisor?"

    D. any of the above

39. Mrs. F. says that she wants a peaceful death, without pain. A DNR order is written. Which of the following statements is NOT true about a DNR order?

    A. It should not be written unless the patient is consulted and approves of the order.

    B. The responsible attending physician writes the order in the chart.

    C. Once a DNR order is written, no further medical treatment is begun.

    D. The DNR order can be rescinded at any time.

$\mathcal{L}$earner Self-Evaluation

Do I fully understand the content? If no, then the areas I need to review are:

I need more information from my instructor on:

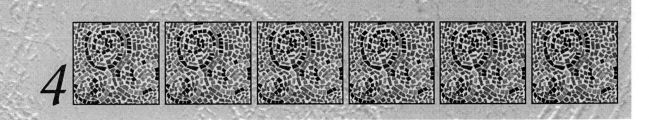

Special Considerations for Nursing Care of Elderly Patients

Objectives

1.0 Demonstrate an understanding of the changes associated with the normal aging process.
  1.1 Identify normal assessment findings in the elderly.
  1.2 Identify changes in the body systems related to aging.
  1.3 Identify nutritional needs of the elderly.
  1.4 Identify important considerations related to drug metabolism in the elderly.

2.0 Plan appropriate interventions for elderly patients with changes related to the normal aging process.
  2.1 Identify some teaching needs of the elderly.
  2.2 Identify nursing interventions to help the elderly cope with changes related to aging.
  2.3 Identify alternative treatment and care settings for elderly patients.
  2.4 Identify nursing interventions that promote wellness in the elderly.

Learning Activities

Short Answers

1. The U.S. Census Bureau projections are that by the year 2030, ____% of the population in the U.S. will be over age 65.

2. _____ is the study of the process of aging and the needs of older people.

3. An understanding of the changes associated with aging allows the nurse to differentiate between _____ and _____ assessment findings.

4. Elderly adults who deal well with changes have usually developed good _____ strategies throughout life.

5. According to the Food and Drug Administration, there should be a ____% reduction in calorie intake after age 76.

6. List three factors that cause increased sensitivity to cold in the elderly.
  1.
  2.
  3.

7. Even though older adults make up 12% of the population, they account for almost

    _____% of all drugs used today.

8. The way that the elderly absorb and metabolize medications alters the action of some drugs. List three reasons that drugs may be more potent and are more toxic in the elderly.
    1.

    2.

    3.

9. Correct administration of medications is very important for the elderly. List five instructions related to administration of medications that the nurse should review.
    1.

    2.

    3.

    4.

    5.

Knowledge Application

10. Which of the following factors would affect the aging process?

    A. heredity

    B. activities of daily living

    C. health habits

    D. socioeconomic factors

    E. all the above

11. Which of the following would be considered to be a functional limitation of aging?

    A. change in lifestyle

    B. loss of mobility

    C. inability to drive

    D. limited resources

12. Alterations in appetite in the elderly are often due to

    A. diminished taste and smell

    B. loss of teeth

    C. poor sight

    D. chronic illnesses

13. The current recommended dietary allowance (RDA) standards for the elderly recommend a diet that contains

    A. 70% carbohydrates, 15% protein, < 15% fat

    B. 60% carbohydrates, 25% protein, < 15% fat

    C. 55% carbohydrates, 15% protein, < 30% fat

    D. 40% carbohydrates, 40% protein, < 20% fat

14. Vitamin deficiencies may occur in the elderly because of poor dietary habits. Symptoms of night blindness would suggest a lack of vitamin

    A. C

    B. A

    C. B_{12}

    D. E

15. Changes in the skin have been related to environmental factors, of which the most significant is

    A. smoking

    B. exposure to cold

    C. exposure to sun

    D. changes in diet

16. Loose, wrinkled skin in the elderly is due to

    A. increase in collagen fibers

    B. changes in pigmentation

    C. loss of subcutaneous adipose tissue

    D. increase in fat cells

17. Knowing that there are visual changes associated with aging, the nurse might suggest which of the following?

    A. turning the head to compensate for loss of peripheral vision

    B. holding reading materials closer to improve vision

    C. avoiding driving in bright sunlight

    D. using low-level lighting

18. Forgetfulness and short-term memory loss in the elderly may be due to

    A. changes in physiologic status

    B. decrease in blood flow to the brain

    C. decrease in the number of neurons

    D. all of the above

19. All of the following are considered part of the normal aging process EXCEPT

    A. inappropriate behavior

    B. forgetting names

    C. occasional confusion

    D. slowing of reaction time

20. Mr. B., age 82, states that even though he goes to bed at 11 PM, he still wakes up at 5:30 AM. He asks for some advice. As the nurse you reply,

    A. "A sleeping pill would probably be helpful."

    B. "This is a normal sleep pattern for your age."

    C. "You should drink wine before you go to bed."

    D. "You should exercise more just before sleep."

21. Because the elderly have a slowed response to the autonomic nervous system, they are at risk for

    A. heart attacks

    B. transient ischemic attacks

    C. orthostatic hypotension

    D. respiratory insufficiency

22. Because constipation is a common problem in the elderly, a recommended treatment might be

    A. eat large meals that are high in fiber

    B. increase fluids, fiber, and exercise

    C. take a laxative daily

    D. increase milk intake and eat bland foods

23. A patient in the hospital is having problems with stress incontinence. The nurse is aware that

    A. loss of urinary control is a normal part of aging

    B. loss of renal function is progressive and irreversible

    C. restricting fluids helps this problem

    D. pelvic exercises can help in treating this problem

24. Changes in skeletal structure occur with aging. Kyphosis produces

    A. increased anteroposterior chest diameter

    B. decreased anteroposterior chest diameter

    C. thinning of joint cartilage

    D. increased elasticity and loss of function of spine

25. Because of the increased incidence of osteoporosis in elderly women, the daily dietary intake of calcium and vitamin D should be

    A. 4 g of calcium, 400 units of vitamin D

    B. 2 g of calcium, 800 units of vitamin D

    C. 1 g of calcium, 400 units of vitamin D

    D. 1 g of calcium, 100 units of vitamin D

26. All of the following statements about the aging process are true EXCEPT

    A. sexual activity gradually decreases and usually ceases after age 85

    B. painful intercourse can result from decreased vaginal lubrication

    C. sperm production will decrease with aging

    D. men have a slower arousal time as they age

27. One of the earliest manifestations of drug toxicity in the elderly may be

    A. nausea and vomiting

    B. diarrhea

    C. mental confusion

    D. dizziness and weakness

True/False

28. _____ Malnutrition is a common problem in the elderly.

29. _____ Dryness of the skin is caused by decreased activity of sebaceous glands.

30. _____ Lotions that contain lanolin are useful for treating dry skin.

31. _____ The appearance of gray hair has nothing to do with genetics.

32. _____ Presbyopia is common in individuals over 50.

Identification and Interpretation

33. It is important to be able to differentiate normal and abnormal assessment data. Check the findings below that are consistent with the normal aging process.
    Mr. M. is 85 years old. He has heart disease, high blood pressure, and peripheral vascular disease. He is currently admitted to the hospital with shortness of breath and chest pain.

During the nursing assessment, the findings are:

A. _____ Color is pale

B. _____ Feet are cool to touch

C. _____ Pulses in feet are weak

D. _____ Breathing is labored

E. _____ Neck veins are distended

F. _____ Heart rate is irregular

G. _____ Breath sounds are slightly diminished

H. _____ Decreased sensation in toes

Mr. M. is diagnosed with congestive heart failure. He is treated successfully and will be discharged on two new medications, Lasix (a diuretic) and Lanoxin (to increase strength of heart contraction).

34. Write a nursing plan that deals with his need to understand how and why to take these medications.

Nursing diagnosis:

Patient outcome:

Nursing interventions:

Case Studies

Case Study No. 1

Mrs. B., age 78, is a recent widow. She has symptoms of depression, loneliness, and lack of motivation following the death of her spouse.

35. An important developmental task of late adulthood for Mrs. B. would be to

    A. reestablish a relationship with a male partner

    B. begin the process of life review

    C. develop dependence on children

    D. understand that social isolation needs to be accepted

Mrs. B.'s daughter asks a local home care agency to assess her mother and offer recommendations for her care.

36. The nurse from the agency notes that Mrs. B. is pale, listless, and has lost 15 pounds. This may be because she

    A. has a chronic illness

    B. lacks the motivation to prepare well-balanced meals

    C. lacks transportation to the store

    D. is exhibiting normal aging traits

37. To help Mrs. B. cope with her loss, the nurse

    A. encourages her to reminisce about her husband

    B. tells her to stop living in the past

    C. plans several new activities to keep her busy

    D. all the above

38. The nurse does a follow-up visit several weeks later. She notices Mrs. B.'s appearance is unkempt, she is unable to follow directions, and keeps asking for her husband. This may be a result of

    A. the normal process of aging

    B. the grieving process

    C. malnutrition

    D. alteration in physiologic status

39. An appropriate nursing intervention would be to

    A. have her evaluated by a physician

    B. have her admitted to a nursing home

    C. call her daughter

    D. take her to the emergency room

Case Study No. 2

Mrs. J. is seen by the nurse from a home health agency to evaluate her ability to care for herself at home. She states that she often gets dizzy when she gets up to go to the bathroom at night. She also has a history of irregular bowel movements with frequent laxative use.

40. The dizzy spells are most likely due to

    A. orthostatic hypotension

    B. congestive heart failure

    C. poor food intake

    D. decreased vision

41. Write three nursing interventions to help solve this problem.
    1.

    2.

    3.

42. The irregular bowel movements may be due to

    A. low fiber in the diet

    B. inadequate fluid intake

    C. lack of exercise

    D. all of the above

43. Write three nursing interventions to help solve this problem.
    1.

    2.

    3.

Physical examination reveals a frail, thin, 82-year-old female with changes consistent with aging. Abnormal findings include reddened areas on the scapula and coccyx.

44. The reddened areas on the bony prominence may be due to

    A.   prolonged bed rest and the inability to turn

    B.   limited mobility and pressure that impairs circulation

    C.   poor vision and potential for fall injury

    D.   poor nutrition and inability to cook

45. Write three nursing interventions to help solve this problem.
    1.

    2.

    3.

46. Mrs. J.'s physical appearance suggests a nutritional problem. This may be due to

    A.   limited resources

    B.   physical limitations

    C.   dental problems

    D.   diminished sense of taste and smell

    E.   any or all of the above

*L*earner Self-Evaluation

Do I fully understand the content? If no, then the areas I need to review are:

I need more information from my instructor on:

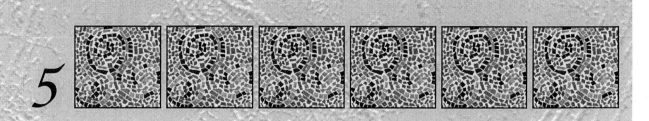

5

Knowledge Base for Patients with Fluid, Electrolyte, and Acid-Base Imbalances

Objectives

1.0 Demonstrate an understanding of extracellular fluid volume deficits (ECFVD).
    1.1 Identify conditions that lead to ECFVD.
    1.2 Identify symptoms of ECFVD.
    1.3 Identify appropriate interventions for a patient with ECFVD.
    1.4 Plan the nursing care for a patient with ECFVD.

2.0 Demonstrate an understanding of extracellular fluid volume excess (ECFVE).
    2.1 Identify conditions that lead to ECFVE.
    2.2 Identify symptoms of ECFVE.
    2.3 Identify appropriate interventions for a patient with ECFVE.
    2.4 Identify a diet appropriate for a patient with ECFVE.
    2.5 Plan nursing care for a patient with ECFVE.

3.0 Demonstrate an understanding of third space volume shift.
    3.1 Identify conditions that can lead to a shift in fluid to the third space.
    3.2 Identify appropriate nursing interventions for the treatment of third space volume shift.
    3.3 Plan nursing care for a patient with a third spacing of fluid.

4.0 Demonstrate an understanding of intracellular fluid volume excess (ICFVE).
    4.1 Identify conditions that lead to ICFVE.
    4.2 Identify symptoms of ICFVE.
    4.3 Identify appropriate nursing interventions for the treatment of ICFVE.
    4.4 Plan nursing care for a patient with ICFVE.

5.0 Demonstrate an understanding of electrolyte imbalances that can occur as a result of fluid shifts.
    5.1 Identify values for normal electrolytes.
    5.2 Identify symptoms of imbalances.
    5.3 Identify treatments for electrolyte imbalances.
    5.4 Plan nursing care for a patient with an electrolyte imbalance.

6.0 Demonstrate an understanding of the acid-base system.
    6.1 Identify normal and abnormal laboratory findings.
    6.2 Identify conditions that can lead to abnormalities in the acid-base system.

Learning Activities

Short Answers

1. A diet ____ in protein and ____ in sodium would be most appropriate for a patient with severe fluid overload.

2. Another name for ECFVD is _____.

3. In an adult, water accounts for about ____ of the body weight.

4. Hyperosmolar fluid deficit occurs when the loss of _____ exceeds the loss of _____.

5. The most common symptom that occurs with ECFVD is _____.

6. The three "Ds" frequently prescribed for iso-osmolar ECFVE are _____, _____, and _____.

7. _____ _____ _____ are considered to be essential tools in diagnosing acid-base disturbances.

Identification and Interpretation

The ability of the nurse to correctly assess and interpret findings is an important skill. Indicate whether each of the signs or symptoms listed below is associated with fluid volume excess (FVE) or fluid volume deficit (FVD).

8. _____ Poor skin turgor

9. _____ Pitting edema

10. _____ Irritability and confusion

11. _____ Full, bounding pulse

12. _____ Low urine output

13. _____ Engorged hand and neck veins

The ability to determine which individuals are at risk for an electrolyte disorder is another important nursing role. For each of the following, fill in which electrolyte disorder would be most likely to occur. (example: hypokalemia)

14. _____ Cushing's disease

15. _____ History of steroid use

16. _____ Malabsorption syndrome

17. _____ Renal failure with low urine output

18. _____ Chronic alcoholism

19. _____ Syndrome of inappropriate antidiuretic hormone (SIADH)

Knowledge Application

20. ECFVD is defined as a loss of fluid from the
    A. interstitial and intravascular spaces
    B. intracellular and vascular spaces
    C. extracellular and extravascular spaces
    D. intracellular and interstitial spaces

21. When extracellular fluid volume loss is present, the patient will probably exhibit signs of
    A. hyponatremia
    B. hypernatremia
    C. hyperkalemia
    D. hypomagnesemia

22. Signs that would alert the nurse to a severe FVD are
    A. thirst, apprehension
    B. hot dry skin, hypotension
    C. thirst, lethargy, cold skin, tachycardia
    D. dyspnea, tachycardia, hypertension

23. A patient exhibits signs of mild FVD. the nurse notices weight loss of 2 kg. This corresponds to a change in fluid balance of

    A. 1 L

    B. 2 L

    C. 3 L

    D. 4 L

24. If a patient has moderate or severe ECFVD, the nurse would expect the patient's orders to include

    A. force 4–6 glasses of water

    B. maintain IV with D_5W at 50 mL/hour

    C. maintain D_5/.9 normal saline at 100 mL hour

    D. administer one unit of whole blood

25. The nurse notices that a patient is dyspneic, has a rapid pulse, elevated blood pressure, and peripheral edema. These symptoms are suggestive of

    A. fluid volume excess

    B. fluid volume deficit

    C. dehydration

    D. metabolic acidosis

26. The nurse is aware that management of a fluid volume excess will probably include

    A. diazepam, digoxin, morphine

    B. diuretics, digitalis, low-sodium diet

    C. intravenous fluids, potassium

    D. morphine, high-sodium diet

27. From the group of individuals listed below, which is most at risk for third spacing of fluid?

    A. patient who had a heart catheterization

    B. patient with cirrhosis and low serum albumin

    C. patient with a urinary infection

    D. patient with a respiratory infection

28. The nurse is assessing a burn patient for signs of fluid shift three to five days after the injury. Which of the signs would alert the nurse of a potential problem?

    A. bradycardia, hypertension

    B. tachycardia, hypotension

    C. dyspnea, crackles in chest, jugular vein distention

    D. peripheral edema, diminished pulses, hypotension

29. The management of a patient with increased secretion of antidiuretic hormone would focus on identifying signs of

    A. ECFVE

    B. third-spacing of fluid

    C. ICFVE

    D. ECFVD

30. Signs of cerebral edema in a patient diagnosed with water intoxication would include

    A. anorexia, projectile vomiting, blurred vision

    B. nausea, hypotension, tachycardia

    C. weight loss, hypertension, tachycardia

    D. weight gain, lethargy, fever

31. An appropriate nursing intervention for the patient with a ICFVE would be to

    A. provide stimulation

    B. maintain seizure precautions

    C. decrease stimulation

    D. force fluids

32. A patient comes to the clinic with severe vomiting and diarrhea. The nurse will draw blood to check for loss of serum

    A. sodium

    B. potassium

    C. albumin

    D. protein

33. Hypokalemia is a frequent problem with patients receiving

    A. Aldactone

    B. digoxin

    C. furosemide

    D. verapamil

34. A patient comes to the hospital with a potassium level of 2.6 mEq/L. The nurse attaches the cardiac monitor, knowing that hypokalemia can cause which of the following rhythm changes?

    A. prolonged PR interval

    B. premature atrial contractions

    C. prolonged ST segment and inverted T wave

    D. atrial fibrillation

35. The nurse would also observe for physical signs of low potassium including

    A. lethargy, confusion, diminished sense of touch

    B. anxiety, hallucinations, convulsions

    C. Hyperactive bowel sounds, diarrhea

    D. dyspnea, edema, vein distention

36. The nurse would anticipate that the physician would order which of the following therapies?

    A. 100 mEq of KCl in 100 cc D$_5$W to run in one hour

    B. IV of D$_5$W at 150 cc/hour

    C. 25 mEq of K-Lyte orally

    D. 50 mEq of KCl in 250 cc of D$_5$W to run over four hours

37. An ominous sign for a patient with low potassium would be

    A. heart rate of 52

    B. blood pressure of 90/60

    C. respirations 12, shallow and irregular

    D. lethargy, cool skin

38. A patient with hypokalemia is receiving digoxin. Before administering the medication, the nurse should check

    A. serum potassium level

    B. serum sodium level

    C. serum magnesium level

    D. serum chloride level

39. In caring for a patient with hyperkalemia, the nurse would carefully assess for any effects on which system?

    A. cardiovascular

    B. renal

    C. respiratory

    D. neurologic

40. In caring for a patient with a serum potassium of 6.0, the nurse would expect to see which treatment ordered?

    A. low potassium diet

    B. blood transfusions

    C. sodium polystyrene

    D. dialysis

41. The nurse would check for hyponatremia if a patient exhibited which of the following symptoms?

    A. headache, drowsiness, confusion

    B. hyperreflexia, spasms of muscles

    C. hypoactive bowel sounds, nausea

    D. lethargy, hypertension, bradycardia

42. A primary nursing goal for the patient with a low sodium level would be to

    A. maintain airway patency

    B. prevent injury

    C. maintain sodium restriction

    D. force fluids

43. Part of the nursing care for the patient with a low sodium level might involve

    A. administering narcotics

    B. maintaining fluid restrictions

    C. administering laxatives

    D. maintaining IV fluid with D_5W

44. When caring for a patient with chronic renal failure, the nurse would expect lab values to show

    A. hypokalemia

    B. hyponatremia

    C. hyperkalemia

    D. hypercalcemia

45. Which nursing action should be included in the plan of care for a patient with a low calcium level?

    A. monitor for signs of tetany

    B. monitor for hypoglycemia

    C. monitor for bradycardia

    D. monitor for constipation

46. A patient with a high serum calcium might develop

    A. vomiting, diarrhea

    B. excessive blood clotting

    C. muscle twitching

    D. renal failure

47. An elevated magnesium level results in a _____ of acetylcholine and a _____ in excitability of the nerve fibers.

    A. decrease, decrease

    B. increase, increase

    C. decrease, increase

    D. increase, decrease

48. Nursing care for a patient who has a nasogastric tube that is putting out 800 mL of fluid each shift would include monitoring for signs of

    A. fluid overload

    B. respiratory acidosis

    C. metabolic alkalosis

    D. metabolic acidosis

49. Nursing care for a patient who has chronic obstructive pulmonary disease would include monitoring for signs of

    A. respiratory acidosis

    B. respiratory alkalosis

    C. metabolic acidosis

    D. metabolic alkalosis

Identification and Interpretation

Identification of alterations in acid-base balance is an important nursing skill. Determine the correct imbalance for the values listed below and identify some signs and symptoms.

   A. Metabolic acidosis

   B. Respiratory acidosis

   C. Metabolic alkalosis

   D. Respiratory alkalosis

		pH	CO_2	HCO_3^-
50.	____	7.30	40	18
51.	____	7.56	30	23
52.	____	7.48	43	32
53.	____	7.18	65	26

54. When a patient has a low pH (acidosis) and a rise in CO_2, the nurse would expect to observe

    A. decrease in respiratory rate and depth

    B. increase in respiratory rate and depth

55. When the patient has a high pH, the nurse would expect

    A.   increase in respiratory rate

    B.   decrease in respiratory rate

56. A patient is admitted for surgery. He is very nervous and begins to pace in the room and hyperventilate. The nurse would monitor for signs of

    A.   respiratory acidosis

    B.   respiratory alkalosis

    C.   metabolic acidosis

    D.   metabolic alkalosis

True/False

57. _____ Hypotonic fluid has low osmolality.

58. _____ Dehydration occurs when loss of water exceeds the loss of sodium.

59. _____ Blood urea nitrogen (BUN) will be low with an FVD.

60. _____ Fluid constantly shifts between the intravascular and interstitial spaces.

61. _____ Excess potassium in the body can be life-threatening.

62. _____ Hyperkalemia is seen more frequently than hypokalemia.

63. _____ Most Americans consume 2–4 grams of sodium daily.

64. _____ Digoxin is more effective when serum potassium is high.

Basic Knowledge

Write the normal lab values for the following

65. Potassium

66. Sodium

67. Serum calcium

68. Ionized calcium

69. Magnesium

Case Studies

Case Study No. 1

A patient is admitted to ICU with extreme shortness of breath, rales in lungs, BP 190/102, pulse 104, respiration 32, pitting edema in legs and positive JVD. A diagnosis of pulmonary edema is made. The following questions relate to this situation.

70. This patient is exhibiting signs of FVE probably as a result of

    A.   left sided heart failure

    B.   emphysema

    C.   renal insufficiency

    D.   sepsis

71. Treatment involves administration of a diuretic and cardiac glycosides. Which would be the drug of choice to remove fluid rapidly?

    A.   HydroDIURIL

    B.   Micronase

    C.   furosemide

    D.   digoxin

72. The purpose of administering digoxin is to

    A.   decrease the force of myocardial contraction

    B.   lower heart rate and increase force of contraction

    C.   raise heart rate and help excrete potassium

    D.   prevent cardiac arrhythmias

73. Write a care plan for this patient.

Nursing diagnosis:

Patient outcome:

Interventions:

Case Study No. 2

A patient is admitted to the hospital with renal failure. On admission he has periorbital and ankle edema. BP is 160/104, pulse 96, respiration 24. BUN is 40 mg/dL, creatinine is 3.2 mg/dL.

74. The nurse would expect which electrolyte to be elevated in this patient?

A. potassium

B. sodium

C. calcium

D. albumin

75. Physical assessment findings indicate that this patient is showing signs of

A. fluid volume excess (extracellular)

B. fluid volume deficit (extracellular)

C. third spacing of fluid

D. intracellular excess

76. Which condition if present would cause a worsening of his condition?

A. metabolic acidosis

B. metabolic alkalosis

C. respiratory acidosis

D. respiratory alkalosis

77. If the serum potassium level for this patient was 7.2 mEq/L, the nurse would be aware that the patient is at risk for

A. respiratory failure

B. total renal shutdown

C. cardiac arrest

D. cerebrovascular accident

Case Study No. 3

A patient is admitted to the hospital with an extracellular fluid overload caused by heart failure. He receives digoxin to strengthen his heart rate and large doses of Lasix to remove fluid. He develops hypokalemia as a result of the treatment. He will be discharged on these medications.

78. The patient should be instructed to eat a variety of foods that are rich in potassium. From the list below, check those foods that would be recommended.

_____ Oranges

_____ Spinach

_____ Potatoes

_____ Yellow squash

_____ Turkey

_____ Fish

_____ Broccoli

_____ Tomatoes

79. Because of its effect on the gastrointestinal system, the patient with a low potassium level would be instructed to

A. eat a low-fiber diet

B. avoid use of laxatives

C. eat a high-fiber diet

D. restrict fluids

80. Signs of low potassium that should be reported at once would include

    A.   muscle cramps

    B.   diarrhea

    C.   anxiety

    D.   tachycardia

81. The physician orders a potassium supplement to be taken orally three times a day. The nurse would explain that side effects might include

    A.   headache, dizziness, hypotension

    B.   nausea, vomiting, GI bleeding

    C.   muscle cramping, spasticity

    D.   diaphoresis

Case Study No. 4

Ms. P. is admitted to the hospital with a sodium level of 150 mEq/L. She appears lethargic and confused. Breathing is rapid and she is diaphoretic. History reveals that she has been sick and not eating for several days. She is admitted and treatment is started.

82. During the initial assessment the nurse finds which of the following symptoms that may be caused by the high sodium level?

    A.   muscle twitching, hyporeflexia

    B.   moist, clammy skin

    C.   increased urine output

    D.   all of the above

83. The nurse would expect this patient to be treated with

    A.   hypotonic IV fluid

    B.   isotonic IV fluid

    C.   hypertonic IV fluid

    D.   tube feedings

84. Which information from the patient's history would be a contributing factor to this problem?

    A.   seizures

    B.   takes prednisone for arthritis

    C.   takes Theo-Dur for emphysema

    D.   takes estrogen replacement

85. Ms. P. recovers and is ready to be discharged. She will need to monitor her sodium intake carefully until she is seen in three weeks by the physician. Foods she should avoid would include

    A.   milk, green and yellow vegetables

    B.   whole grains, cheese

    C.   lunchmeats, snack foods

    D.   all of the above

86. Ms. P. is readmitted two months later with a hip fracture. The nurse would monitor for increase in which lab value?

    A.   potassium

    B.   sodium

    C.   calcium

    D.   magnesium

Case Study No. 5

A patient is admitted to the hospital with acute renal failure. The patient appears acutely ill with a pale color, sacral and peripheral edema, high blood pressure, distended abdomen. He is somewhat confused and irritable. The following questions relate to this situation.

87. This patient appears to be showing signs of

    A.   extracellular fluid volume deficit

    B.   intracellular fluid volume deficit

    C.   extracellular fluid volume overload

    D.   dehydration

88. Which lab value, if elevated, is most significant?

    A.   sodium

    B.   calcium

    C.   potassium

    D.   magnesium

89. The nurse reviews the chart and finds this patient has a high phosphorous level. She would also expect to find low

    A.   calcium

    B.   chloride

    C.   magnesium

    D.   potassium

90. The patient has not had a bowel movement for one week; all of the following could be ordered except

    A.   Colace

    B.   Dulcolax

    C.   Milk of Magnesia

    D.   Metamucil

91. Arterial blood gases for this patient are: pH 7.28, CO_2 45, HCO_3 20, O_2 90%. This would be interpreted as

    A.   respiratory acidosis

    B.   respiratory alkalosis

    C.   metabolic acidosis

    D.   metabolic alkalosis

92. The anticipated treatment for this patient would be

    A.   place on ventilator

    B.   begin dialysis

    C.   give oxygen

    D.   increase IV fluid

*L*earner Self-Evaluation

Do I fully understand the content? If no, then the areas I need to review are:

I need more information from my instructor on:

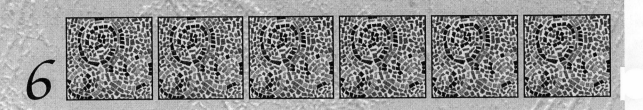

6

Knowledge Base for Patients Undergoing Surgery

*O*bjectives

1.0 Demonstrate an understanding of the legal parameters associated with surgical procedures.
    1.1 Define types of consent required for surgery.
    1.2 Demonstrate understanding of the nurse's role in caring for the surgical patient.

2.0 Identify the needs of the patient during the preoperative period.
    2.1 List diagnostic tests done prior to surgery.
    2.2 Identify teaching needs of the patient having surgery.
    2.3 Identify patients who have increased risk for complications following surgery.

3.0 Demonstrate an understanding of the needs of the patient in the perioperative period.
    3.1 List perioperative medications.
    3.2 Demonstrate an understanding of the types of anesthetic agents.
    3.3 List complications associated with anesthetic agents.

4.0 Demonstrate an understanding of the needs of the patient during the postoperative period.
    4.1 Identify complications that can occur during the postoperative period.
    4.2 Choose appropriate nursing interventions for patients who have had surgery.
    4.3 Demonstrate an understanding of the needs of elderly patients who have had surgery.

5.0 Demonstrate an understanding of the needs of the patient undergoing ambulatory surgery.
    5.1 Identify alternative surgical settings.
    5.2 Identify classification criteria for ambulatory surgery.
    5.3 Identify special considerations for patients using alternative surgical sites.

$\mathcal{L}$earning Activities

Short Answers

1. Today many surgical procedures that used to require hospitalization now take place in

    _____ settings.

2. During the perioperative period, the roles of the nurse are primarily those of patient

    _____ and _____.

3. The _____ is responsible for explaining the benefits and risks of the intended procedure before consent is given.

4. The purpose of the skin preparation is to

    reduce the number of _____ on the skin.

5. All patients should be instructed to

    _____ prior to administration of preoperative medications.

6. A hypermetabolic crisis triggered by administration of certain anesthetic agents is

    known as _____.

7. Developing a respiratory complication such

    as _____ is a major concern during general anesthesia.

8. In an elderly patient, problems such as dehydration or malnutrition should be

    corrected _____.

9. The nurse should carefully monitor an elderly patient who has had surgery because he or she is at greater risk for complications.

    This is due to _____ cardiac output,

    _____ peripheral circulation, and _____ vasculomotor response.

10. _____ _____ _____ allows the patient to control the amount and frequency of self-administered analgesia.

11. _____ is the protrusion of internal organs through a dehisced wound.

Definitions

Written consent must be obtained from the patient before performing surgical procedures. Demonstrate your understanding of this concept by clearly defining the following terms.

12. Informed consent

13. Implied consent

14. Nursing role as it relates to consent

Basic Knowledge

15. List three ways that surgeries have been classified.
     1.

     2.

     3.

16. List several diagnostic examinations that are required prior to surgery.

    1.

    2.

    3.

17. List three types of medications that may be given prior to surgery and explain their use.

    1.

    2.

    3.

18. List the members of the surgical team.

    1.

    2.

    3.

    4.

    5.

19. List three different types of regional anesthesia. Explain how each might be used.

    1.

    2.

    3.

20. List three common complications of general anesthesia.

    1.

    2.

    3.

Identification

Patients undergoing ambulatory surgery are classified into categories that indicate current health status. Match the physical state with the appropriate definition.

    A.   Physical status I

    B.   Physical status II

    C.   Physical status IV

    D.   Physical status V

21. _____ Not a candidate for ambulatory surgery, severe systemic disease exists.

22. _____ Healthy patient with no systemic disease.

23. _____ Not a candidate for ambulatory surgery, moribund patient.

24. _____ Mild systemic disease exists without functional limits.

Knowledge Application

25. Reasons for completing diagnostic tests prior to surgery would include

    A.   establishing baseline values

    B.   screening for preexisting conditions

    C.   evaluation of disease that may affect surgical outcome

    D.   all the above

26. A patient with a poor nutritional status would have increased risk of

    A.   poor wound healing and infection

    B.   fluid volume overload

    C.   decreased peristalsis

    D.   cardiovascular collapse

27. An obese patient has a higher incidence of postoperative complications such as

    A.   urinary retention

    B.   neurologic impairment

    C.   poor wound healing, pulmonary complications

    D.   fluid volume deficit, dehydration

28. A cardiovascular examination and clearance for surgery is necessary because

    A. poor status compromises the patient's ability to adjust to changes in fluid balance

    B. poor status makes it harder to recover from blood loss and shock

    C. poor status may increase the risk of emboli formation

    D. all of the above

29. The nurse knows that a patient who is a heavy smoker is at increased risk after surgery because he or she

    A. is less likely to be able to cough effectively

    B. often has a poor state of nutrition

    C. is usually overweight

    D. has a poor tolerance for pain

30. The patient with liver disease has an increased surgical risk since adequate liver function is needed for

    A. metabolism of carbohydrates

    B. detoxifying drugs and anesthetic agents

    C. eliminating electrolytes

    D. maintaining blood pressure

31. A priority nursing diagnosis for a patient with renal insufficiency who is having surgery would be Potential for

    A. alteration in skin integrity

    B. fluid and electrolyte imbalance

    C. alteration in mobility

    D. injury

32. If the nurse observes nervousness, tremors, insomnia, and agitation in a patient after surgery, he or she may want to consider the possibility of

    A. respiratory insufficiency

    B. nutritional deficit

    C. substance abuse

    D. all of the above

33. The nurse is aware that intravenous fluids may be initiated before or during surgery to

    A. provide calories since the patient is NPO

    B. prevent urinary retention

    C. prevent dehydration because of fluid restrictions

    D. all of the above

34. The purpose of skin preparation prior to surgery is to

    A. facilitate dressing changes

    B. prevent wound contamination

    C. sterilize the skin

    D. reduce the number of microorganisms on the skin

35. Surgery is performed during which stage of anesthesia?

    A. stage 1

    B. stage 2

    C. stage 3

    D. stage 4

36. In the immediate postoperative period, the nurse would promptly report a rapid, thready pulse and drop in blood pressure since these changes may indicate

    A. hypertensive crisis

    B. shock

    C. infection

    D. respiratory distress

37. If, during the postoperative period, the patient exhibits signs of fever, tachypnea, tachycardia, decreased breath sounds, and crackles, the nurse would suspect

    A. atelectasis

    B. aspiration

    C. shock

    D. pulmonary embolism

38. The reason that antiembolic stockings are applied in the immediate postoperative period is to

    A. prevent pulmonary emboli

    B. maintain adequate blood pressure

    C. prevent venous stasis

    D. support surgical incisions

39. The nurse is aware of the high risk for ineffective breathing patterns following surgery. This risk is due to

    A. effects of general anesthesia

    B. postoperative pain

    C. immobility

    D. all of the above

40. If a patient is having respiratory difficulty, the nurse would see signs of

    A. tachypnea, tachycardia, and rapid, shallow breathing

    B. bradycardia, seizures

    C. fever, diaphoresis, hypotension

    D. respiratory alkalosis, hypertension

41. A patient had a thoracotomy three days ago. He still has an IV and PCA for pain. He has been slow to progress. Today he is exhibiting signs of respiratory depression, oversedation, nausea, and urinary retention. The nurse suspects

    A. pneumonia

    B. narcotic side effects

    C. problems from immobility

    D. fluid volume deficit

42. Following surgery, the nurse would monitor for signs of wound infections including

    A. edema, serosanguineous drainage

    B. redness, edema

    C. persistent pain, purulent drainage, delayed healing

    D. partial separation of the wound edges

True/False

43. _____ Corticosteroids will increase the patient's ability to deal with the stress of surgery.

44. _____ Alcohol can interact with preoperative medications.

45. _____ Preoperative medication will usually put the patient to sleep.

46. _____ The elderly patient over age 75 may have three times as many postoperative complications as younger patients.

47. _____ Postoperative confusion is more common in the elderly.

Case Studies

Case Study No. 1

Ms. E. is scheduled for exploratory abdominal surgery in the morning. She is believed to have colon cancer that may have spread. She is anxious and scared about what may be found. The nurse uses the nursing diagnosis Anxiety related to hospitalization, surgery, and outcome of surgery.

48. Write two patient outcomes.
    1.

    2.

49. Write several nursing interventions.
    1.

    2.

    3.

    4.

50. Prior to surgery the nurse would anticipate which of the following orders? (Check all that apply.)

    A. _____ NPO after midnight

    B. _____ laxatives and possible enema

    C. _____ antibiotics

    D. _____ orders for a complete blood count (CBC) and electrolytes

    E. _____ pain medication every four hours

Prior to surgery the next morning, the nurse administers the preoperative medication as ordered. It includes a narcotic and a benzodiazepine.

51. The rationale for these two medications would be to

   A. provide sedation and minimize pain perception

   B. prevent pain and minimize secretions

   C. potentiate sedative effects of anesthesia

   D. provide sedation and reduce secretions

52. For this type of surgical procedure, a general anesthesia will be used. The nurse realizes that this involves

   A. injection of the anesthetic agent in a nerve pathway

   B. injection of the anesthetic agent directly into a vein or by inhalation of gas

   C. both the above are correct methods

53. Knowing the potential complications with this type of surgery, the nurse would be sure to include information about _____ in the preoperative period.

   A. coughing and deep-breathing exercises

   B. chest tubes and heart monitor

   C. intensive care unit

   D. all of the above

54. This patient has a history of diabetes and hepatitis. Knowing this, the nurse is aware that use of _____ would be contraindicated.

   A. nitrous oxide

   B. halothane

   C. isoflurane

   D. methoxyflurane

55. During the surgery, a partial colectomy is performed and the patient is sent to the postanesthesia care unit (PACU). With this type of surgery, the nurse monitors for _____ complications.

   A. cardiovascular

   B. neurologic

   C. respiratory

   D. urinary

When Ms. E. returns to the floor, the nurse attaches her to the cardiac monitor and pulse oximeter and monitors vital signs frequently.

56. Two hours after returning to the floor, the nurse notices that Ms. E. has shallow, rapid breathing; cold, moist skin; skin color is bluish; and there is no urine output. These are manifestations of

   A. respiratory insufficiency

   B. viral infection

   C. shock

   D. stroke

57. Possible causes of this condition may include

   A. reaction to anesthesia

   B. hemorrhage

   C. sepsis

   D. any of the above

58. A priority nursing intervention would be to assess

   A. surgical dressing

   B. bowel sounds

   C. for edema

   D. diet intake

Case Study No. 2

Mr. M. has just returned to the unit from the PACU. He had an appendectomy for a ruptured appendix. He has a history of chronic obstructive pulmonary disease and hypertension. His condition is currently stable.

59. Write four nursing diagnoses that would be important during the immediate postoperative period.
    1.

    2.

    3.

    4.

60. While assessing Mr. M. on the second postoperative day, the nurse notices abdominal distention and an absence of bowel sounds. The patient is not passing any flatus. The nurse would suspect

    A.   wound infection

    B.   bowel obstruction

    C.   paralytic ileus

    D.   stress ulcer

61. Mr. M. is kept NPO and a nasogastric (NG) tube is inserted and attached to low-wall suction. Later that evening, the nurse notices hypotension, tachycardia, decreased level of consciousness, decreased urine output, and poor skin turgor. The nurse suspects

    A.   Ineffective breathing pattern

    B.   Alteration in nutrition

    C.   Fluid volume deficit

    D.   Pain related to surgical incision

62. Mr. M. makes steady progress and is ready for discharge after five days. He will be monitoring the incision and taking antibiotics on discharge. The nurse would

    A.   talk with Mr. M. the day before he leaves

    B.   provide all discharge information in writing

    C.   schedule an appointment with the surgeon in one week

    D.   encourage a full return to normal activities

Case Study No. 3

Ms. P. is scheduled for ambulatory surgery to remove a benign breast lesion. The following questions relate to her pre- and postoperative course.

63. During the office visit, the nurse would be involved in implementing all the following EXCEPT

    A.   preoperative teaching

    B.   establishing time for diagnostic tests

    C.   determining type of anesthesia

    D.   reviewing discharge instructions

64. Ms. P. has a local anesthetic and returns to the recovery room alert and pain-free. Which of the following measures would the nurse implement?

    A.   monitor vital signs every 30 minutes

    B.   monitor vital signs every two hours

    C.   keep Ms. P. flat in bed for 8 hours

    D.   order regular diet

65. Criteria for discharge from the ambulatory surgical unit would include which of the following?

    A.   ability to cough and swallow

    B.   ability to ambulate

    C.   minimal nausea, vomiting

    D.   no respiratory distress

    E.   all of the above

*L*earner Self-Evaluation

Do I fully understand the content? If no, then the
areas I need to review are:

I need more information from my instructor on:

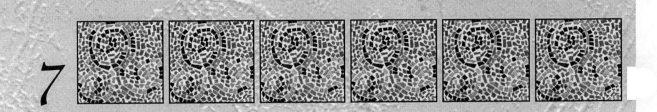

7

Knowledge Base for Patients with Cardiac Dysfunction

Objectives

1.0 Review the anatomy and physiology of the cardiac system.
 1.1 Identify the parts of the heart.
 1.2 Explain the functions of the heart.
 1.3 Explain the three regulatory mechanisms for circulation.

2.0 Demonstrate an understanding of assessment data related to the cardiac system.
 2.1 Identify clinical manifestations of cardiac dysfunction.
 2.2 Match the heart sounds with their specific characteristics.
 2.3 List the cardiac risk factors.
 2.4 Identify tests used to diagnose cardiac disorders.

3.0 Demonstrate an understanding of interventions used to treat patients with a cardiac disorder.
 3.1 Demonstrate an understanding of types of medical treatment used with cardiac disorders.
 3.2 Demonstrate an understanding of types of surgical interventions used to treat cardiac disorders.
 3.3 Plan the nursing care for an adult with a disorder of the cardiac system.

*L*earning Activities

Identification

On the diagram below, identify the parts of the heart.

1. Superior vena cava
2. Right atrium
3. Left atrium
4. Left ventricle
5. Right ventricle
6. Tricuspid valve

7. Mitral valve
8. Pulmonic valve
9. Pulmonary arteries
10. Pulmonary veins
11. Aortic valve

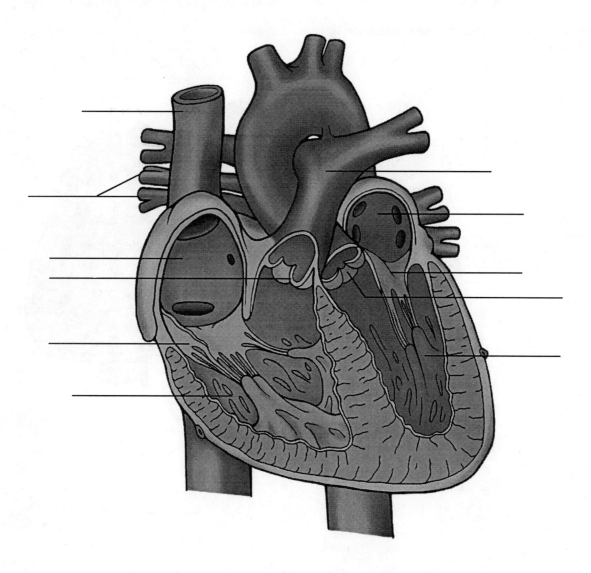

Short Answers

12. The basic function of the heart is:

13. Briefly explain how blood flows through the body.

14. The _____ _____ supply the cardiac muscle with blood, oxygen, and nutrients.

15. Explain the three regulatory mechanisms for circulation.
     1.

     2.

     3.

16. List the cardiac risk factors

     Nonmodifiable
     A.

     B.

     C.

     Modifiable
     A.

     B.

     C.

     D.

17. On the drawing below, label and trace the conductive system through the heart.

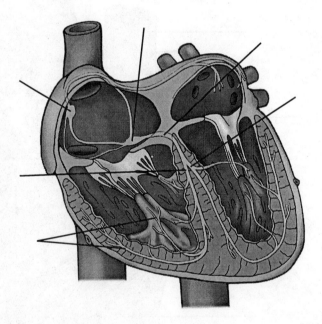

18. Explain what each of the wave forms signify.

    P Wave

    PR interval

    QRS complex

    T wave

19. The _____ is a fibrous sac that surrounds the heart.

20. Cardiac muscle is _____ contractile tissue that requires _____ stimulation in order to contract.

21. Three factors that influence stroke volume are
    1.

    2.

    3.

22. List the five classic signs and symptoms of heart disease.
    1.

    2.

    3.

    4.

    5.

23. Jugular vein distention is associated with:

Identification

The ability of the nurse to correctly assess and interpret findings is a critical skill. Match each of the following heart sounds with the appropriate definition.

   A. S_1

   B. S_2

   C. S_3

   D. S_4

24. _____ Normal in children, but pathologic after the age of 30.

25. _____ Produced by the simultaneous closure of the mitral and tricuspid valves.

26. _____ Produced by high-velocity blood flow during atrial contraction.

27. _____ Produced by the simultaneous closure of the aortic and pulmonic valves.

28. _____ Produced by the rapid, passive atrial filling of a partially filled ventricle.

Define the following terms.

29. Central venous pressure

30. Pulmonary artery pressure

31. Pulmonary wedge pressure

32. Cardiac output

33. Preload

34. Afterload

True/False

35. _____ Any muscle cell within the heart can initiate its own rhythm potential.

36. _____ Cardiac muscle cells carry an electric charge.

37. _____ The atrioventricular valves are closed during ventricle diastole.

38. _____ Dyspnea is a late sign of heart failure.

39. _____ Sharp, midsternal chest pain means a heart attack.

40. _____ Syncope is caused by cerebral hypoxia.

41. _____ Central cyanosis is more serious than peripheral cyanosis.

42. _____ Coronary artery disease is the leading cause of death in women over age 65.

43. _____ A rise in high-density lipoprotein (HDL) cholesterol will protect against heart disease.

Knowledge Application

44. During a cardiac assessment, the nurse counts the apical pulse over the mitral valve, which is located at the

    A.   right second intercostal space

    B.   left second intercostal space

    C.   left sternal border, fifth intercostal space

    D.   epigastric area, at the tip of the sternum

45. A test to record the individual's electrocardiogram during exercise is called a(n)

    A.   fluoroscopy

    B.   stress test

    C.   Holter monitor

    D.   echocardiogram

46. The test that will give the best diagnostic information about the condition of the cardiac valves and the size of the cardiac chambers is a(n)

    A.   Holter monitor

    B.   radioactive image

    C.   stress test

    D.   echocardiogram

47. The type of test where a radiopaque contrast dye is injected into the cardiac chambers and coronary arteries in order to view blood flow is a(n)

    A.   cardiac catheterization

    B.   cardiac stress test

    C.   echocardiogram

    D.   thallium stress test

48. When a cardiac patient has an acid-base imbalance, the nurse would monitor for

    A.   hypoxia

    B.   dysrhythmias

    C.   pain

    D.   respiratory distress

49. When a patient with cardiac dysfunction complains of fatigue, this suggests

    A.   low cardiac output

    B.   hypoxia

    C.   heart failure

    D.   renal dysfunction

50. A patient is admitted to a coronary care unit with chest pain. Later that day, he becomes restless and confused. The nurse notifies the doctor, knowing that these symptoms may indicate

    A.   hypertension

    B.   stroke

    C.   renal failure

    D.   cerebral hypoxia

51. A patient comes to an urgent care center complaining of shortness of breath whenever she lies down. This is known as

    A. orthopnea

    B. paroxysmal nocturnal dyspnea

    C. bradypnea

    D. angina

52. A physician starts the patient on Lasix to help reduce fluid accumulation. She is told to eat a diet high in potassium. Which of the following foods would NOT be included?

    A. green beans

    B. bread and cereal

    C. oranges

    D. liver

53. If a cardiac patient has a high blood urea nitrogen (BUN) and creatinine, the nurse would realize that the patient has

    A. high cardiac output

    B. impaired gas exchange

    C. fluid and electrolyte imbalance

    D. decreased renal perfusion

54. When a patient has had myocardial damage, the first enzyme that will elevate is the

    A. CK

    B. LDH

    C. AST

    D. ESR

55. The blood test that would provide the best diagnostic information about whether a patient has had a myocardial infarction is the

    A. CK-MM

    B. CK-MB

    C. LDH-2

    D. SGOT-BB

56. After extensive testing, a patient is found to have an irregular heart rate of 45–50 bpm. This individual is most likely in need of

    A. open heart surgery

    B. cardiac glycosides

    C. a pacemaker

    D. an implantable defibrillator

57. Cardiac patients often receive medications to slow the transmission of electrical impulses in the heart. An example of this type of drug is

    A. Isordil

    B. digoxin

    C. lidocaine

    D. Lasix

58. When a patient is on a low-sodium diet, which of the following would NOT be permitted?

    A. fresh fruit

    B. cheese

    C. fish

    D. skim milk

59. In caring for a patient with angina, the nurse would instruct him or her to take nitroglycerin when chest pain occurs. Which of the following statements is appropriate?

    A. "If you feel a burning sensation, the medication is no longer effective."

    B. "Replace the medication at least every year."

    C. "If pain is not relieved after three nitroglycerin tablets, seek immediate medical attention."

    D. "When pain occurs, take a tablet every five minutes until it is relieved."

60. When a patient with a cardiac condition has a low cardiac output and is very symptomatic, an appropriate medication would be

    A. dopamine

    B. Lasix

    C. Apresoline

    D. lidocaine

61. During cardiac auscultation, the nurse hears a loud murmur. This is often caused by

    A. increased rate of blood flow

    B. normal blood flow through a narrowed structure

    C. backflow of blood through a valve

    D. blood flow through a dilated structure

    E. any of the above

62. The drug of choice for the treatment of premature ventricular contractions is

    A. digoxin

    B. verapamil

    C. Apresoline

    D. lidocaine

63. The nurse is screening a patient who may be a candidate for thrombolytic therapy. Which of the following would be a contraindication for this therapy?

    A. age over 70

    B. use of estrogen replacement

    C. history of cerebrovascular accident

    D. history of colitis

64. Which nursing action has the highest priority when a patient is receiving thrombolytic therapy? Monitor for

    A. hypotension

    B. arrhythmias

    C. bleeding

    D. pain

65. Elderly persons are more likely to develop heart dysfunction because (Check all that apply.)

    A. _____ the heart muscle loses contractility

    B. _____ vessel walls become less rigid

    C. _____ heart valves become thick and rigid

    D. _____ collateral circulation develops

    E. _____ peripheral vascular resistance develops

66. An 80-year-old male who eats poorly and has a low serum albumin level is likely to develop

    A. peripheral edema

    B. gastritis

    C. cyanosis

    D. angina

67. A serious complication that may occur whenever cardiopulmonary bypass is used is

    A. respiratory arrest

    B. embolus

    C. arrhythmias

    D. sepsis

68. Following open heart surgery, the patient is transferred to a critical care unit. Which of the following findings by the nurse would be considered normal?

    A. hypothermia

    B. hypotension

    C. tachycardia

    D. bradycardia

69. When a patient develops cardiogenic shock, he or she may need intra-aortic balloon pump support. The two main goals of this therapy are

    A. reducing afterload and augmenting diastolic pressure

    B. increasing both preload and afterload

    C. prevention of lethal arrhythmias

    D. increasing the oxygen supply

70. A patient with cardiac disease calls the office complaining of nausea, headache, and visual disturbances. The nurse would ask the patient

    A. what he or she had to eat

    B. what medications he or she is taking

    C. if there has been a change in his or her weight

    D. if he or she is having chest pain

Nursing Care Plans

71. Write a nursing care plan for the patient with an alteration in cardiac output related to mechanical failure.

    Nursing diagnosis: Alteration in cardiac output

    Patient outcome:

    Interventions:

72. Write a nursing care plan for the patient with activity alterations secondary to a cardiac disorder.

    Nursing diagnosis: Activity intolerance related to decreased oxygenation

    Patient outcome:

    Interventions:

73. Determine the teaching needs of the patient who has had coronary artery bypass surgery and is being discharged.

    Nursing diagnosis: Knowledge deficit: signs and symptoms of complications

    Teaching:

Case Studies

Case Study No. 1

Ms. B., age 55, comes to the emergency room with a complaint of substernal, crushing chest pain. It started without warning and is radiating to her right shoulder.

74. The first nursing action for Ms. B. would be to

    A. call a code

    B. apply 100% oxygen

    C. obtain vital signs and basic information about pain

    D. administer pain medication

Ms. B. continues to complain of pain, even after the nurse has administered two nitroglycerin tablets.

75. The nature and description of the pain suggests

    A. angina

    B. heart attack

    C. pericarditis

    D. pneumonia

76. To prevent further tissue damage to the heart, the nurse would

    A. administer morphine

    B. start an intravenous line

    C. administer oxygen

    D. attach a cardiac monitor

77. During the initial assessment, the nurse notes that Ms. B. has crackles in her lung fields and pitting edema in her ankles. This suggests

   A. angina

   B. heart failure

   C. arrhythmias

   D. pleurisy

Case Study No. 2

Mr. M. is having a heart catheterization to determine if he is a candidate for open heart surgery. He has a history of angina that has been worsening over the past six months.

78. Which of the following statements is NOT true about this procedure?

   A. It is painless.

   B. It may produce a warm, tingling sensation.

   C. An allergic reaction is possible.

   D. It is done while the patient is awake.

79. Mr. M. has the catheter inserted in his right antecubital. He returns to the unit in stable condition. The nurse will assess

   A. fluid intake

   B. peripheral pulses

   C. insertion site

   D. all of the above

80. Because Mr. M. is found to have extensive quadruple vessel disease, the most likely treatment will be

   A. oxygen and medication therapy

   B. angioplasty

   C. urokinase

   D. bypass surgery

81. The goal of coronary artery bypass grafting is to

   A. improve blood supply to the ischemic myocardium

   B. decrease the oxygen demand

   C. prevent pain

   D. prolong life

Four weeks after surgery, Mr. M. is scheduled for a stress test.

82. The nurse who schedules the test explains that the purpose of the test at this time is to

   A. detect heart disease

   B. evaluate response to stress

   C. evaluate the effects of surgical treatment

   D. see how effective his new diet is

83. The nurse also describes some of the complications of stress testing, such as

   A. cardiac dysrhythmias

   B. cardiac arrest

   C. myocardial infarction

   D. all the above

Case Study No. 3

Ms. W., age 65, has coronary artery disease. She is 5' 6" and weighs 135 lbs. She has diabetes, hypertension, and smokes one pack of cigarettes per day.

84. What change could Ms. W. make that would bring about the most significant reduction in her cardiac risk factors?

   A. lose weight

   B. control her diabetes

   C. stop smoking

   D. reduce her stress

85. Ms. W. is also started on Isordil (a vasodilator). The nurse is aware that the purpose of this medication is to

   A. help lessen pain

   B. decrease fluid retention

   C. lower cholesterol

   D. increase oxygen supply

86. When a patient is receiving this medication, it would be important for the nurse to monitor

    A. blood pressure

    B. pulse

    C. respiratory rate

    D. temperature

87. The physician decides to do a PTCA. Which of the statements is NOT true about this procedure?

    A. It is usually done when the atherosclerotic disease is limited to one vessel.

    B. The patient needs to sign a consent for coronary artery bypass surgery.

    C. It has a high rate of restenosis.

    D. Activity is limited for four weeks when discharged.

Ms. W. is ready for discharge. Part of her discharge instructions include information about decreasing her risk factors and taking appropriate medications.

88. What information would be appropriate regarding taking nitrates? (Check all that apply.)

    A. _____ Do not drink alcohol while using this medication.

    B. _____ Take sublingual tablets at the first onset of chest pain.

    C. _____ If pain continues after taking four doses, go to the ER.

    D. _____ Keep tablets away from sunlight.

89. Because she is on a diuretic, Ms. W. is instructed to eat food high in potassium. Which foods would you recommend? (Check all that apply.)

    A. _____ raisins

    B. _____ oranges

    C. _____ sardines

    D. _____ broccoli

90. Signs of hypokalemia that the nurse should talk about are

    A. fatigue, anorexia, paresthesia, palpitations

    B. nausea, diarrhea

    C. hypotension, headache

    D. bradycardia, dizziness

*L*earner Self-Evaluation

Do I fully understand the content? If no, then the areas I need to review are:

I need more information from my instructor on:

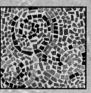

Nursing Care of Patients with Cardiac Disorders

*O*bjectives

1.0 Demonstrate an understanding of infections and inflammations of the cardiac system.

    1.1 Define several cardiac infections and inflammations.

    1.2 Identify the clinical manifestations of several cardiac disorders.

    1.3 Demonstrate an understanding of the medical management of infectious cardiac disorders.

    1.4 Identify the teaching needs of patients with infectious cardiac disorders.

    1.5 Plan the nursing care for patients with infectious cardiac disorders.

2.0 Demonstrate an understanding of other common cardiac disorders.

    2.1 Identify the etiology and clinical manifestations of several common cardiac disorders.

2.2 Identify medical and surgical interventions used with common cardiac disorders.

2.3 Demonstrate an understanding of disorders of the cardiac conductive system.

2.4 Plan the nursing care for patients with common cardiac disorders.

2.5 Identify the teaching needs of patients with cardiac disorders.

2.6 Identify alternative treatments and care settings for patients with cardiac disorders.

2.7 Identify any special considerations for the elderly patient with a cardiac disorder.

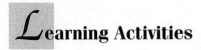

Identification

The ability of the nurse to recognize certain cardiac disorders is important. Match each of these disorders with the best definition.

 A. Endocarditis

 B. Myocarditis

 C. Pericarditis

 D. Congestive heart failure (CHF)

 E. Myocardial infarction (MI)

 F. Cardiomyopathy

1. _____ Inflammation of the endocardium and the heart valves

2. _____ Can occur when the cardiac output is not sufficient to meet body demands

3. _____ Disease of the heart muscle

4. _____ Inflammation of the heart muscle

5. _____ Results from complete obstruction of a coronary artery

6. _____ Inflammation of the sac surrounding the heart

Short Answers

7. An organized method of providing cardiac and/or respiratory support to a victim of cardiac arrest is called _____.

8. Because of trends toward early discharge and management in the home of individuals with cardiac disorders, the nurse knows that early

 _____ and _____ is an essential

 component of the nursing care.

9. Cardiac _____ are abnormalities in the rate and/or rhythm of the heart.

10. Atrial dysrhythmias result when the focus of impulse generation occurs outside the

 _____.

11. When a patient with atrial fibrillation is hemodynamically unstable, the treatment of

 choice is _____.

12. Patients in complete heart block become

 symptomatic because of _____.

13. _____ is unsynchronized cardioversion.

14. List several of the compensatory mechanisms that occur as the heart starts to fail as a pump.

 1.

 2.

 3.

 4.

15. What happens in the kidneys when there is a decrease in renal blood flow?

Interpretation

Using the knowledge from this chapter, identify
the following rhythms. State the rhythm, the rate,
and any specific abnormalities. You may also
calculate the PR and QRS intervals.

16.

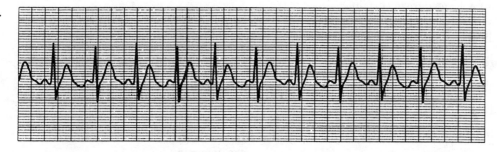

17.

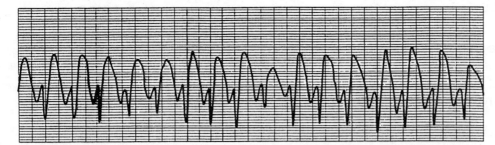

18.

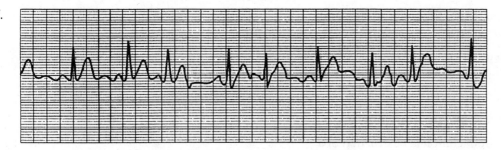

19.

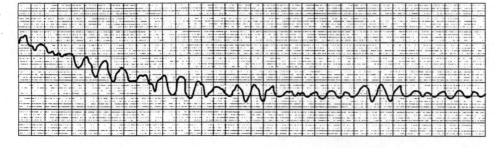

True/False

20. _____ Patients with infective endocarditis typically are managed at home.

21. _____ Tamponade, if not relieved, will lead to cardiac arrest.

22. _____ Patients who have had an MI are kept on bed rest for five days.

23. _____ The exact cause of atherosclerosis is unknown.

24. _____ Patients with mitral valve regurgitation are often asymptomatic.

25. _____ Maximum coronary blood flow at age 60 is about 35% less than that of a 30-year-old.

26. _____ It is often hard to diagnose an MI based on the type of chest pain the patient has.

Basic Knowledge

A basic understanding of cardiac medication is essential for good practice. Match the cardiac medications listed with the correct action.

   A. Digitalis

   B. Beta-adrenergic agonist

   C. ACE Inhibitor

   D. Diuretic

   E. Vasodilator

27. _____ Interferes with the conversion of angiotensin I to angiotensin II

28. _____ Increases the contractility of the myocardium

29. _____ Reverses constriction in heart vessels

30. _____ Increases cardiac output by stimulating beta receptors on the heart

31. _____ Increases urine production, thus reducing volume and pressure of blood to be pumped by the heart

Knowledge Application

32. Adults who develop subacute bacterial endocarditis (SBE) may have had _____ as children.

   A. mononucleosis

   B. rheumatic fever

   C. scarlet fever

   D. chicken pox

33. Assessment findings for the individual who has SBE would include

   A. heart murmur

   B. S_1, S_2, S_3

   C. abnormal breath sounds

   D. peripheral edema, weight gain

34. Medical management of SBE would be aimed at

   A. controlling the inflammatory process

   B. preventing cardiac damage

   C. preventing recurrence

   D. all of the above

35. Surgical management for the individual with SBE and bacterial destruction would involve

   A. angioplasty

   B. valve replacement

   C. bypass graft

   D. commissurotomy

36. If a patient with a cardiac condition were to become dyspneic and the nurse can auscultate rales and wheezes, the patient has probably developed

   A. cardiac tamponade

   B. endocarditis

   C. pleurisy

   D. CHF

37. Which of the following rhythms if seen on a cardiac monitor would the nurse interpret as life-threatening?

    A.   supraventricular tachycardia

    B.   atrial fibrillation

    C.   premature ventricular complexes

    D.   ventricular tachycardia

38. If an individual has chest pain, a pericardial friction rub, and ECG changes, the nurse would suspect

    A.   MI

    B.   SBE

    C.   pericardial effusion

    D.   cardiac tamponade

39. Because elderly individuals have altered pain sensation, their cardiac pain is often

    A.   atypical

    B.   severe

    C.   diffuse

    D.   radiating

40. The nurse is monitoring a patient's lab results and notes that the serum isoenzymes (CPK-MB) are greatly increased. This is due to

    A.   extreme pain and anxiety

    B.   cellular membrane destruction

    C.   inadequate cardiac output

    D.   falling arterial pressure

41. The nurse administers nitroglycerin sublingually to a patient with angina. Which statement best explains the therapeutic action of this medication?

    A.   decreases the myocardial oxygen consumption

    B.   increases the filling pressure (preload)

    C.   causes vasoconstriction of the systemic bed

    D.   increases the systemic blood pressure

42. When a patient has left-sided heart failure, the nurse would consider which goal as primary? Maintaining

    A.   adequate cardiac output

    B.   adequate tissue perfusion

    C.   adequate nutrition

    D.   effective coping skills

43. When a patient has cardiomyopathy, the nurse would monitor carefully for signs of

    A.   infection

    B.   chest pain

    C.   low cardiac output

    D.   heart murmur

44. In a patient with life-threatening cardiomyopathy, the treatment that can offer the best chance of survival is

    A.   bypass surgery

    B.   heart transplant

    C.   pacemaker insertion

    D.   implantable defibrillator

45. The best position for the patient in CHF would be

    A.   prone

    B.   supine

    C.   semi-Fowler's

    D.   Trendelenburg

46. A medication used to treat CHF by providing sedation and reduction of afterload is

    A.   morphine sulfate

    B.   Lasix

    C.   digoxin

    D.   verapamil

47. Treatment for the patient with a cardiac conduction block who is experiencing dizziness and confusion would probably include

    A. open-heart surgery

    B. pacemaker insertion

    C. digoxin, Lasix

    D. angioplasty

48. A cardiac patient is showing premature ventricular contractions (PVCs) on the monitor. Lidocaine is started. He then has a run of ventricular tachycardia followed by ventricular fibrillation. What is the proper nursing action?

    A. set up for pacemaker insertion

    B. prepare for surgery

    C. increase the dose of lidocaine

    D. prepare for defibrillation

49. Streptokinase is given to a patient who is having an MI. The nurse is aware that it is a thrombolytic agent and that it

    A. causes serious allergic reactions

    B. must be administered by the intercoronary route

    C. has the potential to cause systemic bleeding

    D. is a naturally occurring enzyme

50. The pain of an MI differs from that of angina in that it

    A. is retrosternal and radiating

    B. is longer and not relieved by nitroglycerin

    C. occurs with activity

    D. is associated with epigastric distress

51. When a patient has had an MI, the nurse carefully monitors for complications. The most frequent complication is

    A. endocarditis

    B. pulmonary embolism

    C. CHF

    D. cardiac arrhythmias

52. A patient who has had an MI is usually treated with medications that increase

    A. blood pressure

    B. preload and afterload

    C. oxygen supply and demand

    D. oxygen supply and decrease demand

53. The nurse is aware that the most common symptom experienced by patients with coronary artery disease is

    A. angina

    B. intermittent claudication

    C. hypoxia

    D. confusion

54. Which of the following individuals would be the most likely candidate for coronary artery bypass grafting?

    A. male, age 25, with severe cardiomyopathy

    B. male, age 85, with chronic CHF

    C. female, age 48, with chronic angina not amenable to angioplasty

    D. all of the above

55. When a patient has a diagnosis of left-sided heart failure, the nurse might expect him or her to make which of the following statements?

    A. "I am tired at the end of the day."

    B. "I have trouble breathing when I climb stairs."

    C. "My ankles are always swollen."

    D. "I feel bloated after I eat."

56. The most appropriate diet for the patient with CHF is

    A. low sodium, high potassium

    B. low potassium, low sodium

    C. low fat, low calorie

    D. high calorie, low fat

57. The analgesia of choice to control chest pain associated with MI is

    A. Demerol

    B. nitroglycerin

    C. morphine sulfate

    D. lidocaine

58. When lidocaine is not effective in treating ventricular arrhythmias, another drug that is often used is

    A. digoxin

    B. Procan

    C. Isordil

    D. streptokinase

59. A disease that is the result of atherosclerosis is

    A. coronary artery disease

    B. hypertension

    C. peripheral vascular disease

    D. all of the above

60. A medication that causes coronary and peripheral artery dilation as well as increasing myocardial contractility is:

    A. verapamil

    B. Lasix

    C. Inderal

    D. digoxin

61. In a patient with an uncomplicated MI, when would arm and leg exercises be started?

    A. within 4 hours

    B. in 12–24 hours

    C. in 24–48 hours

    D. after 48 hours

62. When valvular problems develop following rheumatic endocarditis, the process involved is

    A. valvular thickening, regurgitation

    B. stenosis, vegetation formation

    C. regurgitation, valvular thickening

    D. vegetation formation, stenosis

63. When a patient is diagnosed with dilated cardiomyopathy, the nurse is aware that symptoms are related to

    A. coronary artery obstruction

    B. increase in contractility

    C. increase in stroke volume and ejection factor

    D. decreased contractility and low cardiac output

64. When a patient has aortic valve stenosis, the nurse would monitor for signs of

    A. angina

    B. left ventricular failure

    C. peripheral edema

    D. cardiac dysrhythmias

65. A patient with mitral valve disease is scheduled for a commissurotomy. The nurse would explain that this means

    A. the valve will be removed and a synthetic valve inserted

    B. the elongated chordae will be shortened

    C. the valve leaflets that have fused together will be separated

    D. a balloon will be inserted and inflated in the valve

66. A patient had surgery to implant a mechanical heart valve and will be discharged on an anticoagulant. Which food would the nurse instruct him or her to avoid?

    A. dairy products

    B. all meat products

    C. green leafy vegetables

    D. bananas

67. Which of the following patients would be a candidate for an implantable cardioverter-defibrillator?

    A. male, age 50, who has survived an episode of sudden death

    B. female, age 60, who has had episodes of ventricular tachycardia even with medication

    C. male, age 35, who has survived a heart attack, but continues to have erratic heart rhythm

    D. any of the above

Nursing Care Plans

68. Write a nursing care plan for the patient in CHF.

    Nursing diagnosis: Altered cardiac output, decreased, related to altered myocardial contractility, alteration in cardiac rhythm.

    Patient outcome:

    Interventions:

69. Write a nursing care plan for the patient who has had an acute MI.

    Nursing diagnosis: Knowledge deficit, nature of MI, treatment, expected outcomes, and lifestyle changes.

    Patient outcome:

    Interventions:

Food for Thought

Do you think the current trend toward managed care will affect the availability of resources for elderly people with cardiac disease?

Case Studies

Case Study No. 1

A patient with a 10-year history of angina is admitted to the hospital with chest pain. He is admitted for a cardiac workup to rule out MI.

70. The diagnosis of MI will be based on

    A. history

    B. lab findings

    C. electrocardiogram

    D. all of the above

71. The nurse notices a run of PVCs on the cardiac monitor. The physician would most likely order

    A. digoxin

    B. lidocaine

    C. Lasix

    D. morphine

72. The patient is determined to have had an acute anterior MI. On the second hospital day, he becomes very short of breath. The nurse would suspect

    A. heart failure

    B. angina

    C. cardiac arrhythmia

    D. extension of the MI

73. He is started on digitalis to help treat this condition. The rationale for this medication is that it will

    A. increase stroke volume and cardiac output

    B. increase peripheral vascular resistance

    C. control irregular heart rhythm

    D. control pain associated with ischemia

74. On the third day, he develops oliguria and edema. Which statement best explains why he has developed oliguria?

    A. He has decreased renal perfusion due to reduced cardiac output.

    B. His kidneys are conserving water because of increased cardiac volume.

    C. He is in renal failure.

    D. His fluid intake has been limited because of chest pain.

75. A cardiac catheterization is scheduled to

    A. revascularize the myocardium

    B. study the action of the heart valves

    C. determine the extent of the MI

    D. administer medications

76. Findings from the heart catheterization show triple vessel disease with narrowing of greater than 60%. The most appropriate treatment would be

    A. angioplasty

    B. medication

    C. exercise program

    D. bypass surgery

Case Study No. 2

Mr. K. is on the open-heart step-down unit. He had coronary artery bypass surgery two days ago.

77. Mr. K. suddenly becomes dyspneic, cyanotic, and has a drop in cardiac output and a paradoxical pulse. These symptoms suggest

    A. cardiac tamponade

    B. pulmonary hypertension

    C. rupture of the graft

    D. pericarditis

78. After calling the physician, the appropriate nursing action would be

    A. set up a chest tube

    B. set up for pericardial tap

    C. call for a ventilator

    D. set up a dopamine drip

79. Mr. K. recovers from this complication but still has some respiratory congestion. The nurse should

    A. encourage the patient to cough and deep breathe every hour

    B. call for respiratory therapy to induce coughing

    C. use splinting when the patient coughs

    D. all of the above

80. Knowing that Mr. K. has severe coronary disease, one of the most important goals of nursing care would be

    A. lower risk factor profile

    B. change occupation

    C. lower simple sugar in his diet

    D. refrain from any exercise in the future

81. Five days later, Mr. K. is discharged. Discharge instruction would include telling him to

   A.   follow a low-potassium diet

   B.   avoid lifting

   C.   avoid any activity

   D.   return to the hospital in one week

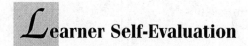

*L*earner Self-Evaluation

Do I fully understand the content? If no, then the areas I need to review are:

I need more information from my instructor on:

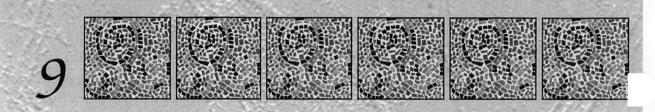

Knowledge Base for Patients with Vascular Dysfunction

Objectives

1.0 Review the anatomy and physiology of the vascular structures.
    1.1 Match the vascular structure with its characteristics.
    1.2 List structural factors that affect blood flow.

2.0 Demonstrate an understanding of the assessment data related to vascular structures.
    2.1 Identify risk factors for vascular disorders.
    2.2 Identify clinical manifestations of peripheral vascular dysfunction.
    2.3 Identify tests used to diagnose vascular dysfunction.
    2.4 Interpret assessment findings that relate to vascular dysfunction.

3.0 Demonstrate an understanding of the interventions used to treat vascular dysfunctions.
    3.1 Demonstrate an understanding of the medical management of the patient with a vascular dysfunction.
    3.2 Demonstrate an understanding of the surgical management of the patient with a vascular dysfunction.
    3.3 Write a nursing care plan for the patient undergoing vascular surgery.
    3.4 Identify special needs for the elderly patient with vascular dysfunction.
    3.5 Identify alternative treatments and care settings within the community for patients with vascular dysfunction.

Learning Activities

Short Answers

1. The three layers of blood vessels are
    1.

    2.

    3.

2. List three of the structural factors that affect blood flow.
    1.

    2.

    3.

3. For many individuals, _____ is always present with vascular dysfunction.

4. Pain that manifests late in the course of arterial insufficiency and is described as a shock-like sensation in the leg and foot is

    called _____.

5. _____ develops in tissues that contain blood deficit in oxygenated hemoglobin.

6. A palliative surgical procedure done to help

    reduce pain is called a _____.

7. The surgical removal of a clot in a vessel is

    called a(n) _____.

8. The surgical removal of fatty plaque from the inner and middle layers of vessel walls is

    called a(n) _____.

9. The only therapeutic option when an extremity is ischemic, painful, and gangrenous is

    _____.

10. The _____ comprise the largest population of persons with peripheral vascular disease.

Basic Knowledge

Match the vascular structure with its characteristics.

    A. Arteries

    B. Capillaries

    C. Veins

    D. Arterioles

    E. Venules

    F. Lymphatics

11. _____ Thin-walled transit tubes that begin the conduit of blood returning to the heart.

12. _____ Blood flow here delivers nutrition and removes waste products.

13. _____ Begins transport of oxygenated blood from the aorta.

14. _____ Serves as an accessory route for the transport of fluid and proteins away from interstitial space.

15. _____ High-resistance vessels that are innervated by sympathetic nervous system.

16. _____ Low pressure unidirectional conduit that relies on muscle contraction to move blood.

Knowledge Application

17. The neural control of blood flow is mediated by the sympathetic branch of the autonomic nervous system. Stimulation results in the release of norepinephrine, causing

    A. an increase in arterial blood pressure

    B. a decrease in arterial blood pressure

    C. a decrease in venous return to the heart

    D. peripheral vasodilation

18. Which of the following is a modifiable risk factor related to peripheral vascular disease?

    A. smoking

    B. age

    C. sex

    D. alcohol use

19. When pain is present in a patient with vascular dysfunction, it is usually related to

    A. decreased blood flow

    B. increased blood flow

    C. tissue hypoxia

    D. tissue injury

20. Cramplike pain felt in the calf muscles that is precipitated by walking is called

    _____.

    A. ischemia

    B. arterial hypoxia

    C. claudication

    D. dysreflexia

21. Resting pain is a sign of acute _____ insufficiency.

    A.   arterial

    B.   venous

    C.   cerebral

    D.   coronary

22. When a person with arterial insufficiency develops permanent dilatation of the arterioles, the extremities will appear

    A.   cyanotic

    B.   pale

    C.   ruddy

    D.   brownish

23. For an individual at home with acute resting pain, the nurse would suggest _____ to gain some relief of pain.

    A.   taking pain medication every four hours

    B.   elevating legs as much as possible

    C.   applying warm, moist compresses to legs

    D.   resting with legs in a dependent position

24. When assessing a patient with arterial insufficiency, the nurse anticipates

    A.   diminished or absent pulses

    B.   adequate capillary refill

    C.   peripheral edema and cyanosis

    D.   irregular pulses

25. A home-care patient tells the nurse that he takes Lovastatin. This would suggest that the patient has

    A.   high blood pressure

    B.   peripheral vascular disease

    C.   high cholesterol

    D.   heart disease

26. An invasive test done to visualize the arteries and assess blood flow is known as a(n)

    A.   venogram

    B.   arteriogram

    C.   Doppler ultrasound

    D.   Perthes' test

27. A noninvasive test that can detect auditory signs of blood flow to detect incompetent valves is known as

    A.   venography

    B.   Doppler ultrasound

    C.   angiography

    D.   impedance study

28. Which test measures resistance in veins related to blood volume and is used to evaluate the presence of iliac or femoral veins?

    A.   ultrasound

    B.   Perthes' test

    C.   arteriography

    D.   digital subtraction test

29. A medication used to treat peripheral vascular disease that works by making red blood cells more flexible is

    A.   Vasodilan

    B.   Trental

    C.   aspirin

    D.   Persantine

30. A medication often used by patients with peripheral vascular disease to help prevent platelet aggregation is

    A.   aspirin

    B.   heparin

    C.   Coumadin

    D.   Trental

31. Peripheral angioplasty may be used to open up an arterial blockage by

    A. vaporizing the plaque

    B. scraping the plaque from the artery

    C. compressing the plaque

    D. dissolving the plaque

32. Complications of angioplasty that the nurse would monitor for include

    A. stenosis

    B. hemorrhage

    C. embolism

    D. all of the above

33. The nurse would explain to a patient that surgical management of peripheral vascular disease is an option when

    A. the patient desires it

    B. medication doesn't work

    C. ischemic pain interferes with activity

    D. all of the above

34. Which of the following changes associated with aging put the elderly population at risk for the development of PVD?

    A. veins lose elasticity

    B. capillary membrane thickens

    C. aorta becomes less elastic

    D. all the above

Nursing Care Plans

35. Use the following nursing diagnosis to write a nursing care plan for the person in the home setting with peripheral vascular pain. Write a specific patient outcome and several nursing interventions.

Nursing diagnosis: Alteration in comfort related to impaired peripheral circulation

Patient outcome:

Interventions:

36. Use the following nursing diagnosis to write a nursing care plan for the patient who has had vascular bypass surgery. Write a specific patient outcome and several nursing interventions.

Nursing diagnosis: Alteration in peripheral tissue perfusion related to thrombus formation or reocclusion

Patient outcome:

Interventions:

Case Studies

Case Study No. 1

Ms. Y. is admitted with severe leg pain. Her left foot is cold and no pulse is present. She is taken for an angiogram. A clot is found in the artery and urokinase is started.

37. The nurse is aware that the purpose of this medication is to

    A. remove the blood clot

    B. stop formation of new clots

    C. dissolve the clot

    D. prevent infection

38. Ms. Y. is observed in the recovery room for 12 hours and then returned to the floor. She is now receiving heparin and Coumadin. Why would she be on both medications?

    A. They have a synergistic effect.

    B. Heparin works faster, Coumadin is slower.

    C. Coumadin works faster, then heparin takes over.

    D. Her condition is severe enough to warrant this.

Ms. Y. will be discharged in approximately 48 hours. It is important to do discharge planning and teaching prior to discharge.

39. Ms. Y. will probably be discharged when

    A. heparin is therapeutic

    B. Coumadin is therapeutic

    C. both are therapeutic

40. The nurse would stress the importance of watching for signs of bleeding while taking Coumadin. Ms. Y. should report

    A. blood in the stools

    B. bleeding gums

    C. epigastric pain

    D. any of the above

41. Upon discharge, it is important for Ms. Y. to recognize the need to

    A. have coagulation studies done frequently

    B. check for any signs of unusual bleeding

    C. practice safety measures to prevent cuts

    D. all of the above

Case Study No. 2

Mrs. R. is admitted with arterial occlusive disease that has not responded to medical treatment. She is undergoing diagnostic testing and possible surgery.

42. Since Mrs. R. has manifestations of arterial insufficiency, you would expect assessment findings to include

    A. brownish discoloration to skin, edema in feet

    B. skin thick and rough, rosy color

    C. feet warm with tissue edema

    D. feet pale and cool, skin dry and smooth

43. Mrs. R. is scheduled for a Doppler ultrasound. You explain that the purpose of this test is to

    A. detect disruption in blood flow in arteries or veins

    B. measure ankle pressure during exercise

    C. determine temperature changes with exercise

    D. visualize the blood flow in veins and arteries

Unfortunately, the results of this test are inconclusive and the physician decides to perform an arterial angiogram.

44. Before the test you would ask about

    A. drug allergies

    B. history of renal problems

    C. status of pulses

    D. all of the above

Mrs. R. is found to have severe stenosis in the right femoral artery. She is scheduled for femoral tibial bypass surgery using an saphenous vein graft from the left leg.

45. She wants to know what the surgery involves. The best explanation would be

    A. a plastic graft will be put in place of the diseased artery

    B. a GoreTex graft will bypass the stenosis and reestablish blood flow

    C. your own vein will be used to bypass the stenosis and reestablish blood flow

    D. a catheter will be inserted into the artery and the clot removed

46. When she returns to the floor, which nursing assessment would be considered a priority?

    A. respiratory status

    B. cardiac arrhythmias

    C. peripheral pulses

    D. fluid status

47. Postoperative orders include bed rest for 24 hours. The nurse realizes the reason for this order is to

    A. prevent trauma to the graft

    B. minimize pain

    C. minimize postoperative edema

    D. prevent risk of hemorrhage

48. Her recovery goes well and Mrs. R. is preparing for discharge. She will be taking Trental when she goes home. The nurse would explain that the action of this drug is to

    A. provide pain relief

    B. promote blood clotting

    C. relax smooth muscle

    D. make RBCs more flexible

$\mathcal{L}$earner Self-Evaluation

Do I fully understand the content? If no, then the areas I need to review are:

I need more information from my instructor on:

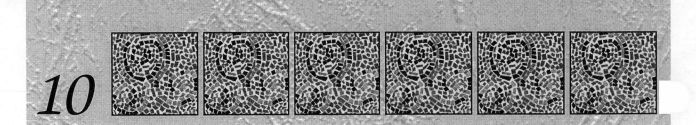

Nursing Care of Patients with Vascular Disorders

*O*bjectives

1.0 Demonstrate an understanding of common arterial vascular disorders.

    1.1 Review the etiology and pathophysiology of several common vascular disorders.

    1.2 Match common arterial disorders with the correct definition.

    1.3 Demonstrate an understanding of the teaching needs of the patient with an arterial vascular disorder.

    1.4 Identify treatment options available for the patient with a common arterial vascular disorder.

    1.5 Write a nursing care plan for the patient with an arterial vascular disorder.

2.0 Demonstrate an understanding of common venous vascular disorders.

    2.1 Review the etiology and pathophysiology of several common venous vascular disorders.

    2.2 Identify the characteristics of venous vascular disorders.

    2.3 Write a nursing care plan for the patient with a venous vascular disorder.

3.0 Demonstrate an understanding of the needs of the patient with an aneurysm.

    3.1 Identify clinical manifestations of aneurysms.

    3.2 Demonstrate an understanding of the medical and surgical interventions used in treating aneurysms.

    3.3 Plan appropriate nursing interventions for the patient with an aneurysm.

4.0 Demonstrate an understanding of the needs of the adult with hypertensive vascular disease.

    4.1 Identify the risk factors associated with hypertensive vascular disease.

    4.2 Demonstrate an understanding of the medical management of hypertensive vascular disease.

*L*earning Activities

Short Answers

1. List five risk factors that are related to the development of atherosclerosis and hypertension.
    1.

    2.

    3.

    4.

    5.

2. Smoking is prohibited for persons with vascular disorders because

    _____.

3. Individuals with arterial occlusive disease

    should be taught to avoid _____ clothing.

4. Most of the cases of arterial thrombus

    formation are related to _____.

5. The reasons that exercise is recommended for individuals with PVD is

    _____.

6. The home health nurse is working with Ms. A., age 30, who has been diagnosed with Raynaud's disease. List information that should be included in the plan of care to prevent vaso-occlusive episodes.
    1.

    2.

    3.

    4.

    5.

7. Arteriosclerosis of the smaller vessels is

    considered to be part of the _____

    process.

8. Dependent _____ is a sign of moderate to severe arterial occlusive disease.

9. Individuals with obstructive vascular disorders are usually managed in the

    _____.

10. When working with a patient who has hypertension, the nurse would emphasize

    the need to make _____.

Identification

Match the disorder with the definition.

    A.   Atherosclerosis

    B.   Raynaud's disease

    C.   Buerger's disease

    D.   Aneurysm

    E.   Arteriosclerosis obliterans

    F.   Thrombophlebitis

    G.   Varicose veins

    H.   Lymphangitis

11. _____ Abnormal dilation of the veins owing to venous insufficiency.

12. _____ An outpouching of a vessel wall or sac.

13. _____ Inflammation of the lymph system.

14. _____ Walls of the arteries become calcified from fatty plaque.

15. _____ Induced by cold or stress and characterized by paroxysmal, bilateral, digital ischemia.

16. _____ Caused by atherosclerosis; results in fatty plaque that blocks large vessels.

17. _____ Development of a clot in a vein.

18. _____ Chronic inflammatory process that involves medium-sized arteries and veins.

Knowledge Application

19. Which of the following diets would be recommended for the individual with atherosclerosis?

    A. fat 30%; protein 15%; carbohydrates 55%

    B. fat 10%; protein 35%; carbohydrates 55%

    C. fat 20%; protein 15%; carbohydrates 65%

    D. fat 30%; protein 25%; carbohydrates 45%

20. Intermittent claudication is a symptom that results from

    A. dorsiflexion of the foot when phlebitis is present

    B. inadequate blood flow to the muscles after exercise

    C. inadequate blood flow to the skin after exposure to cold

    D. stenosis of the veins

21. Ms. P. complains of burning and numbness in her hands. Her hands appear very red. A likely diagnosis is

    A. carpal tunnel syndrome

    B. arterial occlusion

    C. Raynaud's disease

    D. intermittent claudication

22. One of the most common and severe manifestations of thromboangiitis obliterans is

    A. cyanosis

    B. inflammation

    C. pain

    D. fatigue

23. Which procedure might be recommended to promote vasodilation for the patient with Buerger's disease?

    A. angioplasty

    B. bypass surgery

    C. sympathectomy

    D. laser surgery

24. _____ would be contraindicated for patients who have vascular occlusive disease.

    A. caffeine

    B. smoking

    C. vigorous exercise

    D. alcohol intake

25. A patient with Raynaud's disease would exhibit which of the following clinical manifestations?

    A. Hands appear cool and cyanotic.

    B. Numbness, edema, and decreased sensation may be present.

    C. Throbbing pain is felt at the end of an episode.

    D. Any of the above.

26. The nurse would teach a patient with Raynaud's disease that it may be possible to end vasospastic episodes by

    A. taking antispasmodic medications

    B. taking analgesics every day

    C. following an exercise routine

    D. placing fingers in warm water

27. Mr. T., age 45, is newly diagnosed with hypertension. His resting blood pressure was 180/100. The physician wants him to have a chest x-ray, ECG, urinalysis, and renal function studies. He asks the nurse why these tests are necessary. The best response is

    A. "These tests are always part of the workup."

    B. "These tests can determine cardiac changes and possibly the cause of your hypertension."

    C. "If you have a urinary infection, we will know what caused your hypertension."

    D. "You might have had a heart attack."

28. A patient with a peripheral vascular disease and a history of rheumatic heart disease may be at risk for _____.

    A. pulmonary embolism

    B. thrombus formation

    C. cardiac failure

    D. cerebral hypoxia

29. A patient is admitted to the hospital with a possible embolus in the brachial artery. The nurse would expect which of the following orders?

    A. bed rest, heparin therapy

    B. analgesic, force fluids, Coumadin therapy

    C. radiology examination and possible angioplasty

    D. narcotic analgesics and vasodilators

30. A patient is receiving a continuous heparin infusion for therapeutic management of thrombophlebitis. Which lab value would the nurse monitor?

    A. hemoglobin

    B. prothrombin time

    C. partial thromboplastin time

    D. erythrocyte sedimentation rate

31. If a patient with atherosclerosis exhibits symptoms of dizziness, confusion, and transient ischemic attacks, the area affected is most likely the

    A. cerebral vein

    B. carotid arteries

    C. coronary arteries

    D. peripheral vessels

32. When reviewing the lab results for a patient with hypertension and atherosclerosis, the nurse would expect to find high levels of

    A. potassium

    B. sodium

    C. cholesterol

    D. blood urea nitrogen (BUN)

33. Because adults with vascular occlusive disorder should avoid factors that cause vasoconstriction, the nurse would recommend

    A. a smoking cessation program

    B. a Weight Watchers program

    C. referral to a psychologist

    D. a cardiac support group

34. If a patient with an abdominal aneurysm were to suddenly develop hypotension, mottled extremities, and absent pulses, the nurse would

    A. prepare the patient for surgery

    B. elevate the legs

    C. medicate the patient for pain

    D. reassure the patient that this is normal

35. A patient with hypertension is to follow a low-sodium diet. Which of the following foods should be avoided?

    A. turkey breast

    B. eggs

    C. sausage

    D. low-fat milk

36. In a patient with severe arterial occlusive disease, which of the following symptoms would be evident?

    A. dependent rubor and pallor when extremity is elevated

    B. pallor and cyanosis in extremity

    C. peripheral edema, cyanosis, and numbness

    D. brownish discoloration, edema

37. In caring for a patient with arterial occlusive disease, the nurse would position him or her with legs

    A. elevated above heart

    B. level with heart

    C. in dependent position

    D. in any comfortable position

38. Cerebrovascular manifestations of hypertension would include

    A. chest pain, dizziness when arising

    B. vertigo, light-headedness, blurred vision

    C. peripheral edema, weight gain

    D. fatigue, palpitations

39. The treatment of choice for a patient with a 6 cm aortic aneurysm would probably be

    A. medical management

    B. angioplasty

    C. surgery

    D. anticoagulants

40. Patients with hypertension might be treated with any of the following medications EXCEPT

    A. beta blockers

    B. calcium channel blockers

    C. anticoagulants

    D. antispasmodics

41. A patient is admitted with mild back pain and a throbbing sensation in the abdomen. The nurse auscultates a bruit over the abdomen. These symptoms suggest

    A. renal thrombosis

    B. aortic aneurysm

    C. heart attack

    D. pulmonary embolism

42. In caring for a patient following resection of a thoracic aneurysm, the nurse would consider which goal as primary?

    A. maintaining systolic blood pressure < 120 mm Hg

    B. medicating the patient for pain

    C. preventing infection

    D. maintaining adequate nutrition

43. Which nursing action would prevent venous stasis in a patient with a history of varicose veins?

    A. apply elastic stockings

    B. increase fluid intake

    C. maintain activity restrictions

    D. keep legs in dependent position

44. In caring for a patient with a history of a vascular disorder who is on bed rest, the nurse would take appropriate precautions to

    A. avoid venous stasis

    B. provide nutrition

    C. provide relaxation therapy

    D. prevent infection

45. A patient with a thrombophlebitis develops sudden chest pain, dyspnea, diaphoresis, and cyanosis. The nurse suspects

    A. heart attack

    B. cerebrovascular accident

    C. pulmonary embolism

    D. pneumonia

46. A nurse should teach a patient with chronic venous insufficiency to do all of the following EXCEPT

    A. sit with legs in a dependent position

    B. sit with legs above the level of the heart

    C. avoid constricting garments

    D. sleep with the foot of the bed elevated

47. Treatment for the patient with venous stasis ulcers would most likely include

    A. Betadine compresses, antibiotics

    B. bed rest, analgesics

    C. saline compresses, local corticosteroid

    D. narcotics, vasodilators

48. Mr. E. has been given a prescription for prazosin (Minipress) to help treat his peripheral vascular disease. You explain that this works by

    A. increasing peripheral vascular resistance, causing vasodilation

    B. decreasing peripheral vascular resistance, causing vasodilation

    C. relaxing smooth arteriolar muscle

    D. decreasing cardiac output by sympathetic stimulation

True/False

49. _____ The most common occlusive disorder of the arteries is atherosclerosis.

50. _____ Drug therapy is the treatment of choice for most aneurysms.

51. _____ Atherosclerosis has been found in adults as young as 20 years old.

52. _____ Aneurysms are most frequently located in the femoral artery.

53. _____ Primary hypertension is caused by smoking.

54. _____ A false aneurysm is often the result of trauma to the vessel wall.

55. _____ Most older adults have some degree of atherosclerosis.

Nursing Care Plans

56. Use the following nursing diagnosis to write a nursing care plan for the patient with an obstructive arterial vascular disorder. Write a specific patient outcome and several nursing interventions.

    Nursing diagnosis: Altered tissue perfusion, peripheral

    Patient outcome:

    Interventions:

57. Use the following nursing diagnosis to write a nursing care plan for the patient who will be discharged following a recurrent thrombophlebitis. Write a specific patient outcome and several nursing interventions.

    Nursing diagnosis: Knowledge deficit: nature of the disease treatment and measures to reduce risk

    Patient outcome:

    Interventions:

Food for Thought

Develop a teaching plan that could significantly change the risk factors for a patient at risk of developing PVD. How would you realistically motivate him or her to change risk factors such as smoking, diet, exercise habits, and so forth?

Why don't individuals make changes in behavior when they know it is in their best interest to do so?

Case Studies

Case Study No. 1

Mr. Y. is admitted to the hospital with severe peripheral vascular disease. On admission, he states he has severe claudication in his left leg which greatly limits his activity. The nurse cannot palpate the left pedal pulse and notes that both extremities are pale and cool. The following questions relate to this situation.

58. Because the nurse is unable to palpate any pulses, the next step would be to

   A.   chart the findings

   B.   call the physician

   C.   use a Doppler probe

   D.   medicate for pain

59. The cause of claudication in a patient with peripheral vascular disease is

   A.   too much exercise

   B.   tissue ischemia

   C.   lack of adherence to medications

   D.   all of the above

Mr. Y. is scheduled for a femoral-popliteal bypass operation with a synthetic graft.

60. Mr. Y. is wondering what a bypass operation entails. The nurse would explain the procedure by stating

   A.   "The diseased part of your artery is removed and a graft is inserted."

   B.   "A vein from your leg will be used to provide circulation."

   C.   "A synthetic graft will be inserted above and below the area of stenosis."

   D.   "The diseased part of your vein will be cleaned out and a graft placed around it."

61. The evening after surgery, Mr. Y. complains of numbness, pain, tingling, and burning in his leg. The nurse would

   A.   assess pulses

   B.   medicate for pain

   C.   notify the physician

   D.   chart this information

62. Later in the evening, Mr Y. has severe pain in the leg and foot. The physician cannot find the left peripheral pulses. A probable cause of these symptoms is

   A.   thrombus

   B.   embolus

   C.   vasospasm

   D.   infection

63. The most likely intervention at this time would be

   A.   angioplasty

   B.   medicate with narcotics

   C.   embolectomy

   D.   x-ray the extremity

Following the procedure, Mr. Y. is stabilized. He will be discharged in two days.

64. Based on his history and postoperative complications, the nurse would anticipate that he would receive _____ when discharged.

    A. narcotics

    B. anticoagulants

    C. vasodilators

    D. antibiotics

65. Mr. Y. will also be taking clonidine (Catapres) after discharge. The nurse would discuss side effects of this medication, including

    A. headache, vertigo

    B. loss of libido

    C. orthostatic hypotension

    D. all the above

Case Study No. 2

Mrs. R. has been hospitalized for several weeks following a back injury. She has a history of hypertension, cardiac disease, and adult-onset diabetes.

66. Because the nurse recognizes problems that can result from immobility, she would be sure to assess _____ in this patient.

    A. Trousseau's sign

    B. Homans' sign

    C. pain response

    D. neurologic status

67. Late in the day, Mrs. R. complains of pain and warmth in her right calf. Which of the following tests would be ordered?

    A. blood culture

    B. venogram

    C. arteriogram

    D. heart catheterization

68. A diagnosis of thrombophlebitis is confirmed. The patient is started on heparin therapy at 1000 units/hour. A nursing priority would be to

    A. monitor for bleeding

    B. monitor coagulation studies

    C. avoid the use of aspirin

    D. all of the above

69. The lab calls the floor and tells the nurse that the partial thromboplastin time is 120 seconds. The nurse would

    A. stop the infusion and call the physician

    B. increase the infusion based on standing orders

    C. do nothing; recheck the level in eight hours

    D. decrease the rate by one-half

70. Since Mrs. R. is to be discharged on Coumadin, the nurse would provide the following instructions EXCEPT

    A. take the medication until discontinued by the physician

    B. notify the dentist if any work is to be done

    C. continue to take all previous medications

    D. return to medical lab for follow-up studies

*L*earner Self-Evaluation

Do I fully understand the content? If no, then the areas I need to review are:

I need more information from my instructor on:

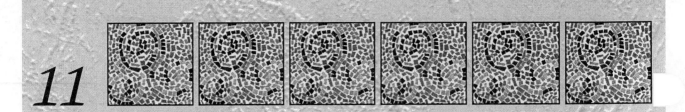

11

Knowledge Base for Patients in Shock

Objectives

1.0 Review the etiology of the three types of shock.
    1.1 Identify hemodynamic principles affected by shock.
    1.2 Identify signs and symptoms of shock.

2.0 Differentiate three types of shock according to their etiologies and pathologic alterations.
    2.1 Demonstrate an understanding of the etiology and management of hypovolemic shock.
    2.2 Demonstrate an understanding of the etiology and management of cardiogenic shock.
    2.3 Demonstrate an understanding of the etiology and management of distributive shock.

3.0 Demonstrate an understanding of interventions used to treat patients in shock.
    3.1 Demonstrate an understanding of the role of intravenous therapy in the management of shock.
    3.2 Plan the nursing care for a patient in shock.

Learning Activities

Short Answers

1. The three types of shock are
    1.

    2.

    3.

2. Adequate blood flow depends on
    1.

    2.

    3.

3. The two major mechanisms that determine cardiac output are

    1.

    2.

4. When afterload is increased, the heart must

    work _____.

5. In the compensatory stage of shock, vasoconstriction in the kidneys causes

    _____.

6. Colloid solutions increase serum colloid

    osmotic pressure in the _____

    compartment.

7. Crystalloid solutions expand the

    _____ volume.

8. The most common cause of septic shock is

    _____.

9. Anaphylaxis is a hypersensitivity reaction to

    an _____.

Basic Knowledge

List the normal value.

                                    Value

10. Cardiac output   _____

11. Central venous pressure _____

The ability of the nurse to know correct medical terminology is important. Match the following.

    A. Cardiac output
    B. Cardiac index
    C. Central venous pressure
    D. Stroke volume
    E. Systemic vascular resistance

12. _____ Pressure created by volume in the right side of the heart.

13. _____ Resistance to blood ejected from left ventricle.

14. _____ Volume of blood pumped by ventricles per minute.

15. _____ Amount of blood ejected per heartbeat.

16. _____ Cardiac output/body surface area.

Knowledge Application

17. A patient comes to the emergency department bleeding profusely after a fall. He would be at risk for

    A. hypovolemic shock
    B. cardiogenic shock
    C. septic shock
    D. neurogenic shock

18. The diagnosis of hypovolemic shock is based primarily on

    A. vital signs
    B. amount of blood lost
    C. history and clinical manifestation
    D. level of consciousness

19. Major goals in treating hypovolemic shock are

    A. control the source of blood loss
    B. reverse the loss of blood
    C. restore tissue perfusion
    D. all of the above

20. The most appropriate solution to increase the extracellular volume for the patient in Class II hemorrhagic shock would be

    A. Ringer's lactate

    B. whole blood

    C. dextran

    D. 5% dextrose in water

21. When a patient develops cardiogenic shock, medications are used to increase cardiac output. Which of the following will increase preload and afterload?

    A. dobutamine (Dobutrex)

    B. dopamine (Intropin)

    C. amrione (Inocor)

    D. norepinephrine (Levophed)

22. The early stage of septic shock is characterized by

    A. a rise in blood pressure

    B. severe vasoconstriction

    C. massive venous and arterial vasodilation

    D. an increase in preload and afterload

23. A patient in the hyperdynamic phase of septic shock would exhibit which of the following symptoms?

    A. normal cardiac output, full bounding pulse, disorientation, rise in temperature

    B. drop in cardiac output, weak thready pulse, disorientation, rise in temperature

    C. low cardiac output, weak pulse, tachycardia, disorientation, rise in temperature

    D. rise in cardiac output, bradycardia, tachypnea, decrease in temperature

24. Which of the following sets of arterial blood gas values would be consistent with progressive shock?

    A. pH 7.45 PaO_2 95% $PaCO_2$ 28%

    B. pH 7.52 PaO_2 65% $PaCO_2$ 40%

    C. pH 7.25 PaO_2 60% $PaCO_2$ 60%

    D. pH 7.30 PaO_2 88% $PaCO_2$ 35%

25. Afterload would probably be increased in an adult with

    A. aortic stenosis

    B. mitral valve prolapse

    C. hypotension

    D. anemia

26. During the compensatory stage of shock, most of the clinical manifestations are due to a

    A. decrease in dopamine

    B. decrease in epinephrine

    C. release of catecholamines

    D. decrease in blood glucose

27. If the patient in shock enters the progressive stage, the primary cause must be corrected quickly or

    A. an increase in oxygen consumption will occur

    B. hypoperfusion of organs will lead to multisystem failure

    C. intracellular dehydration occurs and severe electrolyte imbalances occur

    D. metabolic alkalosis and hypoglycemia occur

28. The nurse is reviewing lab values of an individual in septic shock. Which values are consistent with acute tubular necrosis?

    A. increase in white blood cell count (WBC), decrease in platelets

    B. decrease in hemoglobin and hematocrit

    C. increase in SGOT and LDH

    D. increase in BUN and creatinine

29. The reason that the person in shock loses consciousness is

    A. low blood pressure

    B. decreased cerebral blood flow

    C. respiratory alkalosis

    D. hypotension

30. The widespread tissue responses seen with anaphylaxis are caused by the release of

    A. epinephrine

    B. serotonin

    C. adrenaline

    D. histamine

31. The drug of choice for treating anaphylactic shock is

    A. epinephrine

    B. Benadryl

    C. histamine

    D. dopamine

Nursing Care Plan

32. Use the following nursing diagnosis to write a nursing care plan for the patient in cardiogenic shock. Write a patient outcome and several nursing interventions.

    Nursing diagnosis: Decreased cardiac output related to fluid volume deficit secondary to changes in myocardial contractility

    Patient outcome:

    Interventions:

Case Study

Mr. P. is admitted to the coronary care unit with an acute anterior wall myocardial infarction. He is pale and diaphoretic. His pain is severe. Vital signs are BP 90/60; apical 112; respirations 28; temperature 99° F. He seems confused at times. The physician inserts a central line to monitor CVP, and the reading is low. A diagnosis of cardiogenic shock is made.

33. Based on the initial symptoms, what stage of shock is Mr. P. exhibiting?

    A. compensatory shock

    B. progressive shock

    C. refractory shock

    D. irreversible

34. The physician orders dobutamine started as a continuous infusion at 10 mcg/kg/min. The purpose of this medication is to

    A. lower the heart rate

    B. relieve the pain

    C. improve the cardiac output

    D. increase preload and afterload

35. During this stage of shock, the nurse is aware that

    A. there is a decrease in cardiac output and tissue perfusion

    B. there is an increase in cardiac output and heart rate

    C. the autonomic nervous system causes arteries to dilate

    D. respirations slow and get deeper

36. The most likely cause of Mr. P.'s shock is

    A. aortic aneurysm

    B. dysrhythmias

    C. blood loss secondary to myocardial tear

    D. loss of contractility of myocardium

Medical treatment does not seem to be helping the condition. Mr. P. worsens, becoming more confused, with BP 60/50; apical 128; respirations 40. Pulse is very weak and thready.

37. The physician orders a nitroglycerin infusion. The main purpose of this medication is to

    A.   improve cardiac output

    B.   dilate coronary arteries and increase blood flow

    C.   constrict peripheral vessels

    D.   relieve pain

Because Mr. P. is not improving, the cardiologist decides to insert an intra-aortic balloon pump (IABP). Mr. P.'s wife is very distraught and asks the nurse for an explanation. "I don't want to prolong his suffering," she says.

38. The best explanation of the IABP is that a

    A.   balloon is inserted through an artery and positioned near the subclavian artery; it inflates and deflates to improve cardiac output

    B.   balloon is inserted surgically into the heart where it inflates and deflates mimicking the normal pumping action of the heart

    C.   small window is cut into the heart to decrease the workload

    D.   catheter is inserted into the pulmonary artery to obtain hemodynamic measurements

Learner Self-Evaluation

Do I fully understand the content? If no, then the areas I need to review are:

I need more information from my instructor on:

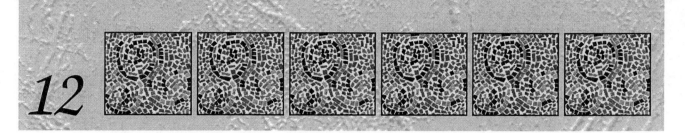

Knowledge Base for Patients with Hematologic Dysfunction

Objectives

1.0 Review the anatomy and physiology of the hematologic system.
    1.1 List the components of the hematologic system.
    1.2 List the functions of the hematologic system.

2.0 Demonstrate an understanding of assessment data related to the hematologic system.
    2.1 Identify clinical manifestations of hematologic dysfunction.
    2.2 Review the health history of a patient with a hematologic disorder.
    2.3 Identify normal laboratory values.
    2.4 Identify tests used to diagnose hematologic disorders.

3.0 Demonstrate an understanding of interventions used to treat patients with hematologic disorders.
    3.1 Demonstrate an understanding of medical management and surgical treatment of hematologic disorders.
    3.2 Demonstrate an understanding of the use of blood transfusions in the treatment of hematologic disorders.
    3.3 Plan the nursing care for a patient with a disorder of the hematologic system.
    3.4 Identify special considerations for the elderly patient with hematologic dysfunction.

Learning Activities

Short Answers

1. List the components of the hematologic system.
    1.

    2.

    3.

    4.

    5.

2. Blood transports _____ to the cells and carries _____ away from the cells.

3. The process by which blood cells are formed is known as _____.

4. _____, a part of the red blood cell, is important in transporting oxygen to the tissues.

5. When a blood vessel is injured,

   _____ occurs.

6. List several functions of the spleen.
   1.

   2.

   3.

   4.

7. Signs of reduced oxygen-carrying capacity of

   the blood are _____, _____,

   _____, and _____.

8. The white blood cells that destroy bacteria

   are called _____.

9. The _____ _____ is used to diagnose
   and assess the extent of bleeding disorders.

10. The _____ _____ test detects the pres-
    ence of antibodies against red blood cells.

Basic Knowledge

The nurse must have a basic knowledge of the
functions of the blood and blood-forming organs.
Correctly match each of the following.

   A. Red blood cells (RBCs)

   B. White blood cells (WBCs)

   C. Platelets

   D. Lymph nodes

   E. Bone marrow

   F. Spleen

11. _____ Serve as filters

12. _____ Protect the body against microorgan-
    isms

13. _____ One of the larger organs of the body

14. _____ Carry oxygen to the cells

15. _____ Remove old or injured red blood cells
    and platelets

16. _____ Important in the blood clotting process

17. _____ Composed of granulocytes and mono-
    nuclear cells

Fill in the normal lab values.

18. WBC _____ mm^3

19. RBC _____ million/mm^3 (male) _____
    million/mm^3 (female)

20. Hematocrit _____ % (male) _____ %
    (female)

21. Hemoglobin _____ g/100 mL (male) _____
    g/100 mL (female)

22. Platelet count _____ mm^3

23. Prothrombin time _____ seconds

24. Partial thromboplastin time (PTT) _____
    seconds

25. Serum iron _____ μg/dL (males) _____ μg/
    dL (females)

The ability of the nurse to know correct medical
terminology is important. Match the following.

   A. Leukocytosis

   B. Anemia

   C. Polycythemia

   D. Leukopenia

   E. Thrombocytopenia

26. _____ Low white blood cell count

27. _____ Increase in red blood cells

28. _____ Decrease in platelets

29. _____ Often seen with infections

30. _____ May occur with decreased cardiac
    output

31. _____ Occurs with aplastic anemia

32. _____ Can lead to shortness of breath

33. _____ May be seen with bone marrow failure

Knowledge Application

34. The older adult is prone to certain blood disorders. The reason is

    A.   change in mental status

    B.   loss of mobility

    C.   increase in infections

    D.   decrease in immunologic defense

35. When a patient with a blood disorder exhibits symptoms of fatigue, weakness, and pallor, it is often due to

    A.   decrease in erythrocytes

    B.   decrease in leukocytes

    C.   decrease in platelets

    D.   all of the above

36. When a patient has low platelet count, the nurse would monitor for

    A.   fatigue, weakness, pallor

    B.   temperature, infection

    C.   bruising, ecchymoses, petechiae

    D.   all of the above

37. Symptoms of joint pain and deformities are often associated with

    A.   leukemia

    B.   hemophilia

    C.   anemia

    D.   leukopenia

38. A patient with leukemia has a cough, dyspnea, and fever. The nurse would suspect

    A.   respiratory infection

    B.   bleeding disorder

    C.   anemia

    D.   sepsis

39. Hemolysis of red blood cells in a patient with a hematologic disorder may lead to

    A.   infection

    B.   bleeding tendency

    C.   nutritional deficit

    D.   jaundice and pruritus

40. A surgical patient who has developed a venous thrombosis has an increased risk of developing

    A.   anemia

    B.   decreased platelet aggregation

    C.   increased platelet aggregation

    D.   increased prothrombin time

41. A patient who has decreased intake and absorption of vitamin K has a risk for developing a(n)

    A.   increase in prothrombin time

    B.   decrease in prothrombin time

    C.   decrease in platelet aggregation

    D.   decrease in bleeding time

42. The home-health nurse is visiting Mr. M., who has been diagnosed with pernicious anemia. When reviewing his lab data, the nurse would look for

    A.   thrombocytopenia

    B.   low hematocrit

    C.   low prothrombin time (protime)

    D.   leukocytosis

43. Which of the following tests is most specific in diagnosing pernicious anemia?

    A.   urobilinogen test

    B.   serum folic acid test

    C.   indirect Coombs' test

    D.   Schilling test

44. Ms. K., age 18, has been diagnosed with aplastic anemia secondary to treatment for leukemia. Which of the following tests would the nurse monitor carefully?

    A.   protime

    B.   sickle-cell test

    C.   bleeding time

    D.   erythrocyte sedimentation test

45. A patient is receiving heparin therapy. The nurse would realize that the heparin is therapeutic when the PTT is

   A. 25–35 seconds

   B. 35–45 seconds

   C. 45–60 seconds

   D. 60–90 seconds

46. A patient is admitted with a diagnosis of multiple myeloma. The nurse would expect laboratory tests to show an increase in _____ cells in the bone marrow.

   A. white blood

   B. plasma

   C. red blood

   D. platelets

47. If a patient has an elevated reticulocyte count, this means an

   A. increased rate of WBC production but low leukocyte count

   B. increased rate of erythrocyte production with premature destruction of mature RBCs

   C. decreased production of platelets and increased destruction of mature RBCs

   D. increase in production of WBCs, RBCs, and platelets

48. A patient is admitted with possible leukemia. The test that would provide the best diagnostic information is

   A. Schilling test

   B. ultrasonogram

   C. CBC

   D. bone marrow aspiration

49. The best explanation of a computed tomography (CT) scan would be

   A. a noninvasive procedure to visualize soft tissue structures

   B. a three-dimensional view of body tissue

   C. a radiation test that visualizes organs

   D. an invasive test where tissue samples are taken

50. When a patient with anemia has a hemoglobin of 9.6 g/100 mL and slight fatigue, which therapy would the nurse expect to be ordered?

   A. oxygen therapy

   B. blood transfusions

   C. IV therapy

   D. vitamin therapy

51. The type of transfusion that would be most appropriate for the patient who is hemorrhaging is

   A. whole blood

   B. packed red cells

   C. frozen red cells

   D. platelets

52. When a transfusion reaction occurs, which of the following nursing actions would be implemented?

   A. Stop the transfusion.

   B. Keep vein open with primary solution.

   C. Monitor vital signs.

   D. Notify the physician and blood bank.

   E. All of the above.

53. To stop the bleeding in a patient with hemophilia, the most appropriate type of transfusion is

   A. whole blood

   B. packed red cells

   C. clotting factors

   D. plasma

54. With severe dehydration, the nurse would expect to see a rise in

   A. white count

   B. hematocrit

   C. BUN

   D. platelets

55. To help determine what type of anemia a patient has, the _____ would give the best information.

    A. hemoglobin and hematocrit

    B. red blood cell indices

    C. platelet count

    D. prothrombin test

Identification

Explain the following types of blood reactions.

56. Hemolytic reaction

57. Nonhemolytic reaction

58. Allergic reaction

59. Anaphylactic reaction

60. Septic reaction

True/False

61. _____ Blood should be administered within one hour of receipt on the unit.

62. _____ Prime the blood tubing with a dextrose solution.

63. _____ All blood should be administered with a pump.

64. _____ Blood should be warmed when given for massive blood loss.

65. _____ Tachycardia and dyspnea are signs of a transfusion reaction.

66. _____ A delayed transfusion reaction can occur days or weeks after the transfusion.

Nursing Care Plans

67. Use the following nursing diagnosis to write a nursing care plan for the patient with symptoms of fatigue, dyspnea and weakness secondary to a hematological dysfunction. Write two patient outcomes and several nursing interventions.

    Nursing diagnosis: Activity intolerance related to fatigue and dyspnea secondary to decreased oxygen-carrying capacity of the blood

    Patient outcomes:

    Interventions:

68. Use the following nursing diagnosis to write a nursing care plan for the patient with a bleeding disorder. Write two patient outcomes and several nursing interventions.

    Nursing diagnosis: Alteration in tissue perfusion

    Patient outcomes:

    Interventions:

Case Studies

Case Study No. 1

A patient with hemophilia is admitted to the hospital with the following symptoms: fatigue, weakness, pallor, bruising, and swelling in the knees.

69. Which of the following laboratory studies would the nurse expect to be abnormal?

    A. WBC, RBC, platelets

    B. RBC, HgB, Hct, platelets

    C. WBC, PTT, PT

    D. leukocytes, CBC

70. Because of the patient's symptoms, an important nursing intervention would be to prevent

    A. bleeding episodes

    B. infection

    C. fluid and electrolyte imbalance

    D. falls

71. If the patient were to exhibit signs of dyspnea and shortness of breath, the nurse would expect to administer

    A. antibiotics

    B. anticoagulants

    C. oxygen

    D. IV fluids

72. An important part of the nursing care with this patient is teaching, including

    A. staying in bed as much as possible

    B. limiting fluid intake

    C. taking antibiotics on a routine basis

    D. carrying an identification card

Case Study No. 2

A patient has been receiving chemotherapy for leukemia. She is admitted to the hospital with shortness of breath, loss of appetite, and weight loss of 20 pounds.

73. The reason for the shortness of breath in this patient is probably

    A. anemia

    B. thrombocytopenia

    C. leukopenia

    D. leukocytosis

74. On assessment, the nurse notices that the patient has ulcerations of the mouth. An appropriate nursing diagnosis would be

    A. Alteration in fluid and electrolytes

    B. Alteration in nutrition

    C. Alteration in elimination

    D. Ineffective coping

75. To treat the mouth ulcers, the nursing actions are to

    A. provide good mouth care and bland, soft foods

    B. start the patient on tube feedings

    C. have meals brought in from home

    D. keep patient NPO until ulcers heal

The patient's WBC is 2000/mm³ today. Because of her low leukocyte count, the nurse realizes that the patient is at risk for infection.

76. The nurse uses a nursing diagnoses of High risk for infection secondary to compromised immunity. An appropriate outcome would be that the

    A. patient reports that pain is controlled with analgesics

    B. patient displays no fever, chills, tachycardia, tachypnea, or pain or burning on urination

    C. patient's oral cavity and legs are free from ulcerative lesions

    D. patient can ambulate 50 feet without fatigue

Unfortunately, the patient's condition worsens and the physician plans a bone marrow transplant.

77. The most important nursing diagnosis related to the bone marrow transplant would be

    A.   Knowledge deficit

    B.   Alteration in nutrition

    C.   Potential for infection

    D.   Alteration in tissue perfusion

Case Study No. 3

A patient who has had recent surgery has a HgB 7.2 g/mL, Hct 27.9%. Because she has symptoms of hypoxia, the physician decides to order a blood transfusion.

78. The most appropriate type of transfusion for this patient would be

    A.   whole blood

    B.   packed red cells

    C.   plasma

    D.   platelets

79. The morning after the transfusion, another HgB and Hct is drawn. The nurse would expect to see

    A.   HgB up 1 gram, Hct up 3%

    B.   HgB up 2 grams, Hct up 6%

    C.   HgB up 3 grams, Hct up 8%

    D.   HgB up 4 grams, Hct up 10%

80. The patient is still symptomatic, so another transfusion is ordered. If this patient were to develop a rash, itching, or a low-grade fever, the nurse would suspect

    A.   hemolytic reaction

    B.   nonhemolytic reaction

    C.   circulatory overload

    D.   septic reaction

81. The most appropriate nursing action would be to

    A.   stop the infusion and notify the physician

    B.   continue the infusion, but monitor the patient carefully

    C.   slow down the infusion and notify the physician

*L*earner Self-Evaluation

Do I fully understand the content? If no, then the areas I need to review are:

I need more information from my instructor on:

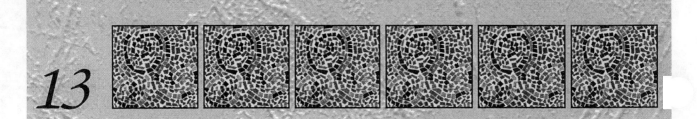

Nursing Care of Patients with Hematologic Disorders

Objectives

1.0 Demonstrate an understanding of the common hematologic disorders.
   1.1 Match erythrocyte-related disorders to their defining characteristics.
   1.2 Identify the clinical manifestations of several of the hematologic disorders.
   1.3 Identify nursing interventions appropriate for the patient with a hematologic disorder.
   1.4 Identify medications used for patients with hematologic disorders.

2.0 Demonstrate an understanding of the neoplasms that affect the hematologic system.
   2.1 Identify the characteristics of several neoplasms of the hematologic system.
   2.2 Identify medical treatments used for patients with neoplasms of the hematologic system.

3.0 Demonstrate an understanding of bleeding disorders.
   3.1 Match several of the bleeding disorders with their defining characteristics.
   3.2 Identify medical management of bleeding disorders.
   3.3 Plan the nursing care for the patient with a bleeding disorder.

Learning Activities

Short Answers

1. Anemia can result from _____ or _____ blood loss.

2. A deficiency in folic acid results in defective

_____ _____ _____ production.

3. In the hemolytic anemias, the red blood cells

   (RBCs) have a _____ life span.

4. The _____ are a group of disorders that have increased RBCs and hemoglobin concentration.

5. Infectious mononucleosis is caused by

   _____.

Identification

The nurse must have a basic knowledge of common hematologic disorders. Correctly match each of the following.

A. Iron deficiency anemia

B. Aplastic anemia

C. Sickle-cell anemia

D. Spherocytosis

E. Pernicious anemia

F. Thalassemia

G. G-6-PD deficiency

H. Immune hemolytic anemia

6. _____ Characterized by thin, fragile RBCs known as target cells

7. _____ Chronic hereditary hemolytic disorder found mainly in black Americans

8. _____ Often related to poor nutrition

9. _____ Characterized by small, ball-shaped RBCs that swell from accumulation of sodium and water

10. _____ Inherited sex-linked disorder involving a deficiency of an enzyme important in glucose metabolism

11. _____ Caused by impaired red blood cell development within the bone marrow

12. _____ Treatment involves taking vitamin B_{12}

13. _____ Caused by the lysis of blood cells

Knowledge Application

14. Anemia in an adult can result from

    A. blood loss

    B. decreased RBC production

    C. RBC destruction

    D. all of the above

15. The adult with severe anemia may become confused and disoriented because of

    A. impaired gas exchange

    B. ineffective breathing patterns

    C. cerebral anoxia

    D. hemorrhagic loss

16. The most common sign of anemia in adults is

    A. dyspnea

    B. fatigue

    C. anorexia

    D. bruising

17. When a patient has anemia secondary to blood loss, the nurse would monitor carefully for signs of

    A. hypovolemia

    B. diarrhea

    C. vomiting

    D. hypertension

18. If a patient with severe anemia and blood loss were to become hypotensive; have rapid, deep respirations; low urine output; and disorientation, the nurse would realize this is due to

    A. low cardiac output

    B. fluid shifts

    C. increased plasma volume

    D. dehydration

19. The management of the patient with hemorrhagic anemia is primarily to

    A. arrest blood loss

    B. replace lost fluid

    C. prevent recurrence

    D. all of the above

20. A patient complains of fatigue, weakness, sensitivity to cold, and dysphagia. The nurse notes he has mouth ulcers and a red tongue. This suggests

    A.   hemorrhagic anemia

    B.   iron deficiency anemia

    C.   aplastic anemia

    D.   pernicious anemia

21. Patients on iron therapy should be taught to take their medication with _____ to increase absorption.

    A.   milk

    B.   orange juice

    C.   water

    D.   none of the above

22. The nurse would suggest that the patient with an iron deficiency should eat foods high in iron. The best sources would include

    A.   milk and dairy products

    B.   bread and grains

    C.   red meat, green vegetables

    D.   chicken, fish, dried fruit

23. Impaired vitamin B_{12} absorption can lead to

    A.   iron deficiency anemia

    B.   aplastic anemia

    C.   pernicious anemia

    D.   macrocytic anemia

24. An elderly individual with a history of past and current alcohol abuse is admitted to the hospital. The nurse is aware that this patient is at risk for developing

    A.   anemia

    B.   folic acid deficiency

    C.   sickle-cell crisis

    D.   aplastic anemia

25. Treatment for aplastic anemia may include

    A.   blood transfusions

    B.   myelotoxic drugs

    C.   bone marrow transplant

    D.   any of the above

26. A side effect that may occur from excessive blood transfusions in individuals with certain anemias is

    A.   dehydration

    B.   elevated iron levels

    C.   sluggish circulation

    D.   rise in hemoglobin

27. Symptoms that might be evident in the individual with polycythemia vera include

    A.   fatigue, shortness of breath

    B.   increased blood pressure and pulse, headaches

    C.   decreased blood pressure, weakness

    D.   dizziness, cyanosis of extremities

28. Emergency management for the individual with polycythemia vera would include

    A.   oxygen therapy

    B.   fluid replacement

    C.   phlebotomies

    D.   antiarrhythmics

29. The most appropriate diet for the individual with polycythemia vera would be

    A.   low sodium

    B.   low cholesterol

    C.   low potassium

    D.   high potassium

30. The most common hematologic disorder found in older adults is

    A.   anemia

    B.   leukemia

    C.   hemophilia

    D.   multiple myeloma

31. A malignant disease that is characterized by the growth of plasma cells invading bone marrow, lymph nodes, liver, and spleen is

    A.   leukemia

    B.   Hodgkin's Disease

    C.   non-Hodgkin's lymphoma

    D.   multiple myeloma

32. Which type of leukemia has symptoms of long bone pain, anemia, and splenomegaly, and is most common in individuals aged 40 to 60 years?

    A.   acute lymphocytic leukemia

    B.   acute myelogenous leukemia

    C.   chronic lymphocytic leukemia

    D.   chronic myelogenous leukemia

33. The primary treatment for patients with acute leukemia would be

    A.   antibiotics

    B.   analgesics

    C.   chemotherapy

    D.   radiation therapy

34. Which of the following statements best describes the prognosis of adults with Hodgkin's disease?

    A.   outcome is uncertain, with many remissions

    B.   over 50% will be cured with chemo-therapy

    C.   over 95% will be cured if treated early

    D.   approximately 25% will live five years

35. If a patient with Hodgkin's disease has respiratory changes, edema, and cyanosis, the nurse would realize that this results from

    A.   deficiency of the immune system

    B.   pressure from enlarging lymph nodes

    C.   RBC destruction

    D.   overwhelming infection

36. For a patient with Stage III Hodgkin's disease, treatment would involve

    A.   chemotherapy

    B.   radiation therapy

    C.   radiation and chemotherapy

    D.   bone marrow transplant

37. If a patient with a neoplasm of the hematologic system has thrombocytopenia, it would be important for the nurse to monitor for signs of

    A.   infection

    B.   bleeding

    C.   dehydration

    D.   confusion

38. A patient with multiple myeloma who has limited activity would be at risk for developing

    A.   kidney stones

    B.   hypocalcemia

    C.   polycythemia

    D.   dehydration

39. Presence of Reed-Stembury cells would indicate to the nurse that a patient might have

    A.   chronic leukemia

    B.   Hodgkin's disease

    C.   aplastic anemia

    D.   infectious mononucleosis

40. Presence of Bence-Jones protein in a patient's urine would indicate to the nurse that a patient might have

    A.   multiple myeloma

    B.   hemophilia

    C.   leukemia

    D.   thalassemia

41. When a patient with a neoplasm is being treated with an alkylating agent such as Alkeran, the nurse would monitor for signs of

A.   polycythemia

B.   leukocytosis

C.   iron deficiency anemia

D.   pancytopenia

Identification

The nurse must have a basic knowledge of common bleeding disorders. Correctly match each of the following.

A.   Purpuras

B.   Disseminated intravascular coagulation (DIC)

C.   Hemophilia

42. _____ Hereditary coagulation disorder

43. _____ Bleeding into the tissue

44. _____ May result from thrombocytopenia

45. _____ A common acquired coagulation disorder

46. _____ Sex-linked recessive disorder

47. _____ Characterized by widespread coagulation in body

Nursing Care Plans

48. Use the following nursing diagnosis to write a nursing care plan for the patient with leukemia. Write two patient outcomes and several nursing interventions.

Nursing diagnosis: High risk for infection related to the compromised immune response

Patient outcomes:

Interventions:

49. Use the following nursing diagnosis to write a nursing care plan for the patient with Hodgkin's disease. Write two patient outcomes and several nursing interventions.

Nursing diagnosis: Ineffective breathing patterns related to obstruction from enlarged lymph nodes

Patient outcomes:

Interventions:

Case Studies

Case Study No. 1

Ms. M., age 24, is admitted to the hospital in sickle-cell crisis. She has had the disease since age 2. She is complaining of severe pain in her knees and abdomen.

50. Which of the following statements best explains the etiology of sickle cell anemia?

A.   a fatal disease occurring after a blood transfusion

B.   a disease characterized by acute bleeding episodes

C.   a chronic hereditary disorder characterized by an abnormal hemoglobin

D.   an acute disease that is easily treatable

51. Which of the following events in Ms. M.'s history may have precipitated the current crisis?

A.   recent divorce

B.   recent intestinal virus

C.   promotion at work

D.   change in medication

52. The reason for the pain in Ms. M.'s knees is

    A. occlusion of the circulatory system

    B. bleeding into the joints

    C. traumatic fall

    D. lack of intrinsic factor

53. Medical management primarily consists of

    A. diet therapy

    B. hydration and pain control

    C. bed rest and immobilization of extremities

    D. antibiotics and anti-inflammatories

54. The nurse is aware that a primary goal is to prevent complications such as

    A. cerebral hemorrhage

    B. renal failure

    C. cardiac disorders

    D. all of the above

Case Study No. 2

Mr. C., age 18, was recently diagnosed with acute myelocytic leukemia. He is admitted with an extremely low WBC and signs of infection. He recently finished a course of chemotherapy.

55. Because of Mr. C.'s low WBC and possible infection, he should be admitted to

    A. a semi-private room

    B. a private room

    C. intensive care

56. Lab results show that Mr. C. also has anemia and thrombocytopenia. The nurse would monitor him closely for signs of

    A. bleeding

    B. confusion

    C. activity intolerance

    D. visual impairment

57. Mr. C. is complaining of a sore mouth. The nurse notices several mouth ulcers. An appropriate nursing intervention would be

    A. lemon glycerin swabs

    B. NPO status

    C. rinse with hydrogen peroxide and water

    D. rinse with Cepacol mouthwash

58. Since Mr. C. is receiving chemotherapy, he is anxious about his prognosis. Which statement by the nurse would be most appropriate?

    A. "The average survival time with treatment is five years."

    B. "With chemotherapy, complete remission occurs in 50–75% of all patients."

    C. "Chemotherapy does not increase life span but does decrease symptoms."

    D. "A complete remission is achieved in about 90% of all patients."

Case Study No. 3

Mr. S., age 21, has hemophilia A. He is in the hospital to control an acute bleeding episode.

59. Individuals with this type of hemophilia are known to be deficient in

    A. Factor VI

    B. Factor VII

    C. Factor VIII

    D. Factor IX

60. Which statement best describes this disorder?

    A. It is a sex-linked recessive disorder transmitted by females.

    B. It is a sex-linked dominant disorder transmitted by males.

    C. It is a bleeding disorder occurring equally in males and females.

    D. It is an acquired coagulation disorder.

61. Medical management of Mr. S.'s bleeding episode would involve administration of

    A. plasma

    B. cryoprecipitate

    C. antihemophilic factor

    D. any of the above

62. Mr. S. has had several episodes of hemarthrosis. The most appropriate treatment for this would be to

    A. apply direct pressure

    B. pack the involved area in ice

    C. administer analgesics

    D. administer antibiotics

Learner Self-Evaluation

Do I fully understand the content? If no, then the areas I need to review are:

I need more information from my instructor on:

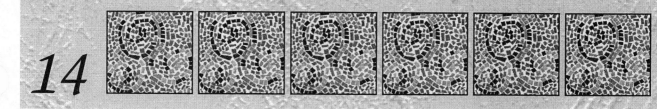

Knowledge Base for Patients with Respiratory Dysfunction

*O*bjectives

1.0 Review the anatomy and physiology of the respiratory system.
   1.1 Identify the parts of the respiratory system.
   1.2 Explain the process of breathing.
   1.3 Demonstrate an understanding of the process of ventilation.

2.0 Demonstrate an understanding of assessment data related to the respiratory system.
   2.1 Identify clinical manifestations of respiratory dysfunctions.
   2.2 Identify data essential to the assessment of respiratory function.
   2.3 Identify normal and abnormal breath sounds.
   2.4 Identify tests used to diagnose respiratory alterations.

3.0 Demonstrate an understanding of interventions used to treat adults with respiratory dysfunction.
   3.1 Identify nonsurgical methods of treating adult respiratory dysfunction.
   3.2 Identify the needs of a patient on a ventilator.
   3.3 Identify the parts of an intrapleural drainage system.
   3.4 Use the nursing process in planning care for the adult having thoracic surgery.
   3.5 Demonstrate an understanding of nursing interventions appropriate for patients with respiratory dysfunction.

$\mathcal{L}$earning Activities

Basic Knowledge

1.   Label the parts of the respiratory system on
      the diagram below.

    A.   Larynx

    B.   Left bronchus

    C.   Visceral pleura

    D.   Parietal pleura

    E.   Diaphragm

    F.   Trachea

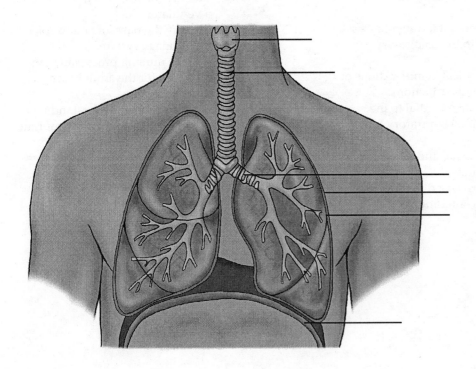

Short Answers

2. List the structures of the lower airway.

3. List the structures of the upper airway.

4. Inspiration is the _____ phase of ventilation.

5. Expiration is the _____ phase of ventilation.

6. During inspiration, the diaphragm

    _____. During expiration, the

    diaphragm returns to its normal position.

7. Lung tissue is _____.

8. Lung compliance is a measure of how easily

    the lung can be _____.

9. External respiration takes place at the

    _____ and internal respiration

    takes place at the _____.

10. Oxygen is transported by _____ in the blood.

11. _____ is a protective mechanism for clearing the lower airways.

12. _____ is a sign of hypoxemia.

13. A technique that involves applying manual compression and tremor to the chest wall

    during exhalation is called _____.

14. A technique that uses the effect of gravity to assist in draining secretions from the lungs is

    _____.

Interpretation

The ability of the nurse to correctly assess and interpret findings is an important skill. Match the normal breath sounds with the appropriate definition.

A. Bronchial

B. Bronchovesicular

C. Vesicular

15. _____ Quiet, low-pitched

16. _____ High-pitched, loud, over trachea

17. _____ Medium-pitched, between trachea and lung

Match the abnormal breath sounds with the appropriate definition.

A. Rales

B. Friction rub

C. Wheezing

18. _____ Creaking, grating sound

19. _____ Discrete, noncontinuous sound

20. _____ Continuous musical sound

Understanding medical terminology is essential when interpreting assessment findings related to respiratory dysfunction. Match the following terms with the correct definition.

A. Hypoxia

B. Hypercapnia

C. Hypocapnia

D. Anoxia

21. _____ Low level of carbon dioxide

22. _____ High level of carbon dioxide

23. _____ Low level of oxygen

24. _____ Absence of oxygen

Define the following terms.

25. Hyperpnea

26. Hyperventilation

27. Kussmaul's breathing

28. Cheyne-Stokes respirations

29. Biot's breathing

30. Pigeon breast

31. Barrel chest

Match each diagnostic test with the appropriate explanation.

A. Sputum test

B. Angiogram

C. Thoracentesis

D. Lung scan

E. Mediastinoscopy

F. Bronchogram

32. _____ Visualizes pulmonary vessels

33. _____ Determines presence of infection

34. _____ Removes fluid from the lung

35. _____ Evaluates pulmonary perfusion

36. _____ Visualizes lymph nodes

37. _____ Radiopaque material is inserted into trachea to allow visualization

Knowledge Application

38. When ventilation is present without perfusion, no gas exchange occurs. This is known as

A. dead space

B. shunting

C. hypoxia

D. hypercapnia

39. When capillaries are perfused but no ventilation occurs it is known as

A. shunting

B. dead space

C. third spacing

D. anoxia

40. Signs and symptoms of a respiratory dysfunction that a nurse would look for when assessing a patient would include

    A. coughing

    B. excessive nasal secretions

    C. dyspnea

    D. fatigue

    E. all the above

41. The purpose of a surfactant is to

    A. stimulate respirations

    B. minimize friction during respiration

    C. prevent collapse of the alveoli

    D. assist with all of the above

42. How much total body energy is used for normal breathing?

    A. 2–3%

    B. 5–10%

    C. 10–15%

    D. 15–25%

43. Which of the following is an example of a shunt-producing condition?

    A. atelectasis

    B. adult respiratory distress syndrome

    C. pneumonia

    D. all of the above

44. Which diagnostic test is the most reliable indicator of hypoxemia?

    A. chest x-ray

    B. ventilation studies

    C. hemoglobin and hematocrit

    D. arterial blood gases

45. The nurse would be alert to a possible hypoxic condition if a patient exhibited which of the following symptoms?

    A. decrease in heart rate and blood pressure

    B. changes in level of orientation

    C. change in urinary output

    D. increase in respiration, coughing

46. When assessing the respiratory system, the nurse is aware that the main respiratory stimulus is

    A. hypocapnia

    B. hypoxemia

    C. hypercapnia

    D. anoxia

47. An adult with chronic hypoxemia might exhibit which of the following symptoms?

    A. cyanosis, palpitations

    B. fatigue, apathy, muscular twitching

    C. confusion, irritability

    D. low heart rate and respiratory rate

48. A patient exhibits a sudden loss of consciousness. The nurse is aware that this may be due to

    A. hypercapnia

    B. hypocapnia

49. A patient who shows signs of hyperventilation is at risk for developing

    A. hypocapnia

    B. hypercapnia

    C. hypoxemia

50. A patient comes to the local clinic complaining of hemoptysis. This symptom may be related to

    A. tuberculosis

    B. emphysema

    C. asthma

    D. pneumonia

51. When obtaining the history for a patient with a respiratory disorder, the nurse would be sure to obtain information on which of the following areas?

    A.   smoking history

    B.   exposure to occupational pollutants

    C.   exposure to carcinogens

    D.   presence of cough, pain

    E.   all of the above

52. Which of the following postures in a patient would indicate a respiratory problem?

    A.   lying prone

    B.   sitting in chair with feet elevated

    C.   sitting up in bed with arms on table

    D.   walking in hall with slow gait

53. Breath sounds are heard as a result of

    A.   vibrations produced in the larynx that are transmitted to the chest wall

    B.   transmission of vibration of air from the larynx to the alveoli

    C.   transmission of the air exchange in the alveoli

    D.   none of the above

54. Adventitious breath sounds can be defined as

    A.   extra sounds heard during inspiration

    B.   harsh sounds heard during expiration

    C.   abnormal sounds superimposed over breath sounds

    D.   abnormal sounds heard instead of normal breath sounds

55. An example of an adventitious breath sound would be

    A.   rales (crackles)

    B.   rhonchi (gurgles)

    C.   wheezing

    D.   any of the above

56. The purpose of pulmonary function studies is to

    A.   measure the tidal capacity

    B.   measure the functional ability of the lungs

    C.   measure the ventilation capacity of the lungs

    D.   evaluate the diaphragmatic excursion

57. Arterial blood gases are used to measure the blood oxygenation. Abnormal blood gases would indicate

    A.   respiratory dysfunction

    B.   cardiac dysfunction

    C.   metabolic imbalance

58. A painless, noninvasive procedure that can monitor arterial oxygen saturation is called

    A.   pulse oximetry

    B.   arterial blood gas measurement

    C.   venous blood sampling

    D.   pulmonary function testing

59. When assessing a patient admitted with hyperglycemia and diarrhea, the nurse is aware that the patient is at risk for

    A.   metabolic acidosis

    B.   respiratory alkalosis

    C.   metabolic alkalosis

    D.   respiratory acidosis

60. A patient with a history of emphysema who has pneumonia is at risk for developing

    A.   metabolic acidosis

    B.   respiratory alkalosis

    C.   metabolic alkalosis

    D.   respiratory acidosis

61. The following set of ABGs are called to the nurse—pH 7.22, $PaCO_2$ 60, HCO_3 29. This indicates

    A.   respiratory acidosis

    B.   respiratory alkalosis

    C.   metabolic acidosis

    D.   metabolic alkalosis

62. To determine adequate tissue oxygenation, what should be examined when evaluating arterial blood gases?

A. oxygen gas tension

B. oxyhemoglobin saturation

C. tissue capillary pressure

D. carrying capacity of the body

63. Nursing care of a patient receiving a perfusion lung scan would include all of the following statements EXCEPT

A. "You will be required to lie still and breathe quietly."

B. "You will receive less radiation than with a chest x-ray."

C. "You will have no discomfort during the procedure."

D. "You may be required to use a mouthpiece and nose clip."

64. The most appropriate diagnostic procedure for the adult who is suspected of having a foreign body in the respiratory tract would be

A. lung scan

B. thoracentesis

C. bronchoscopy

D. pulmonary function test

65. A diagnostic test that is used primarily in the diagnosis of bronchiectasis is called a

A. bronchoscopy

B. bronchogram

C. laryngogram

D. esophagoscope

66. Following a bronchoscopy, the nurse would observe for possible complications such as

A. hyperventilation

B. infection

C. aspiration

D. desaturation

67. Following a thoracentesis, the physician orders a chest x-ray. What is the rationale for this order? To

A. assess for pneumonia

B. check for a pneumothorax

C. evaluate lung perfusion

D. visualize the pulmonary vessels

68. Following a thoracentesis, the nurse would monitor for

A. change in vital signs

B. faintness, vertigo

C. uncontrolled cough

D. blood-tinged mucus

E. all the above

69. The type of oxygen therapy where oxygen is administered through a small catheter inserted directly into the trachea through the lower neck is

A. tracheostomy

B. laryngoscopy

C. transtracheal

D. pericardial

70. The advantages of the above method over continuous oxygen therapy would include that it

A. decreases work of breathing

B. doesn't interfere with eating

C. doesn't lead to sore throat

D. all of the above

71. In caring for the patient with an endotracheal tube, which part of the assessment is a priority?

A. heart rate

B. bilateral breath sounds

C. peripheral pulses

D. ascites

72. A rationale for the insertion of a tracheo-stomy tube is to

    A. allow for long-term ventilation

    B. decrease the respiratory effort

    C. facilitate removal of secretions

    D. prevent aspiration of gastric secretions

    E. all of the above

73. The nurse is aware that the presence of a cough, sharp chest pain, and tachycardia after insertion of a tracheostomy tube may be an indication of

    A. cardiac tamponade

    B. cardiac arrhythmias

    C. pneumothorax

    D. pneumonia

74. Signs of dizziness after a patient has received an IPPB treatment are most likely related to

    A. hypoxemia

    B. hypoventilation

    C. hyperventilation

    D. hypercapnia

75. Following emergency intubation, the nurse auscultates breath sounds. There is no air moving on the left side. This may mean that the

    A. endotracheal tube needs to be reposi-tioned

    B. patient has a pleural effusion.

    C. tube is the wrong size.

76. An appropriate nursing intervention would be to

    A. call physician at once

    B. reposition the tube

    C. recheck tube in one hour

    D. remove the tube

77. A patient with scattered coarse rhonchi requires suctioning. Pre- and postoxygenation is done to

    A. prevent complications of hypoxia

    B. prevent increase in secretions

    C. stimulate the cough reflex

    D. all of the above

78. The physician changes the ventilator mode from assist control (AC) to intermittent mandatory ventilation (IMV). The main difference between AC and IMV is that with IMV the

    A. patient's respiratory effort triggers the machine

    B. volume is delivered at a constant rate

    C. ventilator responds to every patient effort

    D. patient can breathe spontaneously as desired

79. Which ventilator mode is used during weaning?

    A. assist

    B. assist control

    C. intermittent mandatory ventilation

    D. positive end expiratory pressure (PEEP)

80. The nurse notes a patient is restless and confused. This may indicate

    A. hypoxia

    B. hypercapnia

    C. hypocapnia

    D. hyperventilation

81. When a patient is on PEEP the nurse is aware that it is important to observe for signs of decreased cardiac output such as

    A. hypertension, tachycardia

    B. weak pulses, slow capillary refill, low urine output

    C. cyanosis, chest pain

    D. lethargy, diaphoresis, headache

82. Following thoracic surgery, the nurse is aware that it is important for the patient to cough frequently to bring up secretions. This is done to prevent

    A.   hemorrhage

    B.   bronchopleural fistula

    C.   empyema

    D.   atelectasis

83. Nursing care of the patient having a mediastinoscopy includes prevention of complications. These can include

    A.   gastrointestinal bleeding

    B.   myocardial infarction

    C.   thrombophlebitis

    D.   cerebrovascular accident

84. The key parts of an intrapleural drainage system are

    A.   chest tube, collection bottle, suction

    B.   chest tube, one-way mechanism, collection bottles

    C.   collection bottles, one-way mechanism, suction

    D.   drainage tube, air vent, bottle

85. The main reason that a suction is added to an intrapleural drainage system is

    A.   to remove the air faster

    B.   to help patient breathe easier

    C.   when the gravity system is not effective

    D.   when the patient has had thoracic surgery

86. Chest tubes are used to allow for lung reexpansion following thoracic surgery. A chest tube would not be inserted following

    A.   pneumonectomy

    B.   lobectomy

    C.   open-heart surgery

    D.   wedge resection

87. Label each part of the thoracic drainage system.

    A.   Drainage tube

    B.   Suction control device

    C.   Underwater seal chamber

    D.   Drainage collection chamber

    E.   Tube-to-suction device

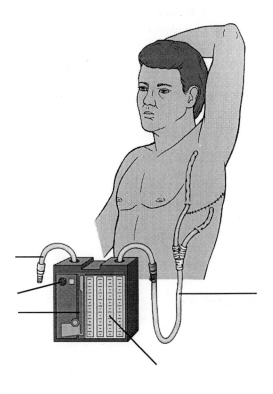

Nursing Care Plans

88. One of the priorities in caring for the patient on a ventilator is to assure effective breathing patterns. Write a nursing care plan that addresses this need.

Nursing diagnosis:

Patient outcome:

Interventions:

89. The patient who had a chest tube inserted following thoracic surgery has a problem with decreased lung expansion. Write a nursing care plan that addresses this problem.

Nursing diagnosis:

Patient outcome:

Interventions:

90. Plan the nursing care for the patient after a pneumonectomy. Keep in mind the information that the patient needs to ensure recovery.

Nursing diagnosis:

Patient outcome:

Interventions:

Case Studies

Case Study No. 1

Mrs. R. had a right upper lobectomy to remove a lung mass. She returns to the unit after surgery. She has a right pleural chest tube to 20 cm suction, oxygen at 2 L/minute via nasal cannula, an IV to KVO. During assessment, the nurse notices fluctuation in the chest tube with respirations. The surgical dressing is dry and intact. Vital signs are stable. She has no complaints at present.

91. The physician has ordered arterial blood gases to be drawn. The lab calls and reports values as follows: pH 7.32, pCO_2 48%, pO_2 90%, HCO_3 25, O_2 sat. 92%. The nurse is aware that this patient is in

A.   respiratory alkalosis

B.   respiratory acidosis

C.   metabolic alkalosis

D.   metabolic acidosis

92. When checking the patient's intrapleural drainage system, the nurse notes bubbling in the suction control chamber. This most likely indicates

    A. the system is malfunctioning

    B. the system is set up correctly

    C. there is a large air leak

93. The physician orders respiratory therapy to start breathing treatments with cool aerosol. Mrs. R. asks why she has to have these treatments. The nurse replies

    A. "You need the treatment to promote ventilation."

    B. "You need the treatment because you may have pneumonia."

    C. "You need the treatment since you can't ambulate yet."

    D. "You need the treatment to remove secretions."

94. On the second postoperative day, the nurse feels crepitus around the chest tube insertion site. This finding indicates:

    A. hemorrhage into the tissue

    B. presence of a fistula

    C. persistent air leak into the tissue

    D. presence of infection

95. Mrs. R. wants to know if she will be able to walk to the bathroom while she has the chest tube in place. The nurse replies

    A. "No, it is too dangerous; the bottle could break."

    B. "Yes, if we clamp off the chest tube."

    C. "Yes, if proper safety measures are taken."

96. It is now three days after surgery, and there is no longer fluctuation in the tubing when the patient breathes. This may mean

    A. the system has malfunctioned and you should call the doctor

    B. the lung is expanded and the tube can be pulled

    C. the patient is lying on the tubing

Case Study No. 2

The nurse is assigned to Mr. B., age 78, who is in acute respiratory failure. He has had chronic obstructive pulmonary disease (COPD) for many years. He was admitted, intubated, and placed on a ventilator with settings of IMV 12; FIO_2 40%; TV 700. He is confused and combative. Lab results confirm pseudomonas in his sputum. He is placed on antibiotics.

97. Which of the following nursing diagnoses would be the most relevant at this time?

    A. Alteration in nutrition related to lack of food intake

    B. Ineffective breathing patterns related to an inflammatory process

    C. Self-care deficit related to impaired thought process

    D. Alteration in tissue perfusion related to disease process

98. Which of the following statements is NOT true about the type of ventilator support Mr. B. is receiving ?

    A. The patient can initiate his own respirations.

    B. This setting is often used to wean patients.

    C. The ventilator delivers a TV of 700 each time the patient breathes.

    D. The ventilator has alarms built in to detect malfunctions.

99. Which of the following would give you the best indication that you should suction this patient?

    A. It has been four hours since you suctioned him.

    B. The alarm on the ventilator goes off.

    C. You hear wheezing during auscultation.

    D. You hear coarse rales during auscultation.

100. The suctioning procedure should not take more than

    A.   10 seconds

    B.   15 seconds

    C.   25 seconds

    D.   40 seconds

101. Suction is applied when the catheter is

    A.   introduced

    B.   removed

    C.   inserted and removed

102. Mr. B. is scheduled to have a bronchoscopy to determine if he is retaining secretions. Nursing responsibilities prior to the procedure would include all of the following EXCEPT

    A.   restricting food or fluid intake for six hours

    B.   obtaining suction equipment for the room

    C.   explaining to the patient that biopsies may be taken

    D.   explaining that the procedure is not uncomfortable

103. Mr. B.'s wife is very concerned that having this procedure will be very painful. What does the nurse say to reassure her?

    A.   "This is an easy and painless procedure."

    B.   "This procedure is done under general anesthesia."

    C.   "This is done with a local anesthesia."

104. After the procedure, which finding by the nurse would be indicative of a complication that should be reported immediately?

    A.   hypotension

    B.   respiratory stridor

    C.   tachycardia

    D.   any of the above

Mr. B. recovers and soon will be discharged to an assisted-living facility. He will need oxygen and assistance with daily activities. The nurse will be responsible for doing the discharge teaching and the continuity of care.

105. Which of the following nursing interventions could help improve the quality of Mr. B.'s breathing?

    A.   doing pursed-lip breathing

    B.   doing diaphragmatic breathing

    C.   exhaling forcibly

    D.   any of the above

*L*earner Self-Evaluation

Do I fully understand the content? If no, then the areas I need to review are:

I need more information from my instructor on:

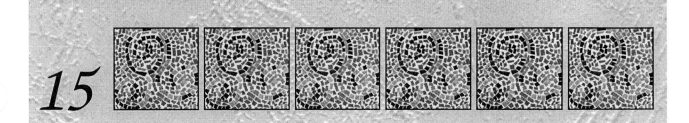

15

Nursing Care of Patients with Upper Respiratory Disorders

Objectives

1.0 Demonstrate an understanding of the infections and inflammations of the upper respiratory tract.

    1.1 Identify the etiology and clinical manifestations of common upper respiratory disorders.

    1.2 Recognize diagnostic procedures and types of medical treatment used for patients with common upper respiratory disorders.

    1.3 Identify complications that can occur for the patient with an upper respiratory infection.

    1.4 Identify nursing interventions for the patient with a common upper respiratory infection.

    1.5 Identify special considerations for the elderly patient with an upper respiratory disorder.

2.0 Demonstrate an understanding of the obstructive disorders of the upper respiratory tract.

    2.1 Identify several obstructive disorders.

    2.2 Identify treatment options for the patient with an obstructive disorder.

    2.3 Identify nursing interventions when caring for the patient with an obstructive disorder.

    2.4 Review the emergency treatment of laryngeal trauma.

3.0 Demonstrate an understanding of the types of neoplasms that can affect the upper respiratory tract.

    3.1 Identify clinical manifestations of laryngeal cancer.

    3.2 Review the surgical interventions used in the treatment of laryngeal cancer.

    3.3 Plan the nursing care for the patient with cancer of the larynx.

$\mathcal{L}$earning Activities

Short Answers

1. Upper respiratory infections rarely require

   _____.

2. Allergic rhinitis is the single most common

   _____ _____.

3. Symptoms of acute sinusitis are a result of

   _____ of drainage.

4. Peritonsillar abscess is a secondary infection

   related to _____.

5. *Epistaxis* is another word for _____.

6. Benign tumors in the nasal mucosa that are freely moveable are known as

   _____.

7. An operative procedure to straighten and reduce the nasal septum is known as a

   _____.

8. An operative procedure that involves surgical reconstruction of the nose is known

   as a _____.

9. Two risk factors associated with laryngeal

   cancer are _____ and

   _____.

10. Danger of _____ is a significant risk following total laryngectomy.

Identification

Match the following common disorders with the correct explanation.

   A. Laryngitis

   B. Sinusitis

   C. Rhinitis

   D. Common cold

   E. Tonsillitis

   F. Pharyngitis

11. _____ Infectious process of the upper respiratory tract that can be caused by any of 100 viruses

12. _____ Caused by an obstruction of the drainage tracts

13. _____ Caused by a bacteria and often seen secondary to an upper respiratory infection

14. _____ Inflammation of the throat

15. _____ An inflammation of the mucous membrane of the nose

16. _____ Inflammation of the vocal cords

True/False

17. _____ Medical management is required for a cold.

18. _____ Pharyngitis is often caused by a streptococcal organism.

19. _____ Tetracycline is the drug of choice for treating hemolytic streptococcal infections.

20. _____ Warm saline irrigations are used to treat pain associated with a peritonsillar abscess.

21. _____ Another name for allergic rhinitis is hay fever.

22. _____ Speech is possible following a partial laryngectomy.

Knowledge Application

23. Why would a geriatric patient with a common cold be more likely to have complications than a young adult?

    A. Atrophy and weakness of respiratory muscles slow the cough reflex.

    B. Hypertrophy of the diaphragm increases susceptibility to infection.

    C. Atrophy of the extremities causes immobility and leads to increased risk of infection.

    D. Changes in white blood cell production cause elderly people to acquire infections easily.

24. The nurse would urge the patient with a cold to seek medical advice if he had which of the following symptoms?

    A. low-grade fever for more than 48 hours

    B. cough productive of yellow sputum

    C. high fever and greenish sputum production

    D. diaphoresis, weakness, and loss of appetite

25. Symptoms of sinusitis such as fever, chills, and pain over the affected sinuses are a result of

    A. obstruction of drainage

    B. bacterial infection

    C. surgery

    D. ineffective antibiotic therapy

26. The most appropriate medication to treat the symptoms of sinusitis would be

    A. Tylenol

    B. Darvocet

    C. phenylephrine

    D. Phenergan

27. When an adult has pharyngitis caused by group A beta-hemolytic streptococcus, the nurse would carefully monitor for complications of which systems?

    A. respiratory and cardiac

    B. cardiac and renal

    C. gastrointestinal and neurologic

    D. endocrine and respiratory

28. Presence of which of the following symptoms would indicate to the nurse that an adult has a complication secondary to a group A beta-hemolytic streptococcal infection?

    A. wheezing with breathing

    B. hyperactive bowel sounds

    C. diminished sensation in the lower extremities

    D. systolic heart murmur

29. The most appropriate nursing diagnosis for the patient with acute pharyngitis is Potential for

    A. alteration in cardiac output

    B. fluid volume deficit

    C. impaired tissue perfusion

    D. alteration in gas exchange

30. Why would a vasoconstrictive drug such as phenylephrine be used for an individual with sinusitis? To

    A. prevent postural hypotension

    B. maintain adequate cardiac output

    C. promote drainage of the sinuses

    D. prevent spread of the infection to the brain

31. The nurse is often involved in teaching individuals how to cope with allergic rhinitis. Teaching includes

    A. avoiding the responsible antigen

    B. antihistamine therapy

    C. desensitization

    D. any of the above

32.   A patient calls the physician with persistent headache, chronic cough, and purulent nasal drainage. These are indicative of which of the following conditions?

   A.   meningitis

   B.   bacterial endocarditis

   C.   emphysema

   D.   chronic sinusitis

33.   Presence of persistent postnasal discharge following chronic sinusitis can predispose the patient to

   A.   bronchiectasis

   B.   pneumonia

   C.   sepsis

   D.   meningitis

34.   When caring for a patient with tonsillitis, which of the following goals would be primary? The patient

   A.   sleeps 12 hours per day

   B.   has adequate urinary output

   C.   has understanding of antibiotic therapy

   D.   avoids irritating foods

35.   For the patient with tonsillitis, presence of unilateral pain radiating to the ear with swallowing may indicate

   A.   mastoiditis

   B.   peritonsillar abscess

   C.   esophagitis

   D.   laryngitis

36.   A major complication of a tonsillectomy in the immediate postoperative period would be

   A.   hemorrhage

   B.   shock

   C.   sepsis

   D.   infection

37.   Based on your knowledge of the importance of careful assessment of the patient who has had a tonsillectomy, which lab values would you be certain to assess?

   A.   CBC, platelets, clotting time

   B.   CBC, WBC, BUN, creatinine

   C.   CPK, SGOT, LDH, electrolytes

   D.   electrolytes, PT, PTT

38.   Which of the following would be an appropriate nursing intervention to help alleviate pain following tonsillectomy?

   A.   analgesics as ordered

   B.   warm saline gargles

   C.   ice collar as ordered

   D.   all of the above

39.   A common condition caused by the overuse of nose drops is known as

   A.   vasomotor rhinitis

   B.   rhinitis medicamentosa

   C.   medicatisus allergitis

   D.   nasal pharyngitis

40.   Which of the following diseases has been associated with episodes of epistaxis?

   A.   laryngitis

   B.   hypertension

   C.   pneumonitis

   D.   hyperglycemia

41.   The first intervention for an episode of epistaxis that the nurse would implement would be to

   A.   administer an anticoagulant

   B.   apply ice compresses

   C.   apply pressure to the nares for 10 minutes

   D.   insert nasal packing

42. A patient is admitted to the emergency room after a motorcycle accident. His neck is swollen and bruised. Hoarseness and respiratory stridor are present. What is a probable cause of these symptoms?

    A. laryngeal trauma

    B. fracture of the neck

    C. pneumothorax

    D. esophageal trauma

43. Because of the possible complications of this condition, what equipment would the nurse have available?

    A. endotracheal tube

    B. tracheostomy set

    C. chest tube

    D. nasogastric tube

44. Which of the following would be a late symptom of laryngeal cancer?

    A. dyspnea

    B. dysphagia

    C. weight loss

    D. all of the above

45. The nursing care of the patient with a nasal fracture is aimed at

    A. preventing bleeding

    B. maintaining a patent airway

    C. maintaining hydration

    D. preventing infection

Nursing Care Plan

46. Write a care plan for a patient who has had a total laryngectomy.

    Nursing diagnosis: Ineffective airway clearance related to altered airway

    Patient outcome:

    Interventions:

Case Studies

Case Study No. 1

Mr. A. has had sinusitis for several years. He often wakes with headaches and suffers from nasal discharge and chronic fatigue. He is admitted for possible surgery.

47. Although sinusitis may be attributed to a specific organism, other factors may be indicated. These would include

    A. irritating gases

    B. tobacco smoke

    C. irritating dusts

    D. all of the above

48. Which of the following symptoms, if exhibited by this patient, would indicate to the nurse a possible side effect of his medication (Neo-Synephrine).

    A. tachycardia, hypertension, shortness of breath

    B. anxiety, tremors, chest pain

    C. lethargy, confusion

    D. urinary or bowel incontinence

49. Mr. A. has surgery to remove the diseased mucous membrane. After surgery, which of the following would be an appropriate nursing diagnosis in view of the fact that nasal packing is in place?

    A.   Potential for alteration in oral mucous membrane

    B.   Potential for sensory perceptual deficit

    C.   Knowledge deficit related to outcome of surgery

    D.   Alteration in body image

50. Nasal packing after this type of surgery would be removed in

    A.   6–8 hours

    B.   12 hours

    C.   24 hours

    D.   48 hours

51. Which of the following instructions would the nurse give to the patient following the removal of the packing?

    A.   Do not blow your nose.

    B.   Avoid any activity for two days.

    C.   Do not drink hot beverages.

    D.   Do not engage in sexual activity.

Case Study No. 2

Mr. K. has been diagnosed with laryngeal cancer and has just returned to the unit following a total laryngectomy.

52. As a nurse you are aware that many changes will occur to the patient following the surgery. Which of the following would NOT occur? Loss of normal

    A.   speech

    B.   respiratory patterns

    C.   eating habits

    D.   olfactory sensations

53. Which of the following health-care professionals should be consulted since he or she will have a critical role in the recovery of Mr. K.?

    A.   occupational therapist

    B.   speech therapist

    C.   pharmacist

    D.   dietitian

54. Mr. K. wants to know how he will communicate following the surgery. The nurse would explain

    A.   "You will need to use a communication board."

    B.   "Some individuals like to use a computer."

    C.   "You will have to learn esophageal speech."

    D.   "There are several options including esophageal speech or even prosthetic voice-restoration."

The nurse will need to do health teaching for Mr. K. so that he can care for himself after discharge.

55. Which of the following would not be important to teach him? How to

    A.   suction the tracheostomy

    B.   perform tracheostomy care

    C.   care for his feeding tube

    D.   contact a support group

56. Since body image is an important factor, the nurse should

    A.   encourage him to look at the stoma

    B.   do not force him to view the stoma

    C.   suggest ways to change his appearance

    D.   ignore the change in appearance

Case Study No. 3

Ms. O. has had recurrent episodes of tonsillitis and is being evaluated by her physician for the most appropriate treatment.

57. During the physical exam, which of the following would most likely be present?

    A.   Tonsils are red and swollen with white patches.

    B.   Tonsils are whitish or gray with reddish lesions.

    C.   Throat is red and cervical lymph nodes are swollen.

    D.   Tongue and gums are red with white patches.

58. The office nurse would pick which of the following nursing diagnoses as having the highest priority with this patient?

    A.   Pain related to inflammation of the tonsils

    B.   High risk for fluid volume deficit related to inability to swallow

    C.   Knowledge deficit related to treatment of tonsillitis

    D.   Ineffective family coping

59. When Ms. O. is seen in one week for a recheck, she is complaining of a sore throat with pain radiating to her ear. On examination, there is swelling of the soft palate. A possible explanation is

    A.   the antibiotics were not effective

    B.   she has pharyngitis

    C.   she has a peritonsillar abscess

    D.   she has become reinfected

60. Because of her recurrent infections, the physician decides to perform a tonsillectomy. The nurse is aware that a major complication is

    A.   infection

    B.   bleeding

    C.   aspiration

    D.   septicemia

61. In the immediate postoperative period, which of the following nursing diagnoses would have the highest priority?

    A.   Pain related to surgical procedure

    B.   Potential for fluid volume deficit

    C.   High risk for aspiration

    D.   Anxiety related to procedure

*L*earner Self-Evaluation

Do I fully understand the content? If no, then the areas I need to review are:

I need more information from my instructor on:

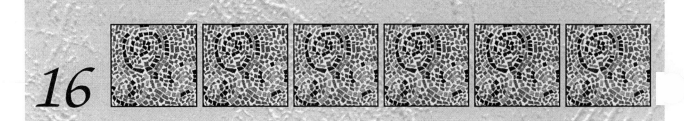

16

Nursing Care of Patients with Lower Respiratory Disorders

Objectives

1.0 Demonstrate an understanding of the infections and inflammations of the lower respiratory tract.
    1.1 Identify several respiratory tract infections.
    1.2 Review the etiology and clinical manifestations of several infectious disorders.
    1.3 Identify the nursing interventions for the adult with an infectious process.
    1.4 Identify the medical management of several types of infectious processes.
    1.5 Plan the nursing care for an adult with an inflammatory disorder.

2.0 Demonstrate an understanding of obstructive disorders of the lower respiratory tract.
    2.1 Review the etiology of several obstructive disorders.
    2.2 Identify the medical management of patients with an obstructive disorder.
    2.3 Plan the nursing care for an adult with an obstructive disorder.

3.0 Demonstrate an understanding of disorders of pulmonary circulation.
    3.1 Identify the pathophysiology of pulmonary embolism.
    3.2 Review the clinical manifestations of disorders of pulmonary circulation.

3.3 Describe the medical management for a patient with a pulmonary embolism.
3.4 Plan the nursing care for an adult with a disorder of pulmonary circulation.

4.0 Demonstrate an understanding of traumatic injuries to the lower respiratory tract.
    4.1 Identify the clinical manifestations of the adult with a chest injury.
    4.2 Describe the medical management of chest injuries.
    4.3 Pick appropriate nursing interventions for the adult with chest trauma.

5.0 Demonstrate an understanding of the types of neoplasms that can affect the lower respiratory tract.
    5.1 Identify clinical manifestations of lung cancer.
    5.2 Identify the medical management of lung cancer.
    5.3 Assess the needs of the adult with lung cancer.
    5.4 Plan nursing interventions for the adult with lung cancer.

*L*earning Activities

Identification

Match the following lower respiratory tract disorders with the appropriate definition.

A. Bronchitis

B. Pneumonia

C. Empyema

D. Emphysema

E. Hemothorax

F. Bronchiectasis

G. Atelectasis

H. Asthma

I. Pneumothorax

J. Silicosis

1. _____ Partial or complete collapse of lung tissue

2. _____ Permanent abnormal dilation and distortion of the bronchi

3. _____ Acute inflammation of the gas-exchanging units of the lungs

4. _____ Presence of blood in the pleural cavity

5. _____ Collection of pus in the pleural cavity

6. _____ Disease that is produced by exposure to silica

7. _____ Chronic disorder where there is enlargement of the air spaces and destruction of the alveolar walls

8. _____ Presence of air in the pleural cavity

9. _____ Inflammation of the larger bronchi

10. _____ Immunologic allergic disease with chronic inflammation of the lower airways

Short Answers

11. The majority of community-acquired pneumonias are believed to be _____ in origin.

12. A lung abscess is a collection of _____ within the substance of the lung.

13. The causative agent of tuberculosis is _____.

14. Tuberculosis is controllable by _____.

15. Tuberculosis requires close _____ contact for transmission.

16. The highest death rate for those with asthma is among the _____.

17. _____ _____ is a severe asthma attack that lasts for hours or days and does not respond to usual treatment.

18. In a patient with chronic obstructive pulmonary disease (COPD), _____ are often given at the first sign of any cold symptoms.

19. Sustained _____ can result in pulmonary hypertension.

20. _____ is the cardinal symptom of pulmonary hypertension.

21. Adult respiratory syndrome (ARDS) is manifested by severe _____ and _____ lung compliance.

22. Medical management for the patient with a pneumothorax involves the insertion of a _____ _____ to reestablish the _____ pressure.

23. _____ is often used as a definitive treatment for the person with a localized intrathoracic lung lesion.

24. Metastasis occurs in _____ of the patients with lung cancer.

25. Assessment of the patient with a respiratory infection would include which of the following? (Check all that apply.)

 A. _____ Monitor vital signs

 B. _____ Check results of ABGs

 C. _____ Check for Homans' sign

 D. _____ Assess presence of cough

 E. _____ Assess breathing patterns

 F. _____ Check results of chest x-ray

 G. _____ Check for cyanosis

 H. _____ Assess mucous membranes

Knowledge Application

26. A patient is discharged after therapy for acute bronchitis and pneumonia. Which of the following would alert the nurse to the need for further education? The patient asks

 A. for prescriptions

 B. how long before he can smoke again

 C. for instruction in diet

 D. if there are any activity limits

27. Paroxysmal attacks of coughing and wheezing in acute bronchitis may be precipitated by

 A. exposure to irritants

 B. exposure to heat

 C. exposure to cold

 D. A and C

 E. A,B,C

28. Assessment of the individual with pneumonia would most likely produce which of the following findings?

 A. fever, chills, productive cough

 B. purulent sputum, signs of shock

 C. diminished breath sounds, wheezes

 D. absent breath sounds over involved area

29. Common causes of pneumonia are known to include

 A. viruses

 B. bacteria

 C. aspiration

 D. all of the above

30. Viral and nonbacterial pneumonia result primarily from

 A. droplet inhalation

 B. aspiration of organisms

 C. invasion from bloodstream

 D. improper handwashing

31. Which statement best describes the physiologic changes associated with pneumonia? They result

 A. from specific injury to the cells in the alveoli

 B. in permanent destruction in lung tissue

 C. from reduced functioning of lung volume and alteration of ventilation and blood flow

 D. from aspiration of chemical irritants

32. Nonbacterial atypical pneumonia is most frequently caused by

 A. *Staphylococcus aureus*

 B. *Haemophilus influenzae*

 C. *Mycoplasma pneumoniae*

 D. *Legionella pneumophila*

33. The choice of the proper antibiotic for the adult with a lower respiratory disorder is best determined by

 A. physician orders

 B. patient preference

 C. results of blood culture

 D. all of the above

34. Which individual would have the highest risk for developing influenza?

    A.   18-year-old female

    B.   50-year-old male executive

    C.   70-year-old female with cardiac disease

    D.   65-year-old male, recently retired

35. A 75-year-old lethargic patient with loss of mobility and loss of gag reflex has a fever, chills, and productive cough, and the nurse suspects _____ pneumonia.

    A.   viral

    B.   aspiration

    C.   bacterial

    D.   fungal

36. A patient has developed a lung abscess and is admitted for evaluation and treatment. The nurse would expect to see which of the following medical therapies?

    A.   oral analgesics and antibiotics

    B.   surgical intervention

    C.   intravenous antibiotics, postural drainage

    D.   all of the above

37. The nurse is caring for a patient with empyema. On reviewing the lab results, findings reveal that the pH of the exudate is 7.16. The nurse would be ready to

    A.   assist with chest tube insertion

    B.   start oxygen therapy

    C.   discharge the patient

    D.   start IV antibiotics

38. Empyema is often a recurrent condition. Upon discharge, the nurse instructs the patient and family about signs and symptoms that should be reported. These would include

    A.   cough, expectorating whitish sputum

    B.   shortness of breath, painful breathing

    C.   weight gain, increased appetite

    D.   lack of energy, increased thirst

39. An elderly debilitated patient is receiving tube feeding through a nasogastric tube. Which of the following nursing interventions would NOT prevent aspiration?

    A.   elevating the bed

    B.   checking for proper tube placement

    C.   checking the amount of residual every four hours

    D.   turning every two hours

40. A patient is admitted with fever, right-sided chest pain, dyspnea, and anorexia. He has a recent history of bacterial pneumonia. His symptoms suggest

    A.   empyema

    B.   tuberculosis

    C.   septicemia

    D.   emphysema

41. What is the best method for obtaining a culture and sensitivity of the pleural exudate?

    A.   blood culture

    B.   skin culture

    C.   thoracentesis

    D.   bronchoscopy

42. In caring for a patient with influenza, it is important to be aware that it is transmitted by

    A.   direct contact

    B.   aerosol

    C.   body secretions

    D.   indirect contact

43. To prevent a complication of influenza, the nurse would carefully assess for symptoms of which of the following? (Check all that apply.)

    A.   _____ pneumonia

    B.   _____ renal disease

    C.   _____ cardiac disease

    D.   _____ encephalitis

44. Annual influenza vaccination is recommended for which population group(s)? (Check all that apply.)

   A. _____ over the age of 50

   B. _____ over the age of 65

   C. _____ with a chronic illness

   D. _____ who has already had influenza

45. The clinic nurse is doing health education at a senior citizens' group. Ways to prevent contracting influenza are explained. The nurse realizes that teaching is effective when a participant says

   A. "I never realized that I needed to stay in all winter."

   B. "I shouldn't go to the mall during a flu epidemic."

   C. "I never realized everyone harbors this virus."

   D. "I guess getting the flu is a risk I'll have to take."

46. Individuals in which environment would be most susceptible to developing tuberculosis?

   A. crowded, inner city, lower socioeconomic area

   B. rural areas with septic system and well

   C. inner city, living in apartments

   D. suburbs with crowded school system

47. The main treatment of tuberculosis is chemotherapy. The most effective drug is considered to be

   A. streptomycin

   B. rifampin

   C. isoniazid

   D. penicillin

48. The nurse would make which of the following statements to the patient who is receiving drug therapy for tuberculosis?

   A. "You will take this medication until symptoms subside."

   B. "You may take as many as four different medications for two months."

   C. "You may have intermittent drug therapy for a total of six months."

   D. "You may take a combination of medications for a period of nine months to as long as two years."

49. Knowing the therapeutic regimen required for the treatment of tuberculosis, what is a appropriate nursing diagnosis? Potential for

   A. alteration in mobility

   B. noncompliance

   C. fluid volume overload

   D. alteration in elimination

50. A patient is admitted with a respiratory disorder. During auscultation of breath sounds the nurse hears an audible friction rub. This is most indicative of

   A. pneumonia

   B. lung abscess

   C. influenza

   D. pleurisy

51. Education is paramount for the person with asthma. The nurse would want to discuss well-known triggers such as

   A. cold or dry air

   B. air pollutants

   C. perfumes

   D. chemicals

   E. all the above

52. During the early response to an asthma attack, which of the following occurs?

   A. contraction of the smooth muscle of bronchi and edema of the mucous membrane

   B. activation of the lung's immune system

   C. bronchodilation and mucous production

   D. severe reflexive coughing and decrease in mucous

53. Using the stepped-care approach to asthma treatment, the nurse would anticipate that with mild asthma, the first drug used is

   A. Ventolin

   B. Theo-Dur

   C. prednisone

   D. ampicillin

54. When a patient has chronic obstructive pulmonary disease (COPD), the highest nursing priority should be to prevent

   A. hypoxia

   B. infection

   C. sepsis

   D. altered nutrition

55. Pick the statement that best explains the immediate effect of COPD in a patient.

   A. Expiration is restricted, causing hypoxia.

   B. Alveoli are insufficiently ventilated and cannot provide the normal oxygen to surrounding blood.

   C. Airway obstruction leads to hypoxia and hypocapnia.

   D. Elastic recoil of the alveoli is hampered by excessive secretions.

56. Why is the expiratory phase longer than the inspiratory phase in the individual with COPD?

   A. There is loss of lung recoil and it is harder to get trapped air out.

   B. The drive to breathe has been lost.

   C. The muscles of the diaphragm are beginning to hypertrophy.

   D. The passive process of inspiration and expiration is impaired because of loss of elasticity.

57. The nurse is aware that prolonged hypoxemia causes the body to produce more red blood cells. This condition is known as

   A. anemia

   B. leukopenia

   C. polycythemia

   D. hypercapnia

58. Which of following factors have been implicated in the development of chronic bronchitis?

   A. smoking

   B. air pollution

   C. dust

   D. toxic fumes

   E. all of the above

59. The continual inflammation with chronic bronchitis makes the patient susceptible to

   A. dehydration

   B. infection

   C. cyanosis

   D. hypocapnia

60. Which of the following best describes the pathophysiology involved in pulmonary emphysema?

    A.   Alveoli are insufficiently ventilated because of obstruction.

    B.   Prolonged exposure to irritants results in excessive mucus production.

    C.   Inflammation of large and small airways leads to infection and scarring.

    D.   Alveoli lose elasticity, lungs become stiff, and compliance decreases with loss of lung recoil.

61. What mechanism in the individual with emphysema results in the barrel-chest appearance?

    A.   chronic hypoxia

    B.   pulmonary hypertension

    C.   cor pulmonale

    D.   loss of lung recoil

62. While assessing the patient with emphysema, the nurse would expect to see typical symptoms such as

    A.   dyspnea, pursed-lip breathing, barrel chest, diminished breath sounds

    B.   cyanosis, labored breathing, hyperresonance

    C.   weight gain, edema, rhonchi, and wheezing throughout

    D.   anorexia, weight loss, pallor

63. In emphysema, high levels of carbon dioxide can result in which of the following symptoms?

    A.   anorexia, weakness, lethargy

    B.   headache, lack of ability to concentrate

    C.   dyspnea, cyanosis

    D.   pursed-lip breathing, dyspnea

64. Medical management of the individual with emphysema is designed to

    A.   cause remission of the disease

    B.   control symptoms and prevent further deterioration

    C.   prevent development of pneumothorax

    D.   return the normal respiratory function

65. For the patient with emphysema and chronic bronchitis, there is a risk of developing

    A.   pulmonary hypertension and cor pulmonale

    B.   pneumonia and renal failure

    C.   pleurisy and peripheral vascular disease

    D.   pulmonary embolus and hypoxia

66. The nurse would check which of the following diagnostic tests to determine the severity of a patient's obstructive disease?

    A.   lung function studies

    B.   arterial blood gases

    C.   ventilation and perfusion scan

    D.   chest x-ray

67. Along with influenza, which of the following is the leading infectious cause of death among the elderly?

    A.   bronchitis

    B.   emphysema

    C.   lung cancer

    D.   pneumonia

68. A patient with COPD who is experiencing dyspnea may be taught which of the following to assist in controlling the dyspnea? (Check all that apply.)

    A. _____ how to control the inspiratory to expiratory (I:E) ratio to prolong expiration

    B. _____ how to control the I:E ratio to prolong inspiration

    C. _____ how to do diaphragmatic breathing

    D. _____ how to do pursed-lip breathing

69. Medical management of the patient with an obstructive lung disorder would be designed to prevent further deterioration of the condition. The nurse would expect the patient to be taking

    A. antibiotics

    B. antihypertensives

    C. bronchodilators

    D. beta blockers

70. Which of the following individuals would be at the greatest risk for developing a pulmonary embolus?

    A. male, 20 years old, admitted with pneumonia

    B. female, 28 years old, admitted with asthma

    C. female, 80 years old, with COPD, pneumonia, and cerebrovascular accident

    D. male, 72 years old, in for workup for possible lung CA

71. The nurse should consider which intervention of primary importance to prevent the development of a pulmonary embolus?

    A. bed rest with limited activity

    B. early ambulation and leg exercises

    C. administering antibiotics on time

    D. administering oxygen therapy as ordered

72. Medical treatment for pulmonary embolus involves using heparin therapy. Which of the following shows the desired effect of this treatment?

    A. PT level is 12 seconds

    B. PTT is 25–25 seconds

    C. PTT is 60–80 seconds

    D. PFT tests are normal

73. Which of the following is an adverse effect of thrombolytic therapy?

    A. chest pain

    B. cyanosis

    C. hemoptysis

    D. tachycardia

74. One of the main causes of pulmonary hypertension is

    A. pulmonary edema

    B. cardiac arrhythmias

    C. surgery

    D. pulmonary embolism

75. A condition that may develop following the fracture of several ribs is known as *flail chest*. Symptoms result from

    A. diminished movement of air

    B. pulmonary hypertension

    C. pain caused by the injury

    D. hypoxia

76. Medical management for the patient with a flail chest following a serious traumatic injury might involve which of the following?

    A. endotracheal intubation

    B. surgical intervention

    C. mechanical ventilation

    D. any or all of the above

77. Problems that can occur as a result of chest trauma include which of the following? (Check all that apply.)

    A. _____ pulmonary congestion

    B. _____ atelectasis

    C. _____ lung abscess

    D. _____ pneumothorax

    E. _____ paralytic ileus

78. An open pneumothorax is often the result of which of the following? (Check all that apply.)

   A. _____ thoracentesis

   B. _____ stab wound

   C. _____ paracentesis

   D. _____ insertion of Swan-Ganz catheter

   E. _____ insertion of Dobbhoff tube

79. Which type of bronchogenic carcinoma is the most common?

   A. epidermoid (squamous cell) carcinoma

   B. small cell carcinoma

   C. adenocarcinoma

   D. large cell carcinoma

80. The medical diagnosis of bronchogenic carcinoma is confirmed by which of the following?

   A. chest x-ray and history

   B. sputum cytology and bronchoscopy

   C. chest x-ray and pulmonary function tests

   D. open chest biopsy

81. Treatment for lung cancer involves which of the following forms of treatment?

   A. chemotherapy

   B. radiation therapy

   C. surgical excision

   D. any or all of the above

82. A finding of neck edema in the patient with adenocarcinoma suggests which of the following?

   A. metastasis to the pleural space

   B. metastasis to the brain

   C. metastasis to the mediastinum

Nursing Care Plans

83. Plan the nursing care for an adult with pneumonia using the following nursing diagnosis.

   Nursing diagnosis: Impaired gas exchange related to inflammation and production of exudate

   Patient outcome:

   Interventions:

84. Write a nursing care plan for the patient with active pulmonary tuberculosis using the following nursing diagnosis.

   Nursing diagnosis: High risk for transmission of infection related to lack of understanding of method of spread of disease

   Patient outcome:

   Interventions:

85. Write nursing care plans for the patient with COPD using the following nursing diagnoses.

    A. Nursing diagnosis: Ineffective airway clearance related to excessive secretions

        Patient outcome:

        Interventions:

    B. Nursing diagnosis: Ineffective breathing pattern related to increased work of breathing and need for oxygen

        Patient outcome:

        Interventions:

86. Write a nursing care plan for a patient with a spontaneous pneumothorax using the following diagnosis.

    Nursing diagnosis: Impaired gas exchange

    Patient outcome:

    Interventions:

87. Write a nursing care plan for a patient admitted with a diagnosis of squamous cell cancer r/o metastasis using the following nursing diagnosis.

    Nursing diagnosis: Anxiety related to diagnosis, treatment, and potential for recovery

    Patient outcome:

    Interventions:

Case Studies

Case Study No. 1

Mr. S. has had COPD for 20 years with many hospitalizations. Currently, he is admitted with pneumonia. He shows signs of acute respiratory distress such as dyspnea, cyanosis, and labored breathing. Orders include O_2 at 2 L/min, Cefoxitin 1 g q6h, aminophylline drip, Solu-Cortef 100 mg q6h.

88. On admission, a theophylline level is drawn. The level is 5.5 mEq/mL. An appropriate nursing action would be to

   A. stop the aminophylline drip and call the physician

   B. do nothing; this is a therapeutic range

   C. call the physician; the aminophylline needs to be increased

89. The purpose of the aminophylline is to

   A. treat bronchospasm

   B. treat the infection

   C. prevent further complications

90. In assessing Mr. S., which clinical manifestation would indicate a possible side effect of this therapy?

   A. bradycardia

   B. tachycardia

   C. tachypnea

   D. polycythemia

91. Mr. S. is coughing up green sputum. What organism is probably the cause of this?

   A. *Pseudomonas*

   B. *Klebsiella*

   C. *Candida*

   D. *Staphylococcus*

92. Mr. S. says, "I can't breathe; please turn up the oxygen." What is an appropriate action?

   A. turn the oxygen up to 6 L/min

   B. explain that too much oxygen will decrease his stimulus to breathe

   C. call the physician, because Mr. S. needs a ventilator

   D. check the results of the blood gases

93. An important nursing intervention for Mr S. would be to

   A. teach him to perform breathing exercises correctly

   B. explain that staying in bed will increase his strength

   C. restrict fluids to avoid complications

   D. explain how to avoid irritation of the lungs

94. The rationale for teaching Mr. S. how to do diaphragmatic breathing is to

   A. prolong the inspiratory phase of breathing

   B. help conserve oxygen

   C. help reduce expiration and exhale carbon dioxide

   D. help control breathing and prolong expiration

Case Study No. 2

Mr. B. was involved in a car accident two days ago. He suffered a concussion and fractured four ribs, resulting in a flail chest. He was placed on mechanical ventilation and two chest tubes were inserted.

95. What is the rationale for placing this patient on mechanical ventilation? To

   A. stabilize ventilation internally

   B. prevent the patient from aspirating

   C. prevent a hemothorax

96. The rationale for the placement of the chest tubes is to

    A. prevent infection

    B. remove air and fluid from the chest

    C. administer oxygen

    D. all of the above

97. Which of the following medications might be ordered to keep the patient from bucking the ventilator?

    A. morphine sulfate

    B. Demerol

    C. Pavulon

    D. Valium

98. The morning assessment of this patient reveals dyspnea, cough, fever, and chest discomfort. The nurse would suspect

    A. pneumothorax

    B. atelectasis

    C. pulmonary edema

    D. pulmonary embolus

99. Mr. B. is receiving heparin 5000 units subcutaneously every 12 hours. The nurse is aware that the reason for this is to

    A. prevent embolus formation

    B. prevent a stroke

    C. increase clotting of the blood

    D. help prevent pneumonia

Case Study No. 3

Mrs. P. is 65 years old. On a routine chest x-ray, a spot was noted on her lung. She is admitted for a bronchoscopy and biopsy. She has smoked for 45 years. She is found to have squamous cell carcinoma and is scheduled for a right pneumonectomy.

100. The nurse should include which of the following in the preoperative instructions? (Check all that apply.)

    A. _____ A chest tube will be inserted during surgery.

    B. _____ An IV solution will be maintained.

    C. _____ A nasogastric tube will be inserted.

    D. _____ An order for pain medication will be given.

101. Which of the following would the nurse demonstrate to the patient prior to surgery?

    A. proper ways to cough and deep breathe

    B. how to splint the incision

    C. how to use the call light

    D. all of the above

102. Which of the following symptoms are commonly seen after a pneumonectomy?

    A. hypervolemia

    B. bradycardia

    C. cardiac arrhythmias

    D. nausea

103. Mrs. P. asks you if her smoking had anything to do with her lung cancer. What do you reply?

    A. "You'll have to speak with the doctor."

    B. "Yes, smoking has been linked with this type of cancer."

    C. "Definitely; didn't the doctor tell you not to smoke?"

    D. "No, you were just unlucky."

*L*earner Self-Evaluation

Do I fully understand the content? If no, then the
areas I need to review are:

I need more information from my instructor on:

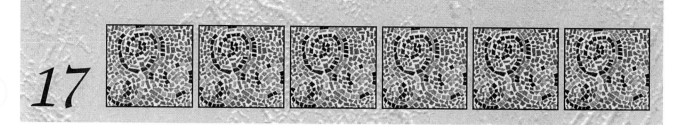

Knowledge Base for Patients with Neurologic Dysfunction

Objectives

1.0 Review the anatomy and physiology of the nervous system.
    1.1 Label the parts of the nervous system.
    1.2 Demonstrate an understanding of nerve impulse transmission.
    1.3 List the functions of the nervous system.
    1.4 Identify causes of altered levels of consciousness.
    1.5 Identify reasons for increases in intracranial pressure.

2.0 Demonstrate an understanding of the assessment data related to the nervous system.
    2.1 Demonstrate an understanding of how to assess the nervous system.
    2.2 Interpret assessment data related to the nervous system.
    2.3 Identify common clinical manifestations of neurologic dysfunctions.
    2.4 Identify dysfunctions of language and speech.
    2.5 Identify several types of diagnostic tests.
    2.6 Plan the nursing care for a patient undergoing diagnostic testing.

3.0 Demonstrate an understanding of the interventions used to manage neurologic dysfunctions.
    3.1 Identify medical/surgical management techniques of the patient with a neurologic dysfunction.
    3.2 Identify ways to treat increases in intracranial pressure.
    3.3 Plan the nursing care of the patient having a craniotomy.
    3.4 Write a nursing care plan for the patient having spinal surgery.
    3.5 Plan the nursing care for a patient with an altered level of consciousness.
    3.6 Write a nursing care plan for the patient with a visual field disturbance.

*L*earning Activities

Basic Knowledge

1. On the figure below, label the following parts
    of the central nervous system.

    A. Cerebrum

    B. Brain stem

    C. Cerebellum

    D. Midbrain

    E. Diencephalon

    F. Pons

    G. Medulla

    H. Spinal cord

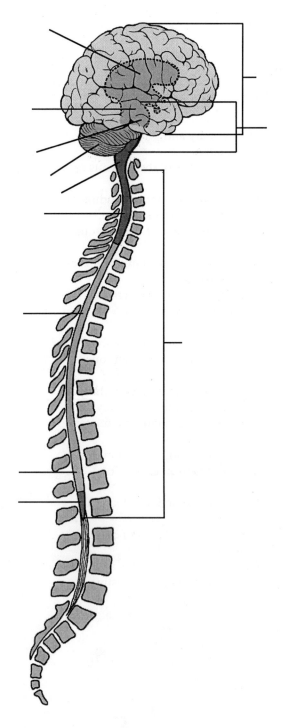

Short Answers

2. The central nervous system is composed of the _____ and the _____.

3. The peripheral nervous system is composed of the _____, _____, and _____.

4. _____ conduct impulses to the cell body and _____ conduct impulses away from the cell body.

5. The membranes that cover the brain and spinal cord and provide support and protection are the _____.

6. Cerebrospinal fluid (CSF) is formed primarily in the _____ _____.

7. The purpose of CSF is _____.

8. CSF is reabsorbed constantly into the _____ _____.

9. In the spinal cord, _____ pathways carry sensory impulses to the brain and _____ pathways carry motor impulses from the brain.

10. Superficial receptors of pain, temperature, and light touch are located throughout the skin in regions known as _____.

Identification

Match each of the common diagnostic tests below with the best definition.

A. MRI

B. CAT scan

C. PET scan

D. EP study

E. EMG

F. Doppler studies

G. Angiogram

H. Lumbar puncture

I. EEG

J. Myelogram

11. _____ Uses a powerful magnet and radio frequency to scan the head and body, then a computer creates pictures

12. _____ Noninvasive procedure to evaluate carotid arterial blood flow

13. _____ Uses an x-ray scanner, computer, and display mechanism to print images of the brain

14. _____ Imaging techniques that use radioactive tracers to produce images that measure physiologic and biochemical activities of the brain

15. _____ Invasive procedure to allow visualization of the intracranial vasculature

16. _____ Performed to determine CSF pressure

17. _____ Measures the electrical impulses of the brain

18. _____ Measures brain waves to determine cerebral response to peripheral sensory stimulation

19. _____ Records electrical impulses of the peripheral nerves

20. _____ Introduces contrast medium into the subarachnoid space to diagnose a herniated disc

Basic Knowledge

Demonstrate your understanding of the nervous system by matching the following.

    A.   Autonomic nervous system

    B.   Sympathetic system

    C.   Parasympathetic system

21. _____ Associated with "fight or flight" response

22. _____ Composed of the sympathetic and parasympathetic systems

23. _____ Associated with a conservation of energy

24. _____ Neurotransmitter acetylcholine is associated with this system

25. _____ Neurotransmitter noradrenalin is associated with this system

Knowledge Application

26. Intracranial pressure (ICP) can be defined as

    A.   pressure caused by changes in fluid volume

    B.   controlled by the central nervous system

    C.   pressure exerted within the cranial cavity by its contents

    D.   all the above

27. Normal ICP is _____ mm of water.

    A.   40–60

    B.   60–80

    C.   80–180

    D.   100–300

28. A decreased level of consciousness is often a result of

    A.   brain tissue damage due to lack of oxygen

    B.   change in pulmonary oxygen

    C.   cardiovascular hypertension

    D.   age-related perfusion deficiency

29. In the event of neuron trauma or injury, which of the nerves have the ability to recover?

    A.   cranial nerves

    B.   spinal nerves

    C.   peripheral nerves

    D.   none

30. During the depolarization process of nerve impulse transmission, which of the following will occur?

    A.   The cell membrane becomes permeable to sodium.

    B.   The neuron has a negative membrane potential.

    C.   An influx of potassium occurs.

    D.   Chloride and potassium ions move into the cells.

31. During neuromuscular transmission of the nerve impulse, which process occurs?

    A.   Neurotransmitters cause repolarization at the neuron junction.

    B.   Acetylcholine binds with acetylcholinesterase at the myoneuron junction causing release of calcium and contraction of the muscle.

    C.   Acetylcholine is released and travels across the synaptic cleft to bind with receptor sites.

    D.   Acetylcholinesterase is released, which stimulates the release of calcium to produce contraction.

32. The protective membrane that adheres to the brain and spinal cord is the

    A.   dura mater

    B.   arachnoid

    C.   pia mater

33. Which part of the cerebral hemisphere is thought to be the seat of abstract thought, judgment, and emotion?

    A.   frontal lobe

    B.   temporal lobe

    C.   parietal lobe

    D.   occipital lobe

34. The area in the cerebral hemisphere responsible for speech is known as

    A. Wernicke's area

    B. Broca's area

    C. Rolando's area

    D. lateral fissure

35. In most individuals, the right hemisphere of the cerebrum is responsible for

    A. understanding speech and expression of speech

    B. sensation of touch, position, and pressure

    C. perception of spatial orientation and perspective

    D. conscious awareness of pain

36. The respiratory centers of the brain are located in the

    A. midbrain

    B. pons

    C. medulla oblongata

    D. cerebellum

37. An activity which can result in an increased ICP is

    A. coughing

    B. performing the Valsalva maneuver

    C. flexion of the head

    D. all of the above

38. The reason that pupil checks are important when a change in ICP is suspected is because

    A. high pressure clouds the vision

    B. pupil changes can be caused by pressure on the ocular nerve

    C. hemorrhages will cause visual impairment

    D. pupil dilation is the first sign of increased ICP

39. The nurse is aware that the most sensitive indicator of increased ICP in a patient is

    A. increase in blood pressure

    B. decrease in level of consciousness

    C. agitation and hostility

    D. rise in temperature

40. Displacement of intracranial components from one compartment to another is called

    A. deceleration

    B. herniation

    C. decortication

    D. tamponade

41. Brain stem compression resulting in a change in vital signs is called

    A. Cushing's response

    B. decerebrate response

    C. hypothalamic response

    D. Glasgow response

42. A patient with an altered level of consciousness exhibits a downward drifting of an extended hand. This may indicate

    A. a developing hemiparesis

    B. increasing ICP

    C. overdose of medication

    D. alteration in electrolytes

43. A patient exhibits the following posturing: rigid spine, flexed and abducted arms, and legs extended. This is called

    A. decerebrate posturing

    B. hyperreflexia posture

    C. decorticate posturing

    D. persistent vegetative state

44. The nurse is assessing a patient with an altered level of consciousness. The assessment reveals eye opening to painful stimuli, abnormal extension of extremities, and no verbal response. The Glasgow coma scale total for this patient would be

    A.   5

    B.   7

    C.   9

    D.   12

45. An impairment of consciousness occurs when there is a disruption in which of the following circuit systems?

    A.   cerebellar area

    B.   reticular activating system

    C.   myoneural junction

    D.   bundle of Hesse

46. An altered level of consciousness can be the result of

    A.   metabolic disorders

    B.   infectious processes

    C.   psychiatric disorders

    D.   all of the above

47. Medical management of increased ICP will include medications such as

    A.   osmotic diuretics

    B.   corticosteroids

    C.   anticonvulsants

    D.   any or all of the above

48. When a patient is receiving mannitol, the nurse would monitor _____ .

    A.   serum osmolarity

    B.   hemoglobin and hematocrit

    C.   serum electrolytes

    D.   arterial blood gases

49. When a patient has an increase in ICP, the nurse would place him or her in the _____ position.

    A.   Trendelenburg

    B.   reverse Trendelenburg

    C.   semi-Fowler's

    D.   supine

50. When a patient has receptive aphasia, the nurse is aware that this is the result of injury to

    A.   Broca's area

    B.   Wernicke's area

    C.   the cerebrum

    D.   the lateral fissure

51. Assessment data of a patient reveals involuntary twisting movements of the body and trunk. This condition is called:

    A.   dystonia

    B.   bradykinesia

    C.   hemiparesis

    D.   torticollis

52. Following a stroke, a patient keeps walking into the wall on the right side. This type of visual field disturbance is known as

    A.   nystagmus

    B.   diplopia

    C.   tinnitus

    D.   hemianopsia

53. Following removal of a brain tumor, the patient is unable to understand spoken language. This is known as

    A.   aphasia

    B.   agraphia

    C.   dyslexia

    D.   alexia

54. The nurse is aware that if a lumbar puncture is performed on a patient who has an increased ICP, the following complication may occur.

    A. herniation syndrome

    B. hydrocephalic syndrome

    C. intracranial hemorrhage

    D. sepsis

55. Nursing care following angiography would involve

    A. monitoring neurologic signs for 24 hours

    B. immobilization of puncture site for 8 hours

    C. assessment of distal pulses

    D. all of the above

56. A patient who has returned from a cerebral angiogram is complaining of an inability to understand questions. The nurse is aware that this may indicate

    A. increase in ICP

    B. cerebrovascular accident

    C. hemorrhage

    D. renal shutdown

57. When a patient is scheduled for a myelogram, which medication should be withheld for several days before the procedure?

    A. calcium channel blocker

    B. diuretic

    C. MAO inhibitor

    D. analgesic

58. Which of the following nursing interventions would be implemented for the patient following a myelogram?

    A. limit fluids

    B. elevate bed to 45 degrees for six hours

    C. keep bed flat for 24 hours

    D. check peripheral pulses hourly for six hours

59. Which of the following symptoms may indicate an allergic reaction to the contrast medium given during a myelogram?

    A. vomiting

    B. raised rash

    C. pain in flank area

    D. anorexia

Identification

Match the test or action that would give you information on the status of each of the following.

    A. Sensory system

    B. Speech and language

    C. Motor function

    D. Abstract thinking

60. _____ Proprioception

61. _____ Arm drift

62. _____ Reflex testing

63. _____ Ask patient to explain a proverb

64. _____ Ask patient to identify objects

65. _____ Check resistance to movement

Nursing Care Plans

66. Write a nursing care plan for the patient who has an intracranial bleed. Use the following nursing diagnosis.

    Nursing diagnosis: Altered tissue perfusion (cerebral)

    Patient outcome:

    Interventions:

67. Write a nursing care plan for the unconscious patient. Use the following diagnosis.

    Nursing diagnosis: Impaired physical mobility related to the inability to participate in movement

    Patient outcome:

    Interventions:

68. Write a nursing care plan for the patient who has expressive aphasia as a result of a stroke. Pick an appropriate diagnosis.

    Nursing diagnosis:

    Patient outcome:

    Interventions:

69. Write a nursing care plan for the patient with a visual field deficit. Use the following diagnosis.

    Nursing diagnosis: Potential for injury related to sensory system dysfunction

    Patient outcome:

    Interventions:

70. Write a nursing care plan for a patient who has had spinal surgery. Use the following diagnosis.

    Nursing diagnosis: Altered comfort related to pain

    Patient outcome:

    Interventions:

Case Studies

Case Study No. 1

The nurse is caring for a 25-year-old male who is the victim of a motorcycle accident. He was not wearing a helmet. Severe head injury is suspected.

71. Assessment of this patient finds he is restless, with inappropriate verbal response. BP is 140/50; pulse is 50. The most likely reason for these signs and symptoms is

    A. hypovolemic shock

    B. hemorrhage

    C. increased ICP

    D. posttraumatic stress syndrome

72. Medical management of this patient would include administration of osmotic diuretics such as

    A. Lasix

    B. mannitol

    C. Dyazide

    D. Aldomet

73. The physician orders Decadron intravenously every six hours. Which of the following symptoms would indicate a side effect of this therapy?

    A. rapid heart rate

    B. hyperglycemia

    C. vomiting and nausea

    D. blurred vision

Nursing care of the patient with a head injury is aimed at preventing any further injury from an increase in ICP.

74. A nursing intervention that would be appropriate would be to

    A. increase fluid intake

    B. keep the patient in a prone position

    C. maintain the head of bed at a 30 degree angle

    D. monitor neurologic status q4h

75. The physician decides to start therapeutic hypothermia. The rationale for this order is that it will

    A. lower the ICP

    B. increase the metabolic demands

    C. lower the pain threshold

    D. decrease cerebral blood flow

76. The nurse's assessment for the last shift states that the patient has shown decerebrate posturing. This means that the patient

    A. withdraws only from painful stimuli

    B. has a rigid spine, flexed and adducted arms, extended and externally rotated legs

    C. has a rigid spine with arms extended and pronated, and extended legs with plantar flexion

    D. shows no response of any kind to verbals or touch

Case Study No. 2

Ms. Y. is admitted with a possible brain tumor. She is 66 years old and has a history of diabetes and heart disease with a pacemaker inserted five years ago. She is scheduled for diagnostic testing and possible surgery.

77. Ms. Y. is scheduled for a complete workup. Which of the following tests would NOT be appropriate for this patient?

    A. cerebral angiogram

    B. CAT scan

    C. MRI

    D. EEG

78. The diagnosis of a cerebral neoplasm is confirmed and Ms. Y. is scheduled for a craniotomy. The physician is likely to order which of the following medications prior to surgery?

    A. Dilantin

    B. Ancef

    C. Lasix

    D. potassium

79. Following the surgery, one of the most important nursing goals would be

   A.   preventing alteration in fluid and electrolytes

   B.   maintaining adequate cardiac output

   C.   maintaining adequate breathing patterns

   D.   preventing increased ICP

80. Which of the following symptoms would indicate a serious complication of the surgery?

   A.   nausea and vomiting

   B.   change in level of consciousness

   C.   rise in temperature

   D.   decrease in urine output

Ms. Y. begins to complain of a severe headache on the second postoperative day. She is also more lethargic.

81. The nurse notifies the physician at once because these symptoms may be related to

   A.   decreasing ICP

   B.   cerebral vasoconstriction

   C.   increase in ICP

   D.   instability of the suture line

82. To prevent impaired gas exchange following surgery, the nurse would implement which of the following interventions?

   A.   deep breathing

   B.   deep coughing

   C.   frequent suctioning

   D.   high-Fowler's position

*L*earner Self-Evaluation

Do I fully understand the content? If no, then the areas I need to review are:

I need more information from my instructor on:

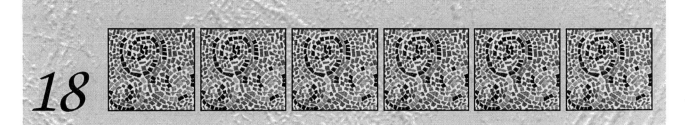

18

Nursing Care of Patients with Neurologic Disorders

*O*bjectives

1.0 Demonstrate an understanding of the infections and inflammations that affect the nervous system.

    1.1 Identify characteristics of the infections and inflammations of the nervous system.

    1.2 Assess clinical manifestations of several of the infectious disorders.

    1.3 Identify nursing interventions and rationales for patients with infectious disorders.

    1.4 Write a nursing care plan that addresses the nutritional needs of the patient with encephalitis.

2.0 Demonstrate an understanding of the degenerative disorders that can affect the nervous system.

    2.1 Identify characteristic symptoms of degenerative disorders of the nervous system.

    2.2 Identify nursing interventions and rationales for patients with degenerative disorders.

    2.3 Identify the pathology of several of the degenerative disorders.

    2.4 Plan the nursing care for the patient with multiple sclerosis.

3.0 Demonstrate an understanding of the functional disorders of the nervous system.

    3.1 Identify symptoms of functional disorders.

    3.2 Plan the nursing care for the patient with a seizure disorder.

4.0 Demonstrate an understanding of the structural disorders of the nervous system.

    4.1 Identify characteristics of structural disorders.

    4.2 Review appropriate medical interventions for the patient with a structural disorder.

    4.3 Write a nursing care plan for the patient with a cerebrovascular accident.

5.0 Demonstrate an understanding of traumatic injuries of the nervous system.

    5.1 Identify symptoms of head injuries.

    5.2 Identify the symptoms of spinal shock.

    5.3 Write a nursing care plan for the patient with a spinal injury.

6.0 Demonstrate an understanding of the neoplasms that affect the nervous system.

    6.1 Assess characteristics of neoplasms of the nervous system.

    6.2 Write a nursing care plan for the patient with a brain tumor.

Learning Activities

Short Answers

1. The medical management for the patient with bacterial meningitis is the administration of _____.

2. The first priority when caring for the patient with a neurologic disorder is _____.

3. Parkinson's disease is related to the availability of _____.

4. Alzheimer's disease is a prominent _____ illness.

5. Cluster headaches are a type of _____ headache.

6. _____ is the major complication of external ventricular shunts.

7. An _____ is a congenital weakness in the wall of an artery.

8. _____ is the leading cause of death in persons younger that 40 years.

9. A progressive impairment of cognitive functioning is called _____.

10. _____ is an acute confusional state.

Identification

Match each of the following neurologic disorders with the appropriate definition.

A. Encephalitis

B. Guillain-Barré Syndrome

C. Amyotrophic lateral sclerosis (ALS)

D. Alzheimer's disease

E. Multiple sclerosis (MS)

F. Parkinson's disease

G. Hydrocephalus

H. Cerebrovascular accident (CVA)

11. _____ Disease characterized by degenerative changes in basal ganglia

12. _____ An inflammation of the brain

13. _____ Condition characterized by demyelination and scarring of sites along the central nervous system

14. _____ Dysfunction in the production, circulation, or reabsorption of cerebrospinal fluid

15. _____ Progressive degeneration and loss of both upper and lower motor neurons

16. _____ Results from interruption of blood flow to the brain

17. _____ Chronic progressive neurodegenerative condition characterized by marked cognitive dysfunction

18. _____ Progressive inflammation and demyelination of the nerve endings of the peripheral nervous system

True/False

19. _____ Herpes simplex encephalitis is the most common form of nonepidemic encephalitis in the United States.

20. _____ Viral encephalitis is treated with antibiotics.

21. _____ Guillain-Barré syndrome is caused by a virus.

22. _____ A diagnosis of ALS can be confirmed with a computed tomography (CT) scan.

23. _____ The cause of Alzheimer's disease is unknown.

24. _____ The mortality rate associated with subarachnoid hemorrhages is > 30%.

25. _____ Cerebral aneurysms are often asymptomatic until rupture.

26. _____ Individuals with arteriovenous malformations may have headaches and seizures.

27. _____ The presenting symptom associated with a subarachnoid hemorrhage is severe dizziness.

28. _____ Dementia and delirium occur more often in the elderly.

Knowledge Application

29. In a patient with suspected meningococcal meningitis, the nurse would assess for
    A. petechial rash or ecchymosis
    B. nausea and vomiting
    C. change in consciousness
    D. pupil changes

30. The nurse is assessing a patient with a neurologic disorder. The nurse performs an assessment and finds that passive flexion of the head results in a flexion of the thighs and legs. This is known as
    A. nuchal rigidity
    B. Kernig's sign
    C. Brudzinski's sign
    D. cortical irritation

31. In order to make a definitive diagnosis of meningitis, the nurse would expect the physician to order a(n)
    A. CT scan
    B. MRI scan
    C. angiogram
    D. lumbar puncture

32. The nurse's responsibility in preventing transmission of herpes simplex virus type 2 would include
    A. testing of all college-age students
    B. determining presence of virus in pregnant women
    C. treating all sexually active men
    D. random screening in drug clinics

33. A patient with a brain abscess exhibits signs of confusion, drowsiness, and irritability. These are signs of
    A. hypotension
    B. hypoxia
    C. increased intracranial pressure (ICP)
    D. increased cerebral perfusion

34. When a patient with herpes simplex encephalitis develops neurologic symptoms such as hemiparesis or behavioral changes, the nurse would monitor closely for
    A. signs of increased ICP
    B. loss of bladder and bowel control
    C. respiratory distress
    D. cardiac arrhythmias

35. Medical management of the patient with herpes simplex encephalitis will include
    A. antibiotics
    B. fluid restrictions
    C. antiviral agents
    D. analgesics

36. An individual who has a severe mastoiditis is at risk for developing
    A. hearing loss
    B. brain abscess
    C. encephalitis
    D. septic shock

37. When assessing a patient who has Guillain-Barré syndrome, the nurse notices asymmetrical facial expressions. This may indicate that there is

    A. cranial nerve involvement

    B. permanent paralysis

    C. an increase in ICP

    D. brain damage

38. Because the patient with Guillain-Barré syndrome often develops flaccid paralysis, the nursing management is primarily directed toward?

    A. preventing dehydration

    B. promoting independence

    C. preventing development of contractures

    D. maintaining bowel and bladder control

39. One of the newer treatments for Guillain-Barré syndrome that is thought to remove antibodies from the bloodstream is

    A. exchange transfusion

    B. hemodialysis

    C. plasmapheresis

    D. immersion therapy

40. The most common motor neuron disease in adults is

    A. MS

    B. ALS

    C. muscular dystrophy

    D. myasthenia gravis

41. The nurse is assessing a patient with a nervous system disorder. All of the following symptoms would indicate ALS EXCEPT

    A. difficulty swallowing

    B. decreased sensation

    C. hyperreflexia

    D. slurred speech

42. In caring for a patient with a diagnosis of ALS, the nurse should be chiefly concerned with

    A. maintaining highest level of functioning of the patient

    B. maintaining adequate nutritional intake

    C. returning the patient to prior activity level

    D. preventing atrophy of muscles

43. The nurse should have which equipment available when feeding the patient with ALS?

    A. cardiac monitor

    B. oxygen

    C. suction machine

    D. oral airway

44. To increase muscle control in the individual with MS, the nurse would administer

    A. Klonopin

    B. Tegretol

    C. Elavil

    D. Cytoxan

45. In the patient with MS, the nurse would anticipate which of the following alterations to be present?

    A. sensory alterations

    B. motor alterations

    C. visual alterations

    D. emotional lability

    E. any or all of the above

46. Which statement best describes the clinical course of MS?

    A. The disease will often go into total remission after aggressive treatment.

    B. The disease is chronic and has a steady downhill course.

    C. The disease is characterized by exacerbation and remissions that are unpredictable.

    D. The disease is curable if recognized and diagnosed early.

47. A patient with MS has severe spasticity of the lower extremities. The nurse would anticipate that _____ would be used.

    A. Lioresal

    B. Tylenol

    C. Decadron

    D. Gantrisin

48. Appropriate nursing interventions for the patient with a neurogenic bladder would include all the following EXCEPT

    A. maintain a schedule for bladder training

    B. monitor intake and output

    C. insert a Foley catheter

    D. use Crédè's maneuver as needed

49. Which description would be most appropriate in explaining the pathophysiology of myasthenia gravis?

    A. It is a hereditary autoimmune disease of the motor neurons.

    B. It is a progressive degeneration of the myelin sheath of the spinal cord.

    C. It is a disease that affects the acetylcholine released at the neuromuscular junction.

    D. It is an acute disease that has effective treatment regimens.

50. The nurse is assisting the physician to make a diagnosis of myasthenia gravis. What is an appropriate nursing action?

    A. have Tensilon ready for administration

    B. explain to the patient this may cure the disease

    C. keep the patient NPO

    D. have the patient sign a consent form

51. The nurse is educating a patient on when to take his Mestinon after discharge. What information should the nurse obtain from the patient?

    A. what time he goes to bed

    B. what time he eats meals

    C. how often he urinates daily

    D. what types of activities he can perform

52. If a patient with myasthenia gravis has a severe infection, the nurse realizes that he or she is at risk for developing which of the following? (Check all that apply.)

    A. _____ cholinergic crisis

    B. _____ myasthenic crisis

    C. _____ septic shock

    D. _____ respiratory arrest

53. A hereditary neurologic condition characterized by progressive degeneration and weakness of the voluntary muscles is known as

    A. MS

    B. Lou Gehrig's disease

    C. muscular dystrophy

    D. Alzheimer's disease

54. When the nurse is assessing a patient with Parkinson's disease, findings would most likely include

    A. tremors, weakness, muscle atrophy

    B. shuffling gait, spastic leg movement

    C. blurred vision, weakness, fatigue

    D. tremors, muscle rigidity, bradykinesia

55. In evaluating a patient for Parkinson's disease, the nurse would expect to see a decreased urine level of

    A. homovanillic acid

    B. uric acid

    C. catecholamines

    D. acetylcholine

56. The medical treatment for the individual with Parkinson's disease would include the use of anticholinergic drugs such as

   A. levodopa

   B. Sinemet

   C. Cogentin

   D. Decadron

57. The nurse is assisting a patient with Parkinson's disease to plan meals. Which foods should be limited?

   A. chicken and turkey

   B. cereal and whole grains

   C. milk and eggs

   D. green vegetables

58. Ms. M., age 63, is admitted to an assisted-living facility with symptoms of forgetfulness, irritability, difficulty following directions, and personal neglect. These suggest which stage of Alzheimer's disease?

   A. early stage

   B. middle stage

   C. final stage

   D. terminal stage

59. An appropriate nursing intervention for the patient with Alzheimer's disease would be to

   A. increase verbal and environmental cues

   B. restrain the individual so they can't harm him- or herself

   C. speak loudly and slowly

   D. involve the patient in new activities

60. A patient is admitted with a possible herniated disc. Which information given by the patient might indicate the cause of the current condition?

   A. "I like to jog in the morning."

   B. "I am 20 pounds overweight."

   C. "I smoke two packs of cigarettes a day."

   D. "I helped my neighbor move his furniture yesterday."

61. A test used to diagnose a herniated disc because it provides clear images of the spinal cord anatomy is the

   A. spinal x-ray

   B. lumbar puncture

   C. magnetic resonance imaging (MRI)

   D. ultrasound

62. The most comfortable position for the patient with herniation of a lumbar disc would be

   A. prone without a pillow

   B. semi-Fowler's

   C. side lying with knees flexed

   D. supine

63. The nurse is assessing a patient who is admitted with seizures. During examination, the patient has a two-minute period of lack of awareness of the environment. This was most likely a

   A. simple partial seizure

   B. complex partial seizure

   C. petit mal seizure

   D. tonic-clonic seizure

64. If a patient developed status epilepticus, the physician might order

   A. Dilantin

   B. Phenobarbital

   C. Valium

   D. any or all of above

65. One of the most important nursing interventions for the patient with a seizure disorder is to

   A. provide a safe environment

   B. maintain effective gas exchange

   C. provide appropriate knowledge of condition

   D. instruct the patient in self-care activities

66. The rationale for treating migraine headaches with medications such as Inderal and
Catapres is to

    A.   promote analgesia and sedation

    B.   promote vasodilatation

    C.   reduce stress and anxiety

    D.   inhibit vasodilation

67. When a patient is admitted with a diagnosis
of communicating hydrocephalus, which
information in the medical history is most
relevant?

    A.   myocardial infarction

    B.   meningitis

    C.   seizures

    D.   adrenal insufficiency

68. Mr. P., 64 years old, is admitted with a
diagnosis of normal pressure hydrocephalus.
Which assessment data is related to this
problem?

    A.   gait disturbance, impaired memory

    B.   mood swings, depression, aphasia

    C.   headache, dizziness, sensory deficit

    D.   hemiplegia, agnosia

69. Mr. P. has a ventricular shunt inserted to
correct the problem. Following the surgery,
the nurse would consider which of the
following to be a serious complication? The
patient

    A.   complains of tenderness at insertion
site

    B.   is incontinent of urine

    C.   is anxious

    D.   is lethargic and hard to arouse

70. The nurse is aware that a CVA is often the
result of

    A.   sudden increase in cardiac output

    B.   interruption of blood flow to the brain

    C.   sudden change in electrolyte balance

    D.   seizure disorder

71. In differentiating between a transient ischemic attack (TIA) and a CVA, the nurse is
aware that a TIA

    A.   has sudden onset and short duration

    B.   has slow insidious onset and lasts up to
48 hours

    C.   is progressive

    D.   is often undetected but will always lead
to a stroke

72. A patient who is admitted with a left-sided
CVA will most likely have

    A.   aphasia

    B.   ataxia

    C.   dyslexia

    D.   quadriplegia

73. Which position would be most appropriate
for the nurse to use for the patient with a
right CVA who is nonresponsive?

    A.   prone position

    B.   right side with knees flexed

    C.   left side with head of bed 30 degrees

    D.   Trendelenburg's position

74. A patient has a CVA with left-sided paralysis.
The nurse positions the bed table on the left
side. The rationale for this is to

    A.   encourage self care

    B.   keep the environment uncluttered

    C.   prevent unilateral neglect

    D.   prevent falls from the bed

75. The treatment of choice for the patient with
an embolic cerebral ischemic event would be

    A.   anticoagulants

    B.   corticosteroids

    C.   antibiotics

    D.   antihistamines

76. Which of the following clinical manifestations is present in a large percentage of the individuals who have brain tumors?

    A.   frontal headache

    B.   projectile vomiting

    C.   papilledema

    D.   seizures

77. Which of the following diagnostic tests may be contraindicated for an individual who is being evaluated for a possible brain tumor?

    A.   CT scan

    B.   lumbar puncture

    C.   angiogram

    D.   MRI scan

78. The nurse is assessing a patient who has a possible skull fracture as a result of an accident. A finding of ecchymosis over the mastoid bone is indicative of a

    A.   linear skull fracture

    B.   scalp laceration

    C.   basilar skull fracture

    D.   leakage of cerebral spinal fluid

79. The nurse is aware that the drug of choice to reduce cerebral edema is

    A.   mannitol

    B.   dexamethasone

    C.   heparin

    D.   cefazolin

80. When caring for the patient with a skull fracture, the nurse would explain to the patient that which of the following activities would be contraindicated?

    A.   blowing his nose

    B.   ambulating in unit

    C.   sitting in a chair

    D.   urinating while standing

81. A traumatic accident that causes the brain to strike the internal surfaces of the skull resulting in bruising of brain tissues is a

    A.   contusion

    B.   concussion

    C.   hematoma

    D.   herniation

82. A patient is admitted with a head injury. Initially he was unconscious for one hour. He wakes later in the hospital, but three hours later he begins to lose consciousness. This suggests

    A.   CVA

    B.   transient ischemia

    C.   epidural hematoma

    D.   subdural hematoma

83. A patient who is admitted with an epidural hematoma is deteriorating rapidly. An appropriate nursing measure would be to

    A.   transfer the patient to intensive care

    B.   prepare the patient for surgery

    C.   notify the code team

    D.   monitor vital signs closely

84. The nurse is assessing a patient with a spinal cord injury. Symptoms indicating spinal shock would include

    A.   flaccid paralysis of skeletal musculature below the level of the lesion

    B.   spastic paralysis of skeletal musculature below the level of injury

    C.   rigidity of the lower extremities with flaccidity of upper extremities

    D.   total lack of sensation and motor activity

85. A patient who has a spinal injury is to be fitted with a Halo device. The nurse realizes one advantage of this device is

    A.   reduction in time of healing

    B.   improvement in mobility

    C.   decrease in complications

    D.   prevention of spinal shock

Nursing Care Plans

86. Write a nursing care plan for a patient with encephalitis who is unable to eat. Write a nursing diagnosis, patient outcome, and several nursing interventions.

Nursing diagnosis:

Patient outcome:

Interventions:

87. Write a nursing care plan for an individual with Parkinson's disease. Focus on problems with mobility.

Nursing diagnosis:

Patient outcome:

Interventions:

88. Write a nursing care plan for a patient who has been admitted with a CVA who is plegic and aphasic. Use the following diagnoses.

Nursing diagnosis: Impaired physical mobility related to plegia

Patient outcome:

Interventions:

Nursing diagnosis: Impaired verbal communication

Patient outcome:

Interventions:

89. Write a nursing care plan for a patient who has sustained a head injury. Use the following diagnosis.

Nursing diagnosis: Altered neurologic function related to acute head injury

Patient outcome:

Interventions:

90. Write a nursing care plan for a patient with a spinal cord injury. Use the following diagnosis.

Nursing diagnosis: Potential for injury related to unstable vertebral column

Patient outcome:

Interventions:

Case Studies

Case Study No. 1

Ms. K., a college-age student, is waiting in the health clinic when she suddenly begins to experience a generalized tonic-clonic seizure.

91. The nurse's first priority should be to

   A. remove everyone from the area

   B. move her to the floor

   C. insert a padded tongue blade between her teeth

   D. ask a bystander what precipitated the seizure

92. The nurse realizes that seizures are a result of

   A. increased ICP

   B. uncontrolled excessive discharge of neurons

   C. cerebral hypoxia

   D. lack of dopamine

93. Immediately following the seizure, Ms. K. is incontinent of urine and difficult to arouse. Based on this information, the nurse should

   A. call the paramedics

   B. do a thorough neurologic check every five minutes

   C. shake her frequently so she doesn't fall asleep

   D. place her on her side and let her sleep

94. After a thorough workup, it is determined that Ms. K. is suffering from epilepsy. She is started on Dilantin. Which information would the nurse emphasize?

   A. Medication needs decrease with age.

   B. Medication should never be stopped suddenly.

   C. Medication should be discontinued if side effects occur.

   D. Medication will probably not totally control seizures.

95. Ms. K. is to be married next year. She wonders if she should have children. Which of the following statements should the nurse make?

   A.   "When you decide to get pregnant, ask your physician to change your medication."

   B.   "Your children won't have any increased risk of having seizures."

   C.   "It is often impossible to become pregnant when a woman has a seizure disorder."

   D.   "Unless you stop having seizures, you shouldn't consider having children."

Case Study No. 2

Mr. S., 75 years old, is admitted with a diagnosis of left hemispheric CVA. He is lethargic and nonverbal.

96. During the acute phase, the nurse is aware that a priority is

   A.   maintaining mobility

   B.   maintaining fluid and electrolyte balance

   C.   maintaining patent airway

   D.   preventing skin breakdown

97. Based on the type of CVA that has occurred, the nurse will anticipate that Mr. S. will have

   A.   language and speech impairment, motor plegia

   B.   left-sided neglect, self-care deficit

   C.   normal speech but plegia on right side

   D.   normal return of function in 6–8 months

98. It is determined that Mr. S. has had an embolic stroke. Knowing this, the nurse would expect what type of treatment to be implemented?

   A.   heparin therapy

   B.   aspirin therapy

   C.   diuretic therapy

   D.   antibiotic therapy

99. The goal of this therapy is to

   A.   prevent secondary infection

   B.   prevent formation of new clots

   C.   control pain

   D.   decrease inflammation

100. After 48 hours, Mr. S. is more alert. He is receiving Coumadin, Minipress, and digoxin. The nurse is reviewing Mr. S.'s lab results. Which lab result shows a therapeutic response to treatment?

   A.   PT of 10.0 seconds

   B.   PT of 16.3 seconds

   C.   PTT of 60.0 seconds

   D.   PTT of 35.3 seconds

After seven days, Mr. S. is transferred to a subacute facility for continued rehabilitation.

101. Which of the following statements best describes the follow-up care for Mr. S.?

   A.   Care for the CVA patient involves a multidisciplinary team.

   B.   Care for the CVA patient involves the physician and the nurse.

   C.   Care for the CVA patient will ultimately become the family's responsibility.

   D.   Care for the CVA patient is always uncertain.

102. Mr. S. has been incontinent of both urine and feces since his stroke. Which nursing measure would be most appropriate to help Mr. S. regain bladder control?

   A.   change the bed pads frequently

   B.   get an order for a Foley catheter

   C.   apply an external urinary catheter

   D.   keep the urinal within easy reach

103. Mr. S. has expressive aphasia. Which technique should the nurse use to facilitate communication with him?

   A.   speak loudly and slowly

   B.   face the patient and speak normally

   C.   use pantomime and gestures frequently

   D.   write down everything and show him

Case Study No. 3

Mr. G., 18 years old, is involved in a climbing accident. He fell from a ledge and a spinal cord injury is suspected.

104. A nurse is in the area and is the first one to find him. Mr. G. is lying on his back and says he can't move his legs. An appropriate action on the part of the nurse would be to

   A.   turn him on his side

   B.   keep him still, call for help

   C.   have him bend his knees to relieve the pain

   D.   carry Mr. G. to the road and summon help

105. While the nurse is awaiting assistance, the priority should be to assess

   A.   for patency of airway

   B.   neurologic status

   C.   for bleeding

   D.   for pain

106. In the emergency room, Mr. G. is alert but anxious. His heart rate and respirations are increasing while his BP is falling. These findings suggest

   A.   autonomic dysreflexia

   B.   hypovolemic shock

   C.   spinal shock

   D.   cardiogenic shock

Mr. G. has a compression injury at the level of T7. Once his condition stabilizes, he is moved to the rehabilitation unit.

107. Which of the following best explains the extent of his injuries?

   A.   He is prone to respiratory failure.

   B.   He will be a quadriplegic.

   C.   He will be a paraplegic.

   D.   He should regain full function.

108. The nurse notices that Mr. G. is uncooperative and hostile. This behavior indicates a

   A.   normal grief reaction

   B.   normal anxiety reaction

   C.   sign of depression

   D.   reaction to being in intensive care

Case Study No. 4

A patient is admitted with a diagnosis of bacterial meningitis. The admitting symptoms include headache, fever, and petechial rash.

109. The nurse is examining the patient. Which of the following signs indicates meningeal irritation?

   A.   severe headache

   B.   seizure activity

   C.   positive Homans' sign

   D.   positive Kernig's sign

110. Medical treatment is initiated immediately. The nurse would anticipate administration of medications such as

   A.   analgesics

   B.   anti-inflammatories

   C.   antibiotics

   D.   antipyretics

111. The nurse realizes it is important to observe the patient for any signs of increased ICP. A sign of increased ICP would be

   A.   difficulty breathing

   B.   irregularity of heart rate

   C.   rapid pulse

   D.   seizure activity

112. Which would be the best method for the nurse to administer Dilantin 100 mg IVP to the patient?

    A. dilute with 100 mL dextrose and administer over 30 minutes

    B. dilute with 10 mL dextrose and give within five minutes to get maximum therapeutic effect

    C. dilute in 100 mL of normal saline and administer over 30–60 minutes

    D. administer cautiously from syringe within 20 minutes and flush with any IV solution

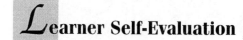

Learner Self-Evaluation

Do I fully understand the content? If no, then the areas I need to review are:

I need more information from my instructor on:

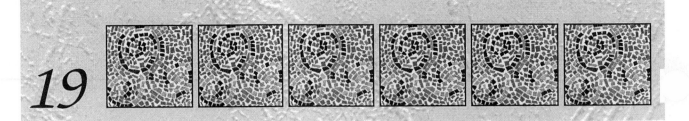

19

Knowledge Base for Patients with Musculoskeletal Dysfunction

*O*bjectives

1.0 Review the anatomy and physiology of the musculoskeletal system.
    1.1 List the parts of the musculoskeletal system.
    1.2 List the functions of the musculoskeletal system.
    1.3 Explain the stages of bone repair.
    1.4 List factors that affect how damaged bone heals.

2.0 Demonstrate an understanding of assessment data related to the musculoskeletal system.
    2.1 Identify symptoms of musculoskeletal dysfunction.
    2.2 Identify common clinical manifestations of musculoskeletal dysfunction.
    2.3 Match diagnostic tests with the appropriate description.

3.0 Demonstrate an understanding of interventions used to treat adults with musculoskeletal dysfunction.
    3.1 Identify types of nonsurgical treatments of musculoskeletal dysfunctions.
    3.2 Demonstrate an understanding of the use of casts in treating musculoskeletal dysfunction.
    3.3 Demonstrate an understanding of the principles of traction.
    3.4 Identify surgical interventions used to treat musculoskeletal dysfunction.
    3.5 Plan the nursing care for an adult with a dysfunction of the musculoskeletal system.

*L*earning Activities

Short Answers

1. List the parts of the musculoskeletal system.
    1.

    2.

    3.

    4.

    5.

2. List the functions of the musculoskeletal system.
    1.

    2.

3. List and briefly explain the five stages of bone healing.
   1.

   2.

   3.

   4.

   5.

4. List six of the factors that can affect how damaged bone heals.
   1.

   2.

   3.

   4.

   5.

   6.

5. The process of bone formation is called

   _____.

6. Axial skeletal growth is completed by the

   end of _____.

7. Throughout life, the _____ deposits newly formed bone while the

   _____ resorb or thin the bone.

8. Bones are enclosed in a tough fibrous tissue

   called _____.

9. The diaphysis of a long bone is made up of

   _____ and the epiphysis is made up of

   _____ bone.

10. Skeletal muscles contract in response to

    impulses from the _____.

11. To produce _____, muscles contract over bones.

12. The primary energy source for muscle activity is the breakdown of

    _____.

13. Muscle activity or movement requires

    _____.

14. A _____ is the point where two or more bones meet.

15. A _____ is a device that is used to measure range of motion.

Identification

Match the following musculoskeletal tissues with their descriptions.

   A. Ligaments

   B. Tendons

   C. Cartilage

16. _____ Strong, nonelastic, fibrous connective tissue cords

17. _____ Smooth, resilient, supporting tissue composed of collagen

18. _____ Fibrous connective tissue bands which bind bones to bones

19. _____ Provides a cushion to absorb shock and reduce joint stress

Match the following diagnostic tests with the appropriate description.

A.   Arthroscopy

B.   Bone scan

C.   Computed tomography (CT) scan

D.   Magnetic resonance imaging (MRI)

E.   Electromyography (EMG)

F.   Thermography

G.   Gallium scan

20. _____ Nuclear scan that uses a radionuclide that is concentrated in areas of inflammation

21. _____ Uses magnetic force to provide three-plane pictures of internal structures

22. _____ Endoscopic examination of a joint

23. _____ Determines the electrical activity of skeletal muscle and its ability to respond to stimulus

24. _____ Combines x-ray with computer technology to produce pictures of internal structures

25. _____ Uses an infrared camera to determine the amount of heat radiating from soft tissue

26. _____ X-ray of skeletal bone using a gamma camera scanner after an injection of a radioactive substance

True/False

27. _____ Muscles can atrophy in a short time from disuse.

28. _____ Without mobility, bone destruction occurs at a greater rate than bone production.

29. _____ MRI can be easily used with all patients.

30. _____ Heat is applied to sore joints to promote circulation.

31. _____ Casts made of plaster of Paris are ready for weight bearing in six hours.

32. _____ Internal fixation devices are usually made of polyethylene.

33. _____ Once a joint has been replaced, it lasts a lifetime.

Knowledge Application

34. Which of the following assessment findings would indicate a possible musculoskeletal disorder?

A.   pain

B.   change in gait

C.   change in elimination

D.   diminished pulses

35. Following a musculoskeletal injury the most appropriate intervention is

A.   application of cold

B.   application of heat

C.   splinting the extremity

D.   transport to emergency room

36. Pain management for musculoskeletal dysfunction may include

A.   anti-inflammatory agents

B.   analgesics

C.   skeletal muscle relaxants

D.   any of the above

37. When caring for the patient in a full body cast, one of the most important nursing responsibilities is to assess for

A.   infection

B.   restricted chest expansion

C.   fluid imbalance

D.   ineffective coping

38. To prevent problems with tissue perfusion when a patient has a full leg cast, the nurse should

A.   maintain bed rest

B.   assess for pulses every shift

C.   keep legs in a nondependent position when not out of bed

D.   keep legs below heart level to increase circulation

39. All of the following are complications of immobility EXCEPT

    A. alteration in elimination

    B. discoloration of the skin

    C. alteration in nutrition

    D. symptoms of infection

40. If the patient in a spica cast develops abdominal distention and vomiting, it may be due to pressure on the

    A. mesenteric artery

    B. aorta

    C. diaphragm

    D. spine

41. When a patient is in traction, the countertraction is usually generated by

    A. weights

    B. pulleys

    C. height of the bed

    D. patient's weight

42. Which of the following conditions would not require the use of traction?

    A. reduction of compound fracture

    B. fracture of the pelvis

    C. nondisplaced fracture of radius

    D. displaced fracture of femur

43. The amount of weight used with the application of skin traction is

    A. 2–4 pounds

    B. 5–7 pounds

    C. 7–12 pounds

    D. 10–15 pounds

44. The amount of weight used with the application of skeletal traction is

    A. 5–7 pounds

    B. 10–15 pounds

    C. 15–25 pounds

    D. 20–30 pounds

45. The reason that skeletal traction is effective in reducing and maintaining alignment of fracture fragments is because

    A. it can be used intermittently

    B. it controls rotation as well as longitudinal pull

    C. it can maintain a position of hyperextension

    D. there is a low rate of infection

46. Skin traction is contraindicated when

    A. there is a fracture of the upper extremities

    B. impaired circulation is present

    C. the patient is over the age of 65

    D. other injuries are present

47. The reason that the halo apparatus is connected to the body jacket when a patient has Crutchfield tongs is to

    A. permit ambulation

    B. prevent infection

    C. prevent rotation of the spine

    D. keep the patient immobilized

48. The purpose of an external fixation device is to

    A. compress bone fragments and maintain alignment

    B. promote external rotation and alignment

    C. prevent infection

    D. promote rapid healing of injuries

49. All of the following would be indications for external fixation therapy EXCEPT

    A. open fracture with nerve damage

    B. leg lengthening

    C. open contaminated fracture

    D. closed fracture with swelling

50. When caring for the patient in traction, which of the following observations by the nurse would be important to report at once?

    A.   low-grade fever

    B.   pain and drainage at pin site

    C.   generalized discomfort

    D.   loss of appetite

51. One of the problems associated with the use of internal fixation devices is

    A.   tissue reaction to a foreign substance

    B.   infection can occur on the surface of the device

    C.   infection can occur long after surgery

    D.   all of the above

52. The purpose of total joint replacement is to

    A.   prevent problems related to immobility

    B.   relieve pain and provide improved joint function

    C.   remove a severely infected joint

    D.   stop further joint degeneration

53. The reason that a patient experiences phantom sensation following a limb amputation is

    A.   the inability to distinguish pain site

    B.   nerve endings in the pathway are still being stimulated

    C.   the intensity of the pain at the site of the amputation

    D.   severe stress increases the pain perception

54. When considering whether a patient is a candidate for an external prosthesis, which of the following factors should be considered?

    A.   general health of individual

    B.   weight and strength of individual

    C.   lifestyle and activity of individual

    D.   potential for rehabilitation

    E.   all of the above

55. Following knee replacement, patients are frequently placed on a continuous passive motion device (CPM). The purpose of this device is to

    A.   put the knee through preset degrees of passive range of motion

    B.   put the knee through a range of passive and active range of motion exercises

    C.   speed up the mobilization of the joint

    D.   reduce pain and inflammation

Nursing Care Plans

56. Write a nursing care plan for the adult experiencing immobility problems. Use the following nursing diagnosis.

    Nursing diagnosis: Knowledge deficit: nature of immobility problems and prevention of complications

    Patient outcome:

    Interventions:

57. Write a nursing care plan for the patient with an external fixation device. Use the following nursing diagnosis.

Nursing diagnosis: Knowledge deficit: nature of care for the external fixation device, pin site care, and mobility management

Patient outcome:

Interventions:

Case Studies

Case Study No. 1

Mr. J. is injured when he is hit by a car. Medics identify a fracture of the leg and possibly the arm. He is assessed, an IV is started, and pain medication is given. He is immobilized and transported to the hospital.

58. The most important measure taken by the medics to ensure no further injury was

A. correct identification of injury

B. immobilization of injuries

C. adequate pain medication

D. transport to proper emergency room

59. Mr. J. is diagnosed with a fracture of the femur, tibia, and clavicle. He is placed in traction. All of the following principles of traction are true EXCEPT

A. sufficient countertraction must be maintained

B. weights must hang free

C. avoid friction on ropes or weights

D. remove weight only when linens are changed

60. His injuries are healed sufficiency to allow a leg cast to be placed. Following the application of a plaster cast, the nurse should

A. dry with a hair dryer

B. ambulate within two hours

C. assess for adequate circulation

D. assess for respiratory distress

61. After casting, the nurse would assess for proper fit of the cast by assessing

A. proximal and distal pulses

B. vital signs

C. pain rating

D. odor or warmth to cast

Mr. J. is discharged and will be monitored by his family physician.

62. Which of the following information would NOT be included in the discharge instructions?

A. cover any rough edges of the cast with tape

B. use emollient lotion on skin around the cast

C. elevate extremity to reduce swelling

D. exercise the joint proximal and distal to cast

63. He returns in six weeks for removal of the cast. Following cast removal, it will be important for the nurse to

A. inspect the limb for atrophy, weakness, and loss of range of motion

B. teach Mr. J. how to use a walker

C. teach Mr. J. proper use of pain medication

D. inspect for signs of infection

Case Study No. 2

Mr. N. is admitted for a below-the-knee amputation because of severe peripheral vascular disease. He refuses to talk about the proposed surgery.

64. The most appropriate nursing diagnosis for this patient is

 A. Alteration in tissue perfusion

 B. Impaired skin integrity

 C. Dysfunctional grieving

 D. Anxiety

65. After the surgery, Mr. N. complains of severe pain in the amputated extremity. The appropriate nursing action is

 A. medicate as needed

 B. reinforce the absence of the extremity

 C. notify the physician

 D. explain that pain is only psychological

66. The proper position for the residual limb immediately following surgery is

 A. elevated on pillow

 B. dependent position

 C. position of comfort

 D. in abduction

67. In preparation for discharge, it would be important for the nurse to instruct Mr. N. in

 A. proper wrapping of the limb

 B. proper skin care

 C. proper nutrition

 D. all of the above

*L*earner Self-Evaluation

Do I fully understand the content? If no, then the areas I need to review are:

I need more information from my instructor on:

20

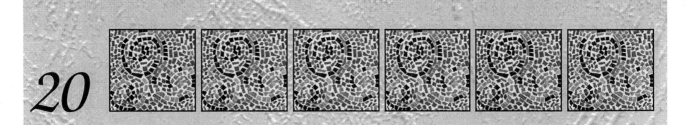

Nursing Care of Patients with Musculoskeletal Disorders

Objectives

1.0 Demonstrate an understanding of the infections and inflammations of the musculoskeletal system.

    1.1 Match common infectious and inflammatory disorders with the appropriate definition.

    1.2 Identify characteristics of infections and inflammations of the musculoskeletal system.

    1.3 Identify common pharmacologic agents used to treat disorders of the musculoskeletal system.

    1.4 Identify nursing interventions used for patients with infectious musculoskeletal disorders.

    1.5 Write a nursing care plan for the patient with an inflammatory musculoskeletal disorder.

2.0 Demonstrate an understanding of structural disorders of the musculoskeletal system.

    2.1 Identify characteristics of specific structural disorders of the musculoskeletal system.

    2.2 Identify the medical management for structural disorders of the musculoskeletal system.

    2.3 Identify nursing interventions used for patients with structural disorders of the musculoskeletal system.

3.0 Demonstrate an understanding of traumatic injuries to the musculoskeletal system.

    3.1 Identify signs and symptoms of musculoskeletal injuries.

    3.2 Identify types of medical management for musculoskeletal injuries.

    3.3 Identify types of surgical treatments of musculoskeletal injuries.

    3.4 Identify nursing interventions used for patients with musculoskeletal injuries.

    3.5 Write a nursing care plan for the patient with a traumatic injury.

4.0 Demonstrate an understanding of the neoplasms that affect the musculoskeletal system.

    4.1 Identify several of the musculoskeletal neoplasms.

    4.2 Identify medical and surgical treatment of musculoskeletal neoplasms.

    4.3 Identify nursing interventions used for patients with musculoskeletal neoplasms.

Learning Activities

Short Answers

1. The cause of rheumatoid arthritis is _____.

2. Rheumatoid arthritis is thought to be an _____ disorder.

3. Rheumatoid factor (RF) is present in approximately ____% of patients with advanced disease.

4. Degenerative joint disease is also called _____.

5. ____ disease is a chronic inflammatory disease that is transmitted by the bite of a flea.

6. _____ is a grating sound heard and felt on joint movement.

Identification

Demonstrate your understanding of the following disorders by matching each one with its definition.

    A.   Osteomyelitis

    B.   Osteoarthritis

    C.   Ankylosing spondylitis

    D.   Gout

    E.   Osteomalacia

    F.   Osteoporosis

    G.   Osteosarcoma

    H.   Fibrosarcoma

    I.   Multiple myeloma

7. ____ Most common malignant bone tumor, characterized by extreme pain, rapid growth, and metastasis

8. ____ Infection of the bone with necrosis of bone and marrow tissue

9. ____ Tumor that arises from fibrous connective tissue

10. ____ Inflammatory joint reaction caused by the accumulation of uric acid crystals in the joints

11. ____ Degenerative nonsystemic joint disease

12. ____ Metabolic bone disorder characterized by bone thinning or porous bone mass

13. ____ Chronic, progressive, inflammatory disease of the spine and sacroiliac joint

14. ____ Primary tumor that arises in the plasma cells in the bone marrow

15. ____ Metabolic bone disorder characterized by a decrease in calcium and phosphorous deposits in bone matrix

True/False

16. ____ Osteomyelitis can only be contracted by direct contamination of the bone.

17. ____ Fractures are more common in geriatric patients.

18. ____ Arthritis is a leading cause of immobility.

19. ____ Osteoarthritis is the most serious form of arthritis.

20. ____ A person can have both rheumatoid arthritis and osteoarthritis.

21. ____ Complications from hip fractures are a leading cause of mortality in the elderly.

Knowledge Application

22. The organism most frequently associated with acute osteomyelitis is

    A.   *Escherichia coli*

    B.   *Staphylococcus aureus*

    C.   *Streptococcus aureus*

    D.   *Pseudomonas*

23. Treatment of osteomyelitis involves

    A.   analgesics

    B.   debridement of necrotic tissue

    C.   antibiotics

    D.   all of the above

24. A complication of acute osteomyelitis that the nurse would monitor for is

    A. meningitis

    B. pulmonary embolism

    C. pneumonia

    D. compartment syndrome

25. A review of an x-ray of a patient with chronic osteomyelitis would reveal

    A. mild inflammation

    B. synovitis

    C. areas of sequestrum

    D. ankylosis

26. Individuals with chronic osteomyelitis are at risk for developing

    A. malnutrition

    B. muscle contractions

    C. septicemia

    D. cardiac arrhythmias

27. If an individual develops fungal or mycotic osteomyelitis the medication of choice would be

    A. amphotericin B

    B. penicillin

    C. isoniazid

    D. streptomycin

28. All of the following risk factors have been associated with the development of osteoporosis EXCEPT

    A. high level of stress

    B. low intake of calcium

    C. Caucasian over the age of 50

    D. immobility

29. The type of diagnostic test that is done to help in determining if a patient has osteoporosis is

    A. CAT scan

    B. nuclear scanning

    C. bone densitometry

    D. chest x-ray

30. Osteomalacia is caused by a lack of

    A. calcium

    B. vitamin A

    C. intrinsic factor

    D. vitamin D

31. From the foods below, which one would have the highest calcium content?

    A. 1 cup low-fat yogurt

    B. 1 oz. Swiss cheese

    C. 1 cup cottage cheese

    D. 1 cup spinach

32. The early joint changes that are evident in the patient with rheumatoid arthritis are caused by

    A. joint calcification

    B. kyphosis

    C. ankylosis

    D. synovitis

33. When a patient has osteoporosis, the nurse would implement interventions to prevent

    A. altered nutrition

    B. cardiac arrhythmias

    C. pathologic fractures

    D. pain

34. A medication that is used by the person with osteoporosis that inhibits osteoclast bone resorption is

    A. calcium

    B. estrogen

    C. Fosamax

    D. vitamin D

35. When a patient is in the second stage of Lyme disease, the nurse would monitor for

    A. cardiac manifestations

    B. musculoskeletal involvement

    C. macular lesions

    D. joint destruction

36. Because of the type of pain experienced by the patient with rheumatoid arthritis, an appropriate nursing intervention would involve

    A. having patient exercise upon rising

    B. have patient take analgesics before rising

    C. use cold compresses to affected joints daily

    D. stay in bed for prolonged periods of time

37. The area that is most often affected when a patient has gout is

    A. ankles

    B. large toes

    C. fingers

    D. spine

38. Which type of arthritis is characterized as being a chronic systemic disease with inflammation of the joints and extra-articular manifestations?

    A. rheumatoid arthritis

    B. osteoarthritis

    C. osteogenic sarcoma

    D. osteochondrosis

39. When a patient with ankylosing spondylitis has developed rigid kyphosis, an important nursing intervention would be to

    A. teach breathing exercises

    B. apply heat

    C. administer NSAIDs

    D. maintain bed rest in supine position

40. Diagnostic testing for the patient with gout would most likely reveal

    A. high blood urea nitrogen (BUN) and creatinine levels

    B. high uric acid level

    C. high white count

    D. low hemoglobin and hematocrit

41. Diagnostic testing for the patient with Paget's disease would most likely reveal an elevated

    A. white count

    B. uric acid level

    C. erythrocyte sedimentation rate

    D. serum alkaline phosphatase level

42. Medical management for the patient with Paget's disease involves administration of medications that inhibit bone resorption such as

    A. calcitonin

    B. vitamin D

    C. allopurinol

    D. Indocin

43. The drug of choice for the patient during an acute episode of gout is

    A. allopurinol

    B. colchicine

    C. probenecid

    D. aspirin

44. A patient is instructed to follow a diet low in purine. Which food should he or she avoid?

    A. bread

    B. ice cream

    C. sardines

    D. green vegetables

45. While examining a patient, the nurse hears crepitus when moving the knees. The patient also has nodules on the fingers. These symptoms suggest

    A. rheumatoid arthritis

    B. osteomyelitis

    C. osteoarthritis

    D. gouty arthritis

46. The type of surgery that might provide some relief of pain for the patient with osteoarthritis is
    A. synovectomy
    B. arthrodesis
    C. incision and drainage
    D. joint replacement

47. A secretary who works on a computer for long hours is complaining of pain, numbness, and tingling in the thumb and middle finger. These symptoms suggest
    A. Paget's disease
    B. carpal tunnel syndrome
    C. Dupuytren's contracture
    D. Volkmann's syndrome

48. Nursing care of the patient who has had a total hip replacement should include
    A. preventing injury
    B. preventing infection
    C. maintaining skin integrity
    D. all of the above

49. Discharge planning for the patient who has had arthroscopic surgery for a tear of the anterior cruciate ligament of the knee should include which of the following?
    A. explanation of cast care
    B. explanation of full-leg immobilizer
    C. explanation of use of a walker
    D. any of the above

50. Fractures may be caused by which of the following?
    A. direct blow to the bone
    B. demineralization of the bone
    C. sudden strong muscle contraction
    D. any of the above

51. Which of the following type of fracture can be considered a life-threatening injury?
    A. closed fracture
    B. comminuted fracture
    C. compound fracture
    D. greenstick fracture

52. The immediate care of the patient with a fracture would include
    A. splinting the injured part in correct alignment
    B. pad or protect the injured area
    C. administer analgesic
    D. all of the above

53. When a patient with a fractured pelvis becomes restless, agitated, and confused, the nurse should assess for
    A. hypovolemic shock
    B. sepsis
    C. compartment syndrome
    D. pulmonary embolus

54. AN early sign of compartment syndrome that the nurse would monitor for in the patient with a cast is
    A. loss of the distal pulse
    B. paresthesia
    C. severe pain in area that is not relieved by narcotics
    D. falling blood pressure and rise in pulse

55. Medical management for the patient with compartment syndrome would include
    A. application of traction
    B. incision and drainage
    C. debridement
    D. fasciotomy

56. When a patient has had an internal fixation for a fractured leg, it is important to monitor for

   A. infection

   B. problems related to immobility

   C. correct traction setup

   D. nutritional deficits

57. A potentially fatal complication of long-bone fractures and multiple trauma is

   A. fat embolism

   B. cardiac arrhythmias

   C. cerebrovascular accident

   D. pulmonary edema

58. A complication of severe trauma that can occur from a lack of circulation to the tissue is

   A. compartment syndrome

   B. septicemia

   C. avascular necrosis

   D. sympathetic dystrophy

59. The treatment of choice for osteosarcoma is

   A. removal of segment of bone

   B. chemotherapy

   C. radiation therapy

   D. amputation

60. The nurse should suspect _____ in a patient who has Bence-Jones protein in the urine.

   A. osteogenic sarcoma

   B. multiple myeloma

   C. leukemia

   D. osteoporosis

61. The most common malignant bone tumor is

   A. osteosarcoma

   B. multiple myeloma

   C. fibrosarcoma

   D. hemangioma

62. A patient is being treated as an outpatient for Ewing's sarcoma. The most successful therapy is

   A. surgical removal

   B. radiation therapy

   C. hormonal therapy

   D. chemotherapy

Identification

Identify information related to these common types of musculoskeletal medications.

   A. NSAIDs

   B. Uricosurics

   C. Oral calcium

   D. Antipagetics

63. _____ Produce an anti-inflammatory, analgesic, and antipyretic effects

64. _____ Inhibit bone resorption and reduce bone vascularity

65. _____ Control serum uric acid levels

66. _____ Used primarily to treat osteoarthritis and rheumatoid arthritis

67. _____ Individuals on these medications should also be on a low-purine diet

68. _____ Supplements are indicated for prevention of osteomalacia and osteoporosis

69. _____ Older adults should be closely monitored for liver impairment when on these medications

Nursing Care Plans

70. Write a nursing care plan for the patient with rheumatoid arthritis. Use the following nursing diagnosis.

    Nursing diagnosis: Impaired mobility related to disease process and pain

    Patient outcome:

    Interventions:

71. Write a nursing care plan for the patient with a compound fracture of the tibia. Use the following nursing diagnosis.

    Nursing diagnosis: Altered tissue perfusion; peripheral, related to trauma

    Patient outcome:

    Interventions:

Case Studies

Case Study No. 1

Mr. W., age 75, has been diagnosed as having chronic rheumatoid arthritis. He has been treated for many years by his family physician. He has been slowly losing mobility.

72. A laboratory value that would increase with this condition is

    A. RBC

    B. ESR

    C. WBC

    D. BUN

73. The office nurse finds deformities in his hands that interfere with ADLs. This is called

    A. subluxation

    B. ankylosis

    C. synovitis

    D. Sjögren's syndrome

74. One goal in the medical management of this condition would be aimed at

    A. curing the condition

    B. preventing recurrence

    C. relieving pain and maintaining mobility

    D. referral to a nursing home in the future

75. A medication prescribed for Mr. W. in the hopes of inducing a remission is

    A. parenteral gold salts

    B. NSAID

    C. enteric aspirin

    D. steroids

76. The nurse would make sure Mr. W. has knowledge of the disease process, treatment, and

    A. stress control techniques

    B. methods to control pain

    C. use of thermal application

    D. all the above

Case Study No. 2

Mr. K. was playing football with some college friends when he fell and injured his shoulder. Clinical manifestations include marked joint deformity, loss of joint function, and ecchymosis.

77. These symptoms suggest

    A. subluxation

    B. dislocation

    C. fracture

    D. ankylosis

78. The usual medical management of this condition would involve

    A. surgical intervention

    B. closed reduction

    C. application of a cast

    D. application of a sling

79. Following the procedure, it is important for the nurse to assess

    A. neurovascular status

    B. cardiac status

    C. mobility status

    D. cerebrovascular status

80. Part of the discharge instructions should include

    A. explanation of need to limit activity

    B. explanation of antibiotic therapy

    C. demonstration of exercise regimen

    D. explanation of cast care

Case Study No. 3

Mrs. M., age 78, fell in the bathroom at the local nursing home. She is admitted to the hospital with a suspected hip fracture.

81. The x-ray studies reveal an intertrochanteric fracture. Typical symptoms associated with this type of injury include

    A. involved limb is of normal length and position with pain radiating to groin

    B. involved limb appears shortened and externally rotated

    C. involved limb is internally rotated and deformed

    D. involved limb appears normal but extreme pain is felt upon movement

82. Mrs. M. has the fracture treated by open reduction and internal fixation under a general anesthesia. Postoperative complications might include (Check all that apply.)

    A. _____ paralytic ileus

    B. _____ disorientation

    C. _____ cardiac arrhythmias

    D. _____ fluid and electrolyte imbalance

    E. _____ thromboembolism

83. Following the surgery, the most important nursing observation includes looking for

    A. impaired skin integrity

    B. signs of confusion

    C. signs of compromised circulation

    D. problems with the traction

On the second postoperative day, Mrs. M. complains of headache and lethargy. She seems confused.

84. During a careful assessment, the nurse notes tachycardia, tachypnea, and dyspnea. The nurse suspects

    A. pneumonia

    B. fat embolism

    C. pneumothorax

    D. atelectasis

85. Arterial blood gases are pH 7.2; PaO_2 50%; $PaCO_2$ 60%; HCO_3 22. The nurse would anticipate

   A. administering oxygen via nasal cannula

   B. administering oxygen via mask, suction frequently

   C. having patient cough and deep breathe every four hours

   D. mechanical ventilation with positive end expiratory pressure

86. A medication the physician would most likely order would be

   A. Coumadin

   B. analgesics

   C. steroids

   D. penicillin

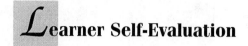

Learner Self-Evaluation

Do I fully understand the content? If no, then the areas I need to review are:

I need more information from my instructor on:

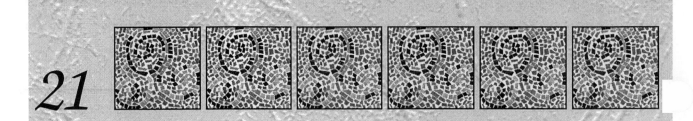

21

Knowledge Base for Patients with Gastrointestinal Dysfunction

Objectives

1.0 Review the anatomy and physiology of the gastrointestinal (GI) system.
    1.1 Identify the parts of the GI system.
    1.2 Identify the purposes of the parts of the GI system.
    1.3 Review the process of digestion.

2.0 Demonstrate an understanding of the assessment data related to the GI system.
    2.1 Identify the clinical manifestations that indicate a GI dysfunction.
    2.2 Identify nursing interventions appropriate for the patient with symptoms of GI dysfunction.
    2.3 Match diagnostic tests with the appropriate description.
    2.4 Demonstrate use of the nursing process when caring for the patient undergoing a diagnostic test.

3.0 Demonstrate an understanding of the medical management of the adult with a GI alteration.
    3.1 Identify the rationale for gastrointestinal intubation.
    3.2 Plan the nursing care for the patient with a GI tube.

3.3 Identify purposes of enteral and parenteral hyperalimentation.
3.4 Demonstrate application of the nursing process to the care of the patient on enteral and parenteral feedings.

4.0 Demonstrate an understanding of the surgical management of the patient with a GI alteration.
    4.1 Identify complications associated with GI surgery.
    4.2 Plan the postoperative care of the patient having a gastric surgery.
    4.3 Demonstrate an understanding of the needs of the patient with a colostomy.
    4.4 Write a nursing care plan for the patient who has had gastric surgery.

Learning Activities

Short Answers

1. The buccal glands, located in the oral cavity, secrete small amounts of _____.

2. The organs of the gastrointestinal (GI) tract below the esophagus are covered by the _____.

3. Food and fluids are moved down the esophagus to the stomach by a process known as _____.

4. The ringlike muscle that controls the opening between the stomach and the duodenum is known as the _____.

5. Intrinsic factor, secreted in the stomach, is essential for absorption of _____ in the terminal ileum.

6. Gastrin secretion is controlled by a _____ feedback mechanism based on the _____ of the stomach contents.

7. Food enters the stomach, is macerated and mixed with gastric secretions, then leaves in the form of a substance called _____.

8. The three segments of the small intestine are the _____, _____, and _____.

9. The principal organ of digestion and absorption is the _____ _____.

10. Adequate production of _____ is necessary to ensure the emulsification of fats into fatty acids and glycerides.

11. The _____ reabsorbs water and electrolytes and stores feces.

12. Three of the functions of the liver are
    1.

    2

    3.

13. The major purpose of the gall bladder is to _____ and _____ bile.

14. The _____ is the primary producer of the digestive enzymes.

Identification

Match the following common symptoms of GI dysfunction with the best definition.

   A.   Anorexia
   B.   Nausea
   C.   Constipation
   D.   Diarrhea
   E.   Hematemesis

15. _____ Vomiting of blood
16. _____ Revulsion toward food
17. _____ Absence of a desire to eat
18. _____ Increased passage of liquid stool
19. _____ Infrequent passage of hard, dry stool

Match the following diagnostic procedures with the best description.

    A.   Gastric analysis

    B.   Upper GI series

    C.   Barium enema

    D.   Oral cholecystogram

    E.   Cholangiogram

    F.   Esophagogastroduodenoscopy (EGD)

    G.   Ultrasonography

20. _____ Aids in the diagnosis of gall bladder disease

21. _____ Direct visualization of esophagus, stomach, and duodenum

22. _____ X-ray examination of the esophagus, stomach, and duodenum

23. _____ Contrast medium outlines the hepatic, cystic, and common bile ducts

24. _____ Allows visualization of structures as patient swallows barium

25. _____ Radiologic examination of the rectum and colon

26. _____ Uses high-frequency sound waves to form images of internal structures

27. _____ Monitors absorption and excretion of orally ingested radiopaque dye tablets

28. _____ Can determine if hydrochloric acid is present in the stomach

Knowledge Application

29. Ms. S. is admitted with a diagnosis of anorexia, vomiting, and weight loss. Which of the following lab results would indicate she is in a state of malnutrition?

    A.   WBC of 8500 mm^3

    B.   HgB of 10.9 g/dL

    C.   albumin of 3.0 g/dL

    D.   potassium of 4.3 mEq/L

30. Before the nurse can establish a nursing care plan for Ms. S., what information should be obtained?

    A.   dietary history

    B.   history and pattern of anorexia

    C.   factors that precipitate vomiting

    D.   general nutritional status

    E.   all of the above

31. Physical findings that indicate malnutrition include

    A.   heart rate of 100, respiratory rate of 22

    B.   dull, thin, brittle nails

    C.   dry skin, edema of the feet

    D.   bruising of the forearms and trunk

32. If, during an abdominal assessment, the nurse finds the patient has a boardlike abdomen, he or she would notify the physician as this might mean

    A.   peritonitis

    B.   GI bleeding

    C.   constipation

    D.   aneurysm

33. The major complication of continuous vomiting is

    A.   weight loss

    B.   cardiac dysrhythmias

    C.   fluid and electrolyte imbalance

    D.   aspiration of vomitus

34. The presence of coffee-ground material in vomitus is often indicative of

    A.   fresh gastrointestinal bleeding

    B.   ingestion of excessive amounts of coffee

    C.   old blood in the GI system

    D.   an obstruction in the biliary system

35. A nursing intervention to provide comfort for the patient who has severe diarrhea would be

    A.   give sitz baths several times daily

    B.   administer analgesics

    C.   administer antidiarrheal

    D.   encourage bed rest

36. When a patient has several episodes of blood mixed with stool, the nurse would suspect

    A.   colon cancer

    B.   inflammatory bowel disease

    C.   malnutrition

    D.   ulcer

37. Absence of gastric acid in a gastric analysis may indicate

    A.   ulcer disease

    B.   malignant disease

    C.   occult bleeding

    D.   pernicious anemia

38. A priority in the management of the patient with GI bleeding is

    A.   take vital signs and reassure patient

    B.   transfer to intensive care unit

    C.   assess blood loss and return to hemo-dynamic stability

    D.   replace blood loss with isotonic IV fluid

39. The nurse would recognize that a severe blood loss (over 40% of total volume) has occurred when a person with a normal BP of 120/80 has which of the following changes?

    A.   systolic pressure < 100 mm Hg and pulse > 100

    B.   systolic pressure < 110 mm Hg and pulse > 120

    C.   systolic pressure < 70 mm Hg and pulse > 130

    D.   systolic pressure is 70–90 mm Hg and pulse 110–120

40. Which of the following conditions could NOT be detected through an upper GI series?

    A.   esophageal tumor

    B.   colon cancer

    C.   diverticula

    D.   gastric ulcer

41. Following the upper GI series, the nurse would

    A.   keep patient flat in bed for four hours

    B.   force fluids

    C.   administer a cathartic

    D.   administer a diuretic

42. As the nurse prepares Mr. M. for an oral cholecystogram, he says that he is allergic to shrimp. An appropriate nursing intervention is

    A.   call the physician and tell him of the allergy

    B.   note the allergy but continue with the procedure

    C.   call radiology and cancel the test

    D.   administer the Telepaque tablets and keep patient NPO

43. Mr. M. is also scheduled for an endoscopy. The most serious complication following this procedure is

    A.   aspiration pneumonia

    B.   perforation of the GI tract

    C.   allergic reaction to dye

    D.   fluid and electrolyte imbalance

44. Following the endoscopy, how soon can Mr. M. resume his diet?

    A.   eight hours after procedure

    B.   as soon as he is alert

    C.   as soon as his gag reflex returns

    D.   as soon as he talks

45. A group of over-the-counter alkaline compounds that neutralize gastric acid are called

   A.   laxatives

   B.   antacids

   C.   antireflux agents

   D.   antidiarrheal agents

46. Which of the following would NOT be a reason for insertion of a nasogastric tube? To

   A.   remove stomach contents

   B.   provide parenteral feedings

   C.   administer medications

   D.   irrigate the stomach

47. Which of the following nasogastric tubes has a double lumen and a small air vent?

   A.   Salem sump

   B.   Levine tube

   C.   Dobbhoff tube

   D.   Blakemore tube

48. What is the correct method to determine the distance to insert a nasogastric tube? Measure the distance from the

   A.   tip of the nose to the earlobe to the xiphoid

   B.   tip of the nose to the earlobe to the xiphoid and add 5 cm

   C.   tip of earlobe to the nose and then to the xiphoid

   D.   nose to the area on the patient's left side just below the diaphragm

49. As the nurse inserts a nasogastric tube, the patient starts to cough. The nurse should

   A.   continue to advance the tube, but more slowly

   B.   have the patient drink water to help him to stop coughing

   C.   withdraw the tube and retry later

   D.   withdraw the tube and call the physician

50. A patient returns from surgery with a NG tube to intermittent suction. One of the nursing diagnoses is Altered oral mucous membrane. An appropriate intervention is to have the patient

   A.   take small sips of water or chew ice

   B.   use lemon and glycerin swabs

   C.   brush his or her teeth and rinse every four hours

   D.   gargle with Cepacol every four hours

51. Which of the following individuals would NOT be a good candidate for enteral feedings? A patient with

   A.   anorexia who has lost 20 pounds

   B.   a bowel obstruction

   C.   a decreased level of consciousness

   D.   malabsorption syndrome

52. An unconscious patient is receiving a continuous tube feeding to provide needed nutrients. Which of the following feedings would NOT meet nutrition needs?

   A.   Ensure

   B.   Isocal

   C.   Osmolite

   D.   Vivonex

53. What is a rationale for using nasoenteric tubes for the administration of tube feedings? They

   A.   are less likely to clog

   B.   help prevent reflux esophagitis

   C.   allow for rapid administration of feedings

   D.   don't have a weighted tip

54. An advantage of a percutaneous gastrostomy over a surgical gastrostomy is that

   A.   general anesthesia is not used

   B.   the procedure is less costly

   C.   recovery is faster

   D.   all of the above

55. A patient with a jejunostomy is receiving continuous tube feeding. All of the following are important nursing interventions EXCEPT to
    A. auscultate bowel sounds
    B. check for placement of feeding tube
    C. aspirate for residual
    D. assess for tolerance of feeding

56. When would total parenteral nutrition (TPN) be the best choice to meet the individual's nutritional needs? When the
    A. patient is older than 75 years
    B. needs cannot be met through the GI tract
    C. patient has a systemic infection
    D. patient is severely dehydrated

57. Which of the following is NOT a major complication of TPN?
    A. infection
    B. hypoglycemia
    C. dehydration
    D. constipation

58. A major complication that can occur during the insertion of a central venous catheter is
    A. pneumothorax
    B. sepsis
    C. hemorrhage
    D. all of the above

59. Why is TPN started at a slow rate and increased gradually? To
    A. prevent infection
    B. allow the pancreas time to adjust
    C. allow the liver time to adjust
    D. prevent hypoglycemia

60. What is the rationale for having a patient receiving TPN perform a Valsalva maneuver during IV tubing changes? To prevent
    A. hemorrhage
    B. infection
    C. an air embolism
    D. speed shock

61. Why is a postoperative patient generally kept NPO until peristalsis returns?
    A. surgical manipulation and anesthetic may result in some degree of paralytic ileus
    B. because of the great risk of wound dehiscence
    C. to reduce the incidence of nausea and vomiting in the first 24 hours
    D. to lower the risk of developing infection

62. Which of the following nursing interventions is important to implement before gastric surgery?
    A. teach patient how to cough and deep breathe
    B. teach patient how to do incision care
    C. teach patient dietary restrictions
    D. all of the above

63. A surgical resection of the bowel has many potential complications. Which complication is more likely to occur about one week after surgery?
    A. wound abscess
    B. wound dehiscence
    C. paralytic ileus
    D. pulmonary edema

64. The most appropriate position for the patient who has had gastric surgery would be
    A. flat with legs slightly elevated
    B. left lateral Sims'
    C. semi-Fowler's
    D. prone

65. In a patient who has had a bowel resection the nurse should take special precaution to prevent

   A. ineffective ventilation

   B. dehydration

   C. thrombophlebitis

   D. all of the above

66. Following gastric surgery, there is an increased risk for an alteration in peripheral tissue perfusion. Choose an appropriate intervention to prevent this problem.

   A. have patient cough and deep breathe every two hours

   B. have patient do leg and foot exercises every two hours

   C. position patient with head of bed up and knees gatched

   D. keep patient on bed rest for at least 72 hours

67. A patient has an ascending colostomy performed. Which description is true about the fecal output? It is

   A. predominantly liquid

   B. tan and mushy

   C. soft and semi-formed

   D. identical to normal stools

68. A temporary colostomy would not be performed for which of the following conditions?

   A. diverticulitis

   B. volvulus

   C. gunshot to abdomen

   D. colorectal cancer

69. When a double-barrel colostomy is created on the abdominal wall, the functioning colon is the

   A. proximal stoma

   B. distal stoma

   C. rectum

70. One of the potential complications of colostomy surgery is stomal necrosis. The cause of this condition is

   A. infection

   B. hemorrhage

   C. impaired circulation

   D. bowel perforation

71. Which emotional response in the patient with a colostomy may indicate grieving because of altered body structure?

   A. anger

   B. depression

   C. denial

   D. withdrawal

   E. all of the above

72. Which comment by the patient with a permanent colostomy would indicate to the nurse that the individual is NOT ready for teaching? The patient says

   A. "This makes me anxious."

   B. "Why did this happen to me?"

   C. "I'm not going to look at that."

   D. "My father also had a colostomy."

73. When teaching the patient who has a sigmoid colostomy, the nurse is aware that control of bowel elimination

   A. never can be totally regulated

   B. may be gained in time by a regular diet

   C. is gained through daily irrigations of the stoma

   D. is so difficult to achieve that it is usually a waste of time to try

74. Individuals with a colostomy are generally taught to avoid foods that cause diarrhea, odor, and excessive flatus. From the foods listed below, which are likely to have these side effects?

   A. cheese, chocolate, milk

   B. fresh broccoli, mushrooms, cabbage

   C. nuts, cereal, pasta

   D. yogurt, buttermilk, parsley

Nursing Care Plans

75. Teaching the patient about the care of the colostomy is an important nursing function. Write an appropriate nursing diagnosis, patient outcome, and several nursing interventions that address this.

    Nursing diagnosis:

    Patient outcome:

    Interventions:

76. Plan the nursing care for the patient scheduled for a subtotal gastrectomy. Use the following diagnoses.

    Nursing diagnosis: Anxiety related to anesthesia and proposed surgery

    Patient outcome:

    Interventions:

Nursing diagnosis: Knowledge deficit related to preoperative preparation and postoperative course

Patient outcome:

Interventions:

77. Plan the nursing care for the patient who has had a bowel resection. Use the following nursing diagnoses.

    Nursing diagnosis: Pain related to surgical trauma to the abdomen

    Patient outcome:

    Interventions:

Nursing diagnosis: Potential for ineffective breathing pattern

Patient outcome:

Interventions:

78. Write a nursing care plan for the patient with anorexia. Use the following nursing diagnosis.

    Nursing diagnosis: High risk for altered nutrition; less than body requirements related to lack of appetite.

    Patient outcome:

    Interventions:

79. Write a nursing care plan for the patient with a gastrointestinal tube. Use the following diagnosis.

    Nursing diagnosis: High risk for altered oral mucous membrane related to mouth breathing

    Patient outcome:

    Interventions:

Case Studies

Case Study No. 1

Mr. F. is admitted with a history of intermittent vomiting for the past two weeks. He also states that he has had some diarrhea and black stools. His blood pressure is 118/78, pulse 88. Initial HgB is 10.8 g/dL and Hct is 40%.

80. Which nursing diagnosis would have a priority as you develop the nursing care plan?

    A. Potential for fluid volume deficit

    B. Alteration in cardiac output

    C. Alteration in comfort

    D. Activity intolerance

After being examined by the physician, Mr. F. is told that he has gastrointestinal bleeding, possibly due to an ulcer.

81. Mr. F. is very restless. His most recent blood pressure is 98/50 and pulse is 100. This suggests he may have a blood loss of approximately

    A. < 25%

    B. 25–40%

    C. > 40%

82. Mr. F. wants to know why they keep drawing blood. You explain that the results of the hemoglobin and hematocrit values do not accurately reflect the amount of blood loss until _____ hours after the onset of bleeding.

    A.   4–6 hours

    B.   6–12 hours

    C.   12–24 hours

    D.   24–36 hours

83. Outcomes that would indicate stabilization of the patient with acute bleeding would be

    A.   increase of BP by 20–30 systolic, decrease in pulse

    B.   return of normal BP, disappearance of vasospasm, urine output of 30 cc/hour

    C.   BP of 100/70, pulse > 50, improvement of cyanosis

    D.   BP returns to normal, pulse > 60 < 120, RR > 12 < 28

84. Which of the following diagnostic tests would be scheduled to determine the presence of an ulcer?

    A.   arteriogram

    B.   insertion of nasogastric tube

    C.   flexible endoscopy

    D.   bronchoscopy

Case Study No. 2

Ms. P. is an 18-year-old who is admitted to the unit with severe anorexia nervosa. She has lost 30 pounds in the last three months. Her current weight is 90 lbs. She is admitted for evaluation and possible enteral feedings.

85. Which of the following statements is true regarding nutritional needs of the normal adult.

    A.   Adults ordinarily need 1500–2000 calories and .5 g/kg of protein per day.

    B.   Adults ordinarily need 1800–2500 calories and 1 g/kg of protein per day.

    C.   Adults need 1500–2500 calories and 2 g/kg of protein per day.

    D.   During illness, the calorie needs and protein needs will always decrease.

86. Ms. P. is started on Osmolite (1 calorie/mL). She is receiving a continuous feeding of 75 mL/hour via pump through a feeding tube. How many calories will this provide per day?

    A.   1500

    B.   1800

    C.   2000

    D.   2400

87. As the primary nurse, you choose a priority nursing diagnosis for Ms. P. Which of the following would be most appropriate?

    A.   Altered nutrition; less than body requirements

    B.   Alteration in fluid and electrolyte balance

    C.   Potential for diarrhea related to formula intolerance

    D.   Potential for ineffective breathing due to feeding tube

88. For the patient receiving enteral feedings, fluid status is always important. How much water would you give Ms. P., knowing her urine output was 2500 cc in the last 24 hours. At least _____ in 24 hours.

    A.   200 mL

    B.   800 mL

    C.   1000 mL

    D.   2000 mL

89. During the morning assessment when checking hte feeding tube, you obtain 100 mL of residual. What is an appropriate nursing action?

    A.   stop the feeding for 60 minutes, then recheck

    B.   stop the feeding for four hours, then recheck

    C.   continue the feeding as ordered, but recheck in one hour

    D.   continue the feeding, but tell the physician when he makes rounds

90. What is a potential complication of high tube feeding residuals?

    A. fluid imbalance

    B. constipation

    C. vomiting

    D. aspiration

Case Study No. 3

Mrs. W. is admitted with a diagnosis of failure to thrive secondary to esophageal cancer. She is having a CVC inserted for the administration of TPN.

91. Following the insertion of the catheter, what would the physician order?

    A. CVC to be checked by a chest x-ray

    B. TPN to be administered at 25 mL/hour

    C. dextrose and water to run at 50 mL/hour

    D. CVC to have a dressing applied daily

92. The physician and the dietitian determine that it is best to start the TPN solution of 10% dextrose at 50 mL/hour. Which of the following complications can occur if administration of the solution is too rapid?

    A. infection

    B. hypoglycemic reaction

    C. hyperglycemic reaction

    D. overhydration

93. To prevent this complication, the nurse would

    A. check blood glucose every six hours

    B. check urine output every four hours

    C. clean the wound daily

    D. give water every four hours

94. Which procedure should the nurse follow when changing the CVC tubing?

    A. with the patient lying flat, have her perform a Valsalva maneuver when the catheter is opened

    B. with the patient in Trendelenburg position, have her breathe in and out slowly to change the catheter

    C. have another nurse present, then always cross-clamp the tubing before changing

    D. change the tubing quickly, but the same as any other IV tubing change

95. Mrs. W. is also to receive 500 cc of 10% lipids twice a week. Which of the statements about lipid administration is NOT true?

    A. keep at room temperature before administering

    B. always administer through a filter

    C. never let the solutions hang longer than 12 hours

    D. run slowly initially and observe for adverse reactions

*L*earner Self-Evaluation

Do I fully understand the content? If no, then the areas I need to review are:

I need more information from my instructor on:

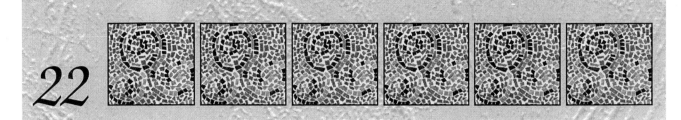

Nusing Care of Patients with Disorders of the Upper Gastrointestinal System

*O*bjectives

1.0 Demonstrate an understanding of the inflammatory processes of the upper gastrointestinal (GI) system.
    1.1 Identify etiology and clinical manifestations associated with inflammatory disorders.
    1.2 Plan nursing interventions for the patient with an inflammation disorder.

2.0 Demonstrate an understanding of the structural and functional abnormalities of the upper GI system.
    2.1 Review the etiology of ulcer disease.
    2.2 Identify medical and surgical treatment of the patient with an ulcer.
    2.3 Demonstrate application of the nursing process when caring for the patient with a functional abnormality.

2.4 Identify the teaching needs of the patient with an ulcer.
2.5 Plan the nursing care for the patient having a surgical resection of the upper GI system.

3.0 Demonstrate an understanding of the types of neoplasms that affect the upper GI system.
    3.1 Identify the clinical manifestations associated with neoplasms of the upper GI system.
    3.2 Identify the medical management for the patient with a gastric neoplasm.
    3.3 Review the surgical management for the patient with a gastric neoplasm.
    3.4 Plan the nursing care for the patient with a gastric neoplasm.

*L*earning Activities

Short Answers

1. Esophagitis is an inflammation of the

    _____.

2. Three factors which may trigger an attack of esophagitis are
    1.

    2.

    3.

3. Daily use of aspirin can result in

_____.

4. The cause of type B chronic gastritis is

_____ _____.

5. The major symptom of uncomplicated peptic

ulcer is _____.

6. The major contributing factor in the development of a hiatal hernia is

_____.

7. _____ is the most frequent symptom
of hiatal hernia.

8. The most common symptom associated with

esophageal cancer is _____.

Identification

Test your basic knowledge of upper GI disorders
by matching each disorder below with the best
description.

    A. Gastritis

    B. Peptic ulcer

    C. Hiatal hernia

    D. Achalasia

    E. Prebyesophagus

    F. Achlorhydria

9. _____ Motor disorder of the lower ⅔ of the
esophagus

10. _____ Absence of hydrochloric acid

11. _____ Protrusion of part of stomach into
thoracic cavity

12. _____ Inflammation of the stomach mucosa

13. _____ Increase in nonperistaltic contractions
and overall weak muscular contraction
in the esophagus

14. _____ Break in the mucosa in any part of the
GI tract

Match the following medication types with the
action.

    A. Antacids

    B. Histamine H_2-receptor antagonists

    C. Proton-pump inhibitors

    D. Prokinetic agents

15. _____ Increase gastric emptying

16. _____ Decrease the basal secretion of gastric
acid

17. _____ Inhibit the enzyme that produces
gastric acid

18. _____ Neutralize acid present in the stomach

Knowledge Application

19. Oral infections may be due to which of the
following? (Check all that apply.)

    A. _____ poor oral hygiene

    B. _____ poor nutrition

    C. _____ stress

    D. _____ systemic disorders

20. Pain from ulcerated areas in the mouth may
be relieved by which of the following?
(Check all that apply.)

    A. _____ topical anesthetic agents

    B. _____ Cepacol spray

    C. _____ soothing foods

    D. _____ viscous Xylocaine

21. Which of the following medications has been
found to irritate the gastric mucosa?

    A. Maalox

    B. aspirin

    C. Tylenol

    D. Carafate

22. Medical management of esophagitis would
include

    A. bland diet

    B. no smoking

    C. antacids

    D. all of the above

23. Gastroesophageal reflux disease (GERD) is caused by

    A. smoking

    B. excessive use of alcohol

    C. reflux of gastric acid

    D. bacterial invasion of the esophagus

24. Treatment of GERD involves use of medications that suppress acid secretion, such as

    A. omeprazole (Prilosec)

    B. metoclopramide (Reglan)

    C. cisapride (Propulsid)

    D. diazepam (Valium)

25. For the patient with chronic esophagitis, surgical resection of the esophagus is indicated if _____ were to occur.

    A. chronic reflux

    B. perforation

    C. stricture

    D. bleeding

26. An undesirable side effect of over the counter (OTC) remedies for treatment of esophagitis is

    A. continued symptoms

    B. hemorrhage

    C. metabolic acidosis

    D. diarrhea

27. Which statement made by Mr. S. could indicate a precipitating factor in his current episode of acute gastritis?

    A. "I recently started drinking coffee."

    B. "I never touch alcohol."

    C. "I started going to Weight Watchers."

    D. "I walk two miles daily."

28. Mr. S. is placed on a medication to inhibit gastric acid secretion. This would most likely be

    A. Carafate

    B. aspirin

    C. cimetidine

    D. ampicillin

29. Mr. S. is given information on the disease and treatment. What is the best indicator that teaching has been effective? He

    A. states he will see the doctor in six weeks

    B. lists foods that he should avoid

    C. states he won't eat after 5 PM

    D. says he has no questions

30. The presence of stomatitis in the patient with chronic gastritis indicates a deficiency of which of the following?

    A. calcium

    B. vitamin K

    C. vitamin B_{12}

    D. histamine

31. Ulcers are a common disorder, accounting for approximately _____ % of hospital admissions.

    A. 10%

    B. 20%

    C. 30%

32. Gastric ulcers are thought to result from

    A. decreased mucosal resistance to the effects of gastric acid

    B. increased exposure of the mucosa to highly acidic materials

    C. increase in the amount of gastric secretion

    D. stress and overactive acid production

33. In the individual with a gastric ulcer, what are two potential complications if it is left untreated?

    A. infection, stricture

    B. obstruction, bleeding

    C. hemorrhage, perforation

    D. sepsis

34. When is the pain of a gastric ulcer more likely to occur?

    A. immediately before meals

    B. immediately after eating

    C. several hours after eating

    D. anytime during the day

35. A diagnosis of a possible peptic ulcer would be confirmed by which of the following diagnostic tests?

    A. endoscopy

    B. sigmoidoscopy

    C. barium studies

    D. angiogram

36. Which particular diet has been found to be effective in the treatment of ulcers?

    A. sippy diet

    B. bland, soft diet

    C. diet low in fiber, roughage

    D. diet that avoids irritating foods

37. Which of the following symptoms indicates a possible obstructive process in the individual with a peptic ulcer?

    A. vomiting of partially digested food

    B. flat, rigid, boardlike abdomen

    C. sudden loss of consciousness

    D. projectile vomiting of blood

38. If on assessment the nurse notices _____, these symptoms indicate a possible perforated ulcer.

    A. tachycardia, hypertension, cyanosis

    B. rigid abdomen, severe pain, symptoms of shock

    C. high fever, lethargy, sudden vomiting

    D. midepigastric pain, diarrhea, vomiting

39. Medical treatment of a perforated ulcer would include which of the following interventions? (Check all that apply.)

    A. _____ nasogastric or gastric suction

    B. _____ fluid and electrolyte replacement

    C. _____ antibiotic therapy

    D. _____ ventilator support

    E. _____ surgical intervention

40. The type of ulcer that might develop in the patient who has experienced a severe burn is known as

    A. Cushing's ulcer

    B. peptic ulcer

    C. Curling's ulcer

    D. duodenal ulcer

41. When assessing the patient admitted with a stress ulcer the nurse would expect to find a history of

    A. chronic pain

    B. nausea and vomiting

    C. hematemesis or melena

    D. acute, sharp pain and reflux

42. Medical management of an acute bleeding ulcer would include which of the following? (Check all that apply.)

    A. _____ preparation for surgery

    B. _____ gastric lavage and vasoconstrictive medication

    C. _____ electrocoagulation during endoscopy

    D. _____ histamine-H$_2$ receptors given IV

43. What is the major contributing factor to the development of a hiatal hernia?

    A. recurrent attacks of stress ulcers

    B. prolonged use of steroids

    C. repeated abdominal surgeries

    D. increase in intra-abdominal pressure

44. When a patient has a hiatal hernia, the nurse would expect him or her to have _____ as the main symptom.

    A. pain when swallowing

    B. heartburn

    C. belching

    D. vomiting

45. The diagnosis of a hiatal hernia is confirmed by which of following diagnostic tests?

    A. barium swallow

    B. sigmoidoscopy

    C. bronchoscopy

    D. chest x-ray

46. The home health nurse is teaching a patient with a hiatal hernia. Which of the following statements would indicate that the patient has a clear understanding of the information?

    A. "I must eat three regular meals daily."

    B. "I should remain sitting after my meals."

    C. "I should lie down and rest for 30 minutes after meals."

    D. "I can eat anything I want, as long as I take my medicine."

47. In the patient who has had a fundoplication for treatment of a hiatal hernia, which of the following nursing diagnoses takes priority?

    A. Potential for alteration in fluid volume

    B. Potential for aspiration

    C. Potential for ineffective airway clearance

    D. Alteration in tissue perfusion

48. Symptoms associated with achalasia are

    A. difficulty swallowing, pain radiating to the jaw

    B. heartburn, vomiting

    C. nausea, vomiting, diarrhea

    D. none of the above

49. Medical management of achalasia aimed at alleviating the obstruction in the esophagus might include

    A. esophageal dilatation

    B. drug therapy

    C. surgery

    D. any of the above

50. Factors that have been identified as causes of oral cancer are

    A. use of tobacco and alcohol

    B. stress and smoking

    C. low-residue diet

    D. OTC drugs such as aspirin, antacids

51. In caring for a patient who has had intermaxillary fixation, the nurse would consider which nursing diagnosis as primary?

    A. High risk for infection

    B. High risk for ineffective airway clearance

    C. Ineffective coping

    D. High risk for altered nutrition

52. Which equipment should the nurse keep at the bedside of the patient having an intermaxillary fixation?

    A. tracheotomy set

    B. large hemostats

    C. wire cutters

    D. Ambu bag

53. A patient who suffered a fractured mandible is being discharged. Home care services are required and should include the expertise of a

    A.   physical therapist

    B.   occupational therapist

    C.   home health aide

    D.   dietitian

54. In caring for a patient having a total glossectomy, the nurse would be chiefly concerned with which patient outcome?

    A.   socializes with other patients

    B.   asks to eat meal in private

    C.   tells friends not to visit yet

    D.   watches television for distraction

55. Which of the following factors have been implicated in the development of esophageal cancer? (Check all that apply.)

    A.   _____ smoking

    B.   _____ alcohol abuse

    C.   _____ poor nutrition

    D.   _____ poor hygiene

56. Diagnosis of esophageal cancer is usually made by

    A.   chest x-ray

    B.   CT scan

    C.   x-ray esophogram with barium swallow

    D.   angiogram

57. The treatment of choice for the individual with cancer of the esophagus would most likely be

    A.   chemotherapy

    B.   surgery

    C.   radiation

58. A frequently fatal development that can result from esophagogastrectomy is

    A.   septic shock

    B.   hemorrhage

    C.   leaking of the anastomosis

    D.   pulmonary emboli

59. You are caring for a patient who has had radiation treatment for esophageal cancer. Which symptom is most indicative of a side effect of radiation therapy?

    A.   continuous vomiting

    B.   alopecia

    C.   diarrhea

    D.   pain on swallowing

60. Which of the following symptoms has been found to be related to gastric cancer?

    A.   abdominal pain

    B.   vague epigastric distress after eating

    C.   sharp midsternal pain two hours after eating

    D.   inability to swallow

61. For the elderly person who suffers from dysphagia, which foods would you instruct him or her to avoid?

    A.   bananas, peanut butter

    B.   apples, raisins

    C.   oatmeal, whole wheat

    D.   lettuce, tomatoes

Nursing Care Plan

62. Write a nursing care plan for the patient who has acute esophagitis. Use the following diagnosis.

    Nursing diagnosis: Pain related to esophageal inflammation

    Patient outcome:

    Interventions:

63. Write a nursing care plan for the patient who has acute midepigastric pain and a possible ulcer.

    Nursing diagnosis:

    Patient outcome:

    Interventions:

64. Write a nursing care plan for the patient with oral cancer who has had a total glossectomy and removal of the mandible. What is the most important aspect of your nursing care? Write this as a nursing diagnosis.

    Nursing diagnosis:

    Patient outcome:

    Interventions:

Case Studies

Case Study No. 1

Mr. W. is a 44-year-old carpenter who is admitted with an episode of acute GI bleeding. He has a history of a peptic ulcer for the past 10 years.

65. Which of the following assessment data would indicate that the patient is bleeding internally?

    A. hypotension, tachycardia, tachypnea

    B. cyanosis, respiratory distress

    C. hypertension, bradycardia, dyspnea

    D. diaphoresis, abdominal pain

66. How would the nurse explain what an ulcer is to Mr. W.?

    A. breaks along the intestinal tract

    B. broken areas throughout the system caused by stress

    C. ulceration of the gastric mucosa resulting from excessive amounts of gastric secretions

    D. opening in the stomach and intestine

67. Which observation on the part of the nurse is most indicative of this particular condition? Patient is

    A. pale and diaphoretic

    B. grimacing in pain

    C. vomiting

    D. lethargic

68. When reviewing the patient's medical history, which of the following medications would have been used in treatment for his peptic ulcer?

    A. Maalox and Zantac

    B. cimetidine and Dyazide

    C. ampicillin and Lasix

    D. Maalox and Reglan

69. Treatment during this episode involves

    A. endoscopy and cauterizing the area

    B. antacids via a nasogastric tube

    C. conservative treatment with proton-inhibitors

    D. surgical intervention

Mr. W. does not respond to traditional medical treatment and is scheduled for a gastric resection in the morning. The nurse's responsibility involves preoperative teaching.

70. Mr. W. asks you what his surgery involves. You know that he is scheduled for a subtotal gastrectomy. You explain

    A. "The entire stomach is removed and the esophagus is attached to the duodenum."

    B. "The distal portion of the stomach including the antrum and pylorus is removed and attached to the duodenum."

    C. "The pylorus is incised and resutured."

    D. "The stomach is resected and the vagus nerve severed."

71. Nursing care of Mr. W. includes observation for postoperative complications. These would include

    A. hemorrhage, projectile vomiting, ileus

    B. GI obstruction, malabsorption

    C. peritonitis, GI bleeding and obstruction

    D. nausea, vomiting, infection

72. Mr. W. has been doing well when suddenly he complains of sudden, sharp midepigastric pain that spreads across the abdomen. Based on your understanding of postoperative complications, these symptoms suggest that he

    A. is hemorrhaging

    B. has developed peritonitis

    C. is overreacting to normal pain

    D. has a GI perforation

73. Mr. W. spends several days in ICU but is finally ready for discharge. Which of the following would you include in your discharge instructions? (Check all that apply.)

    A. _____ ways to cope with stress

    B. _____ foods to avoid

    C. _____ drink 1 quart of water/day

    D. _____ change jobs to avoid stress

Case Study No. 2

Mr. B. is a 60-year-old plumber who has been having difficulty swallowing for two months. He has been diagnosed as having squamous cell carcinoma of the esophagus and is scheduled for surgery.

74. Mr. B. is having an esophagogastrostomy. How would the nurse explain this procedure?

    A. The tumor is resected and the esophagus reanastamosed.

    B. The tumor is removed and the stomach attached to the remaining esophagus.

    C. The tumor is removed and a segment of colon is attached to the esophagus.

75. What would the nurse tell Mr. B. to prepare him for the postoperative course?

    A.   "You will have a nasogastric (NG) tube and be NPO for several days."

    B.   "You will be in intensive care and on a ventilator."

    C.   "You will be started on clear liquid in 48 hours."

    D.   "You will have chest tubes for seven days."

76. Nursing care in the postoperative period is directed toward preventing

    A.   cardiac arrhythmias

    B.   respiratory infections

    C.   fluid volume overload

    D.   diarrhea

77. To prevent this complication, the nurse would

    A.   encourage deep abdominal breathing

    B.   encourage fluids

    C.   watch the cardiac monitor

    D.   administer antacids

Case Study No. 3

Mrs. N. is 48 years old and has a history of chronic gastritis. She lost 20 pounds and has had indigestion for the past six weeks. She is admitted for testing.

78. Mrs. N. is scheduled for a barium study and gastroscopy in the morning. What information would you give to the patient?

    A.   "You will have a liquid diet tonight then nothing by mouth."

    B.   "You can have a regular diet tonight and liquids in the morning."

    C.   "You will have an enema in the morning."

    D.   "You don't have any special preparation for the test."

79. Mrs. N. has had a gastric resection. She is still in intensive care on the second postoperative day. Which of the following findings are abnormal?

    A.   NG tube drains small amount of bloody drainage.

    B.   Chest tube drains 50 mL serosanguineous fluid in eight hours.

    C.   Urinary output is 240 mL in six hours.

    D.   Chest dressing has a moderate amount of pink fluid.

80. Mrs. N. is permitted to take fluids. What would the nurse do to prevent any problems associated with oral intake?

    A.   give liquids only for one week

    B.   give six small feedings daily

    C.   maintain the NG tube for tube feedings

    D.   maintain TPN until caloric intake is adequate

81. Instructing Mrs. N. to lie down for 30 minutes after eating will prevent which of the following problems?

    A.   postural hypotension

    B.   gastric spasm

    C.   dumping syndrome

    D.   gastric reflux

*L*earner Self-Evaluation

Do I fully understand the content? If no, then the areas I need to review are:

I need more information from my instructor on:

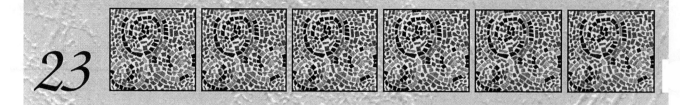

23

Nursing Care of Patients with Disorders of the Lower Gastrointestinal System

*O*bjectives

1.0   Demonstrate an understanding of the inflammatory processes of the lower gastrointestinal (GI) system.

    1.1   Identify several lower GI disorders.

    1.2   Identify clinical manifestations associated with lower GI disorders.

    1.3   Identify medical and surgical interventions used to manage inflammatory processes of the lower GI system.

    1.4   Identify nursing interventions appropriate for patients with an inflammatory bowel disorder.

2.0   Demonstrate an understanding of the functional disorders of the lower GI system.

    2.1   Identify the pathophysiology involved with several of the functional disorders.

    2.2   Identify the medical management of several functional disorders of the lower GI system.

    2.3   Identify several of the functional disorders of the lower GI tract that affect nutrition.

    2.4   Write a nursing care plan for the patient with a mechanical ileum.

3.0   Demonstrate an understanding of the structural disorders of the lower GI system.

    3.1   Identify the pathophysiology involved with several of the structural disorders.

    3.2   Demonstrate an understanding of the medical interventions used to treat structural disorders.

    3.3   Demonstrate an understanding of the surgical procedures used to treat the structural disorders.

    3.4   Write a nursing care plan for the patient with diverticulitis.

4.0   Demonstrate an understanding of the types of neoplasms that affect the lower GI system.

    4.1   Identify the clinical manifestations of the neoplasms that affect the lower GI system.

    4.2   Review the medical and surgical management of the patient with cancer of the colon.

    4.3   Write a nursing care plan for the patient with colon cancer.

$\mathcal{L}$earning Activities

Short Answers

1. The _____ is the thin membrane that lines the abdominal cavity and covers the abdominal organs.

2. In the pathology of appendicitis, an obstruction often results in an increased

    _____ pressure, which predisposes

    to _____ invasion.

3. Appendicitis is always treated

    _____.

4. Treatment for the individual with Crohn's

    disease is _____, as there is no known

    cure.

5. The GI tract has a _____ appearance in the patient with Crohn's disease.

6. _____ are dilated, swollen rectal veins.

7. A paralytic ileus is due to reduced or absent

    _____ and a mechanical ileus is a result of

    a _____.

8. A simple diagnostic test performed to make a diagnosis of lactase deficiency is

    _____.

9. Changes in _____ _____ are often the first symptom of colorectal cancer.

10. Chronic _____ in the elderly can lead to hemorrhoids.

Identification

Match each of the following common lower GI disorders with the best definition.

A. Mechanical ileus

B. Diverticulitis

C. Intestinal hernia

D. Intestinal adhesions

E. Gluten-induced enteropathy

F. Lactase deficiency

G. Malabsorption syndrome

11. _____ Syndrome resulting from impaired passage of nutrients across the intestine and into the circulation

12. _____ Inflammation of mucosal outpouches on the muscular walls of the intestine

13. _____ Condition where movement of intestinal contents is impaired

14. _____ Condition in which there are low levels of lactase in the intestine

15. _____ Bands of fibrous tissue that develop as a result of peritoneal trauma or infection

16. _____ Disorder due to immunologic sensitivity to gluten

17. _____ Peritoneum, omentum, or intestine protrude out of the abdominal cavity through an abnormal opening

True/False

18. _____ Crohn's disease can affect any part of the GI tract.

19. _____ Ulcerative colitis is caused by a viral infection.

20. _____ Diarrhea and rectal bleeding are common with ulcerative colitis.

21. _____ Ulcerative colitis often begins in the ileum and spreads distally.

22. _____ Colon cancer is seen more in men than women.

23. _____ Most GI tract cancers occur in the colon or rectum.

24. _____ There is a poor prognosis with colorectal cancer.

25. _____ Colorectal cancers are primarily adenomas.

26. _____ Inflammatory bowel disorders are not a problem in the elderly.

27. _____ Occlusion of the mesenteric vessels can lead to bowel ischemia.

Knowledge Application

28. The individual with an inguinal hernia should be taught to avoid doing anything that could increase intra-abdominal pressure and result in actual herniation. Which of the following activities would NOT cause an increase in pressure?

    A. strenuous coughing

    B. heavy lifting

    C. becoming overweight

    D. frequent urination

29. The most common cause of peritonitis is

    A. bacterial infection

    B. viral infection

    C. chemical irritation

    D. environmental factors

30. Of the following conditions, which is NOT likely to lead to peritonitis?

    A. perforated peptic ulcer

    B. acute salpingitis

    C. peritoneal dialysis

    D. meningitis

31. The primary symptom of peritonitis is

    A. projectile vomiting

    B. severe abdominal pain

    C. high temperature

    D. anorexia, weight loss

32. When a patient develops peritonitis, the nurse would anticipate treatment with

    A. antiviral drugs

    B. antibiotics

    C. antipyretics

    D. analgesics

33. Because of fluid losses from both the bowel lumen and the peritoneal cavity, the individual with peritonitis has a risk of developing

    A. hypovolemia

    B. hemoconcentration

    C. acute tubular necrosis

    D. all of the above

34. Which of the following would be indications that the treatment for peritonitis is effective?

    A. vital signs, including temperature, are normal

    B. active bowel sounds, passing stool, temperature normal

    C. patient is pain-free, appetite returns, dressing is dry and intact

    D. patient is asymptomatic

35. Perforation is one of the complications of untreated appendicitis. This can result in

    A. peritonitis

    B. hemorrhage

    C. urosepsis

    D. diverticulitis

36. Which of the following signs and symptoms would indicate a possibility of appendicitis in a patient?

    A. rebound tenderness

    B. pain at McBurney's point

    C. anorexia and nausea

    D. any of the above

37. Medical management for the patient with appendicitis might include all of the following EXCEPT

    A. clear liquid diet

    B. intravenous fluids

    C. intravenous antibiotics

    D. diagnostic studies

38. The treatment of choice for acute appendicitis is

    A. antibiotic therapy

    B. analgesics

    C. surgery

    D. laser surgery

39. When assessing a patient following an appendectomy, the nurse notices abdominal distention and an absence of bowel sounds. These findings suggest

    A. peritonitis

    B. diverticulitis

    C. paralytic ileus

    D. septicemia

40. The area of the colon that is most often involved when a patient has Crohn's disease is the

    A. terminal ileum

    B. duodenum

    C. distal part of jejunum

    D. sigmoid colon

41. Which of the following patient data would suggest Crohn's disease?

    A. nausea, vomiting, frequent bloody diarrhea

    B. pain after eating, fever, nonbloody diarrhea

    C. fever, chills, anorexia, constipation

    D. chronic pain, alternating constipation and diarrhea

42. Nursing care of the patient who has Crohn's disease is aimed at preventing complications such as

    A. bowel obstruction

    B. bowel perforation

    C. fistula formation

    D. all of the above

43. When a patient has an acute exacerbation of Crohn's disease, the pharmacologic treatment that takes priority would be the administration of

    A. analgesics

    B. antibiotics

    C. antidiarrheals

    D. corticosteroids

44. When a patient with an inflammatory bowel disorder is admitted with severe diarrhea and vomiting, which nursing action is the priority?

    A. administer analgesics

    B. maintain bed rest

    C. maintain fluid and electrolyte balance

    D. encourage patient to discuss feelings

45. A patient has just had an excision of an anorectal abscess. The nursing diagnosis that would have priority is

    A. Alteration in nutrition

    B. High risk for recurrent infection

    C. Ineffective coping

    D. Ineffective breathing patterns

46. Which of the following conditions can cause a mechanical ileus?

    A. adhesions

    B. hernia

    C. foreign bodies

    D. volvulus

    E. any of the above

47.   Which symptoms in the postoperative patient would indicate a mechanical ileus?

   A.   nausea and anorexia

   B.   sharp knifelike pain at umbilicus

   C.   absence of bowel sounds

   D.   distention and inability to pass stool

48.   Diagnosis of a mechanical ileus is based on history, physical examination, and x-ray findings which would show

   A.   tortuous narrowing of the bowel

   B.   air-fluid levels in the obstructed bowel

   C.   cobblestone ulcers throughout the lumen

   D.   dilatation of bowel from duodenum to rectum

49.   Initial treatment of a bowel obstruction would include insertion of a nasogastric (NG) tube. The rationale for the insertion of the NG tube is to

   A.   provide a route for medication

   B.   allow for tube feedings

   C.   decompress the intestine

   D.   remove liquid stool

50.   Which nursing diagnosis would be a priority in the patient with a mechanical ileus?

   A.   High risk for fluid volume deficit

   B.   Pain related to increased pressure

   C.   Altered health management

   D.   Knowledge deficit related to unknown outcome of treatment

51.   Which of the following conditions is the most likely cause of a paralytic ileus?

   A.   volvulus

   B.   neoplasm

   C.   abdominal surgery

   D.   third-degree burns

52.   The underlying cause of the events leading to a paralytic ileus is thought to be

   A.   excessive sympathetic nervous system activity which decreases peristalsis

   B.   excessive parasympathetic nervous system activity which stops peristalsis

   C.   changes in intraluminal pressure

   D.   severe fluid shifts and electrolyte changes during surgery

53.   The nurse is assessing a postoperative patient. Which of the following findings would be indicative of a paralytic ileus?

   A.   hyperactive bowel sounds, nausea

   B.   hypoactive bowel sounds, increased gastric drainage, abdominal distention

   C.   abdominal pain, projectile vomiting

   D.   increased temperature, hypotension, abdominal pain

54.   When a patient has signs and symptoms of impaired passage of proteins, carbohydrates, fat, and minerals into circulation, he or she is at high risk for

   A.   intestinal cancer

   B.   malabsorption syndrome

   C.   paralytic ileus

   D.   intestinal obstruction

55.   The nurse would instruct the patient with a lactase deficiency to eat foods high in calcium such as:

   A.   milk, red meats

   B.   green and yellow vegetables

   C.   salmon and sardines

   D.   wheat and oat cereal

56.   If, when assessing a patient, the nurse identifies the symptoms of _____, it would be suggestive of malabsorption syndrome.

   A.   weight loss, anorexia, bloating, bulky stools

   B.   nausea, vomiting, abdominal pain

   C.   cramping, passage of clay-colored stool

   D.   fatigue, weakness, confusion, diarrhea

57. Diagnostic testing for the patient with malabsorption syndrome would reveal all of the following EXCEPT

   A.   decreased serum albumin

   B.   decreased potassium

   C.   decreased prothrombin time

   D.   increased stool fat

58. When a person has a lactase deficiency, they are most likely to exhibit which of the following symptoms?

   A.   anorexia, vomiting, weight loss

   B.   abdominal pain, bloating, diarrhea

   C.   nausea, vomiting, abdominal cramps

   D.   intermittent cramps, constipation, lethargy

59. Dietary teaching for the patient with gluten-induced enteropathy requires avoiding all cereal grains EXCEPT

   A.   wheat

   B.   rice

   C.   oats

   D.   rye

60. Which of the following data obtained by the nurse in the health history would indicate a predisposition to the development of diverticular disease? (Check all that apply.)

   A. _____ history of chronic diarrhea, vomiting

   B. _____ history of passing small, scant stools

   C. _____ eats a diet low in fiber

   D. _____ eats a diet high in fiber

   E. _____ history of frequent use of laxatives

61. Medical management of diverticulosis would include

   A.   decreasing fluids, using antidiarrheal drugs

   B.   liquid diet, antispasmodic drugs

   C.   low-fiber diet, anticholinergic drugs

   D.   high-fiber diet, bulk-forming laxatives

62. The nurse would instruct the patient with diverticular disease to avoid foods such as

   A.   apples

   B.   popcorn

   C.   whole-wheat bread

   D.   raw vegetables

63. The nurse should suspect incarceration of a hernia when which of the following symptoms are present?

   A.   severe pain, nausea, vomiting

   B.   left quadrant pain, diarrhea

   C.   fever, hypoactive bowel sounds, anorexia

   D.   rebound tenderness, hyperactive bowel sounds

64. The treatment of choice for an incisional or inguinal hernia is

   A.   diet and exercise

   B.   surgical repair

   C.   analgesics and antispasmodic medications

   D.   antibiotics and use of a truss

65. A patient returns to the unit after an inguinal herniorrhaphy. Which of the following observations is most indicative of a problem following surgery? The patient

   A.   complains of pain

   B.   is nauseated

   C.   has difficulty voiding

   D.   is anxious about getting out of bed

66. Medical management is often possible for uncomplicated hemorrhoids. Which of the following would not be used?

   A.   sitz baths

   B.   witch hazel preparations

   C.   low-fiber diet

   D.   stool softeners

67. Hemorrhoidectomy is the treatment of choice for which of the following? A patient with

    A.   internal hemorrhoids

    B.   prolapsed hemorrhoids

    C.   occasional rectal bleeding

    D.   external hemorrhoids with no symptoms

68. When doing discharge planning for a patient following herniorrhaphy the nurse would stress

    A.   pain can last up to seven days

    B.   resume activity after two weeks

    C.   avoid heavy lifting and sexual activities for six weeks

    D.   follow a low-residue diet and avoid laxatives

69. What is the rationale for having rectal polyps surgically removed? They

    A.   often rupture and bleed

    B.   are potentially malignant

    C.   often become infected

    D.   predispose to diverticulosis

70. Which of the following would NOT be an expected clinical finding 24 hours after a colostomy is performed?

    A.   stoma is bright red and oozing

    B.   NG tube output is 200 mL of green drainage in eight hours

    C.   abdomen is slightly distended with absent bowel sounds

    D.   catheter is in place with urine output of 150 mL in eight hours

71. After abdominal surgery, Penrose drains are often inserted. The nurse explains to the patient that they will be removed when

    A.   the patient can tolerate a liquid diet

    B.   bowel function returns

    C.   drainage is less than 50 mL in 24 hours

    D.   they fall out naturally

Nursing Care Plans

72. Write a nursing care plan for the patient who has had incision and drainage of a rectal abscess. Use the following nursing diagnosis.

    Nursing diagnosis: Pain related to surgical trauma.

    Patient outcome:

    Interventions:

73. Plan the nursing care for the patient with an ileus. Use the following diagnosis.

    Nursing diagnosis: Potential fluid volume deficit related to fluid shifts and vomiting

    Patient outcome:

    Interventions:

74. The nurse is aware that the patient with diverticulitis may have a problem with constipation. Write a nursing diagnosis, patient outcome, and several interventions related to this problem.

    Nursing diagnosis:

    Patient outcome:

    Interventions:

75. A patient is scheduled for an abdominal-perineal resection for colorectal cancer. This patient is exhibiting signs of extreme anxiety. Write a nursing diagnosis, patient outcome, and several interventions that address this need.

    Nursing diagnosis:

    Patient outcome:

    Interventions:

76. Following a hemorrhoidectomy, pain control is important. Since this is often done as same-day surgery, write several nursing interventions that will serve as discharge instruction.

    Nursing diagnosis: Pain related to surgical trauma

    Interventions:

Case Studies

Case Study No. 1

Ms. M. is a 28-year-old legal secretary who has Crohn's disease. She is admitted to the hospital with anorexia and malnutrition because of an inability to eat and frequent diarrhea.

77. All of the following are treatment goals EXCEPT

    A. restoring normal nutritional status

    B. suppressing inflammation

    C. minimizing pain and diarrhea

    D. providing education about surgery

78. The nurse reviews the medication record. She sees that the patient is receiving a medication that is an anti-infective and anti-inflammatory. This is

    A. Azulfidine

    B. prednisone

    C. cefazolin

    D. Valium

79. The nurse performs a thorough assessment, keeping in mind to look for signs of _____ and _____ problems.

    A. skin, hygienic

    B. bowel, bladder

    C. fluid, electrolyte

    D. diet, elimination

80. The nurse should consider which responsibility to be of primary importance when preparing Ms. M. for a colonoscopy?

    A. keep patient on NPO status

    B. medicate prior to procedure

    C. start IV therapy as ordered

    D. ask about allergies to dye

81. Following the colonoscopy, the nurse would expect to administer which medication to Ms. M.?

    A. laxative

    B. stool softener

    C. antacid

    D. analgesic

82. Which goal for Ms. M. will take priority during the initial portion of the hospitalization?

    A. promotion of positive self-image

    B. promoting rest and comfort

    C. maintenance of adequate nutrition

    D. prevention of injury

Ms. M. has symptoms of severely altered nutrition related to limited intake as well as a fear of exacerbating symptoms. The physician decides to start TPN.

83. Which of the following patient outcomes would you select that relates specifically to this problem? The patient

    A. identifies ineffective coping behaviors

    B. is in positive nitrogen balance

    C. maintains intact skin

    D. is free from pain and discomfort

Case Study No. 2

Mrs. N. is admitted to the health-care facility with left-sided pain, abdominal pain, intermittent diarrhea, and blood in her stools. The physician orders diagnostic tests to determine the cause of her symptoms.

84. The nurse is preparing Mrs. N. for a barium enema. The nurse realizes that a colonoscopy is usually contraindicated during an acute illness stage because of the risk of _____.

    A. hemorrhage

    B. infection

    C. perforation

    D. obstruction

85. The test confirms a diagnosis of diverticulitis. The physician opts for medical management first. All of the following medications would be appropriate EXCEPT

    A. narcotic analgesics

    B. stool softeners

    C. antibiotics

    D. antispasmodics

86. Mrs. N. does not respond to the medical management and a decision is made to do a surgical resection of the bowel with a temporary colostomy. The nurse realizes that the patient needs more information when she states

    A. "I don't think I can cope with having a colostomy for the rest of my life."

    B. "I realize that I am going to have to make some diet changes."

    C. "I never realized how important it was to watch my diet and fluid intake."

    D. "I am anxious about the outcome of the surgery."

87. Mrs. N. is ready for discharge and the nurse is reviewing the diet recommendations. The diet is based on the knowledge that

    A. all food high in fiber and roughage should be eliminated

    B. liquids and fluid intake is limited to prevent diarrhea

    C. taking laxatives and prune juice regularly will ensure proper functioning of the colostomy

    D. diet restrictions are often determined individually to avoid gas-forming foods and irritants

Case Study No. 3

Mr. P. has been admitted for diagnostic testing. His symptoms include weakness, anorexia, weight loss, and occasional bleeding with defecation. He also has a chronic cough and back pain.

88. Mr. P. is diagnosed as having a large tumor in the sigmoid colon. He is scheduled for surgery. The surgical procedure that will be performed is most likely

    A. right colectomy with ileotransverse anastomosis

    B. left colectomy with transverse anastomosis

    C. temporary transverse colostomy

    D. abdominal perineal resection

89. Nursing care in the preoperative period is directed toward which of the following?

    A. control of pain

    B. improvement of nutritional status

    C. correction of bowel habits

    D. increasing mobility

90. To reduce the risk of contamination at the time of surgery, the nurse will probably be administering which of the following medications to Mr. P. prior to surgery?

    A. laxatives and anti-infectives

    B. analgesics, antispasmodics

    C. anticholinergics, antispasmodics

    D. analgesics, antibiotics

91. Nursing care in the postoperative period is directed toward preventing

    A. problems related to inactivity

    B. ineffective breathing patterns

    C. imbalances of food and fluids

    D. injury related to weakness

92. Mr. P. is also scheduled for a course of chemotherapy. Which symptom indicates a possible side effect of this therapy?

    A. mucositis

    B. abdominal pain

    C. hiccuping

    D. leg cramps

93. The nurse is teaching Mr. P. how to care for the colostomy. Which of the following statements is most accurate in terms of regulation of bowel habits?

    A. Daily irrigation will keep elimination regular.

    B. Regular bowel elimination is almost impossible.

    C. Control of bowel elimination is often possible by following a dietary regimen and regular habits.

    D. None of the above.

94. Disturbance in body image may be a serious problem following a colostomy. Which of the following reactions by the nurse is inappropriate?

    A. recognize that rejection is a common reaction

    B. permit denial while promoting acceptance

    C. avoid looking at the stoma or calling it by name

    D. encourage good hygiene and grooming

95. Mr. P. says he is ready to learn to care for his colostomy. Which of the following nursing interventions is most likely to be effective in preparing him to look at his colostomy?

   A. Encourage him to verbalize his concerns about the colostomy.

   B. Have a friend who has a colostomy visit Mr. P.

   C. Use prepared materials with illustrations for the first session.

   D. Explain that he will have no problems adjusting.

Case Study No. 4

Ms. B. has chronic renal failure and has been doing home continuous peritoneal dialysis for two years. Today, she came to the clinic complaining of severe abdominal pain, nausea, and vomiting. Her temperature is 101° F. The nurse completes an evaluation.

96. These symptoms suggest

   A. urinary infection

   B. bowel perforation

   C. peritonitis

   D. bowel obstruction

97. To confirm the diagnosis, the physician will probably order

   A. abdominal x-ray

   B. culture of peritoneal fluid

   C. complete blood count

   D. all of the above

98. The management will include

   A. stopping dialysis

   B. fluid restriction

   C. steroids

   D. antibiotics

99. The most important part of the nursing management would be

   A. education to prevent a recurrence

   B. changing the type of dialysis

   C. strict adherence to diet

   D. all of the above

*L*earner Self-Evaluation

Do I fully understand the content? If no, then the areas I need to review are:

I need more information from my instructor on:

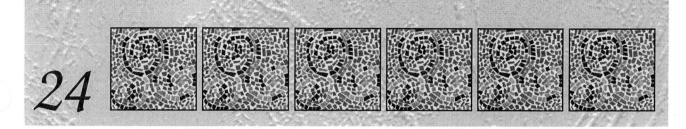

24

Nursing Care of Patients with Disorders of the Accessory Organs of Digestion

*O*bjectives

1.0　Demonstrate an understanding of the inflammatory or infectious disorders of the accessory organs of digestion.

　　1.1　Identify the clinical manifestations of cholecystitis.

　　1.2　Review the medical and surgical management of cholecystitis.

　　1.3　Review the nursing care of the patient having a cholecystectomy.

　　1.4　Review the pathophysiology involved in pancreatitis.

　　1.5　Plan the nursing care for the patient with acute and chronic pancreatitis.

2.0　Demonstrate an understanding of a structural abnormality of the accessory organs of digestion.

　　2.1　Identify the clinical manifestations of a pancreatic fistula.

　　2.2　Identify an inflammatory disorder that can lead to the development of a structural abnormality.

3.0　Demonstrate an understanding of the types of neoplasms that affect the accessory organs of digestion.

　　3.1　Identify the clinical manifestations of pancreatic cancer.

　　3.2　Review the medical interventions used to treat cancer of the pancreas.

　　3.3　Review the surgical management of cancer of the pancreas.

　　3.4　Write a nursing care plan for the patient who has undergone a Whipple procedure.

*L*earning Activities

Short Answers

1.　Cholecystitis is an inflammation of the

　　_____.

2.　Cholelithiasis refers to the presence of

　　_____ in the gall bladder.

3.　One symptom of cholecystitis unique to this

　　condition is _____.

4. Stasis of _____ and imbalances in
    _____ and
    _____ seem to precipitate the
    development of cholecystitis.

5. The basic factor in the onset of acute pancre-
    atitis is the presence of activated

    _____.

6. Approximately _____ % of the cholecystecto-
    mies are performed through the laparoscopic
    approach.

True/False

7. _____ When gallstone dissolution therapy is
    discontinued, stones may recur.

8. _____ Lithotripsy is a procedure that causes
    little discomfort.

9. _____ Laparoscopic cholecystectomy is done
    under general anesthesia.

10. _____ Ambulatory surgical centers are
    performing uncomplicated conven-
    tional cholecystectomies.

11. _____ The patient with acute pancreatitis will
    need oral pancreatic enzymes.

12. _____ Patients with chronic pancreatitis may
    need to take insulin.

13. _____ Pancreatic fistulas are most often a
    result of pancreatic abscesses.

14. _____ Surgery is not recommended for
    treatment of chronic pancreatitis.

15. _____ Cancer of the pancreas is rare in the
    United States.

16. _____ Pancreatic cancers are generally adeno-
    carcinomas.

17. _____ The incidence of gallstones increases
    with age.

Knowledge Application

18. Elevations in which of the following labora-
    tory data would be suggestive of acute
    cholecystitis?

    A. CBC, AST, LDH

    B. WBC, AST, CPK

    C. WBC, alkaline phosphatase, AST, LDH

    D. BUN, creatinine, bilirubin

19. Symptoms associated with cholecystitis
    include (Check all that apply.)

    A. _____ nausea

    B. _____ vomiting

    C. _____ flatulence

    D. _____ elevated temperature

    E. _____ generalized abdominal pain

20. What is one of the drawbacks of use of
    gallstone dissolving drugs such a CDCA
    (chenodiol) and ursodeoxycholic acid
    (UDCA)?

    A. They have serious side effects.

    B. They are very expensive.

    C. They may take up to six months to
        work.

    D. All of the above

21. A patient is scheduled for a cholecystectomy
    and choledocholithotomy. This means that
    the surgeon will remove the gallbladder and

    A. drain the pancreatic duct

    B. explore the common bile duct

    C. remove a stone from the bile duct

    D. remove part of the colon

22. Discharge instruction for the patient who has
    had extracorporeal lithotripsy would include

    A. beginning taking oral bile acids

    B. continuing taking antibiotics

    C. avoiding lifting for six weeks

    D. returning to physician in six months

23. After a choledocholithotomy is performed,
    what is the reason for the placement of a T-
    tube? To

    A. facilitate drainage

    B. prevent infection

    C. maintain patency

    D. prevent stone recurrence

24. How much bile would the nurse expect the T-tube to drain during the first 24 hours after surgery?

A. 50–100 mL

B. 150–250 mL

C. 300–500 mL

D. 500–1000 mL

25. Which of the following findings indicates a possible surgical complication within the first 24 hours following a cholecystectomy?

A. T-tube has stopped draining.

B. NG tube drains 100 mL in four hours.

C. Penrose drain falls out.

D. Respirations are 20 and shallow.

26. Potential complications of laparoscopic cholecystectomy include

A. bowel puncture

B. bladder puncture

C. uncontrolled bleeding

D. all of the above

27. When the patient has had a laparoscopic cholecystectomy a nursing intervention that is unique to this procedure is

A. administer narcotics as needed

B. place patient in Sims' position

C. keep patient in prone position with abdominal binder

D. instruct patient to gradually resume normal activities

28. The most prominent symptom of acute pancreatitis is

A. left upper quadrant pain radiating to the mid-back

B. right lower quadrant pain radiating across abdomen

C. mid-abdominal pain referred to left shoulder

D. back and shoulder pain

29. All of the following have been indicated in the development of pancreatitis EXCEPT

A. excessive use of alcohol

B. use of antibiotics

C. biliary tract disease

D. metabolic disorders

30. Because of systemic vasodilation and increased vascular permeability, the individual with pancreatitis is predisposed to

A. hypovolemic shock

B. sepsis

C. adult respiratory distress syndrome

D. hypertensive crisis

31. Which of the following laboratory results would be consistent with acute pancreatitis?

A. WBC of 15,000

B. BUN of 32, creatinine of 1.2

C. LDH of 40, CPK of 100

D. serum amylase of 520

32. Medical management of acute pancreatitis during the critical stage would include all of the following EXCEPT

A. nasogastric tube to suction

B. clear liquid diet

C. narcotics for pain control

D. IV therapy

33. In caring for the patient with acute pancreatitis during the critical stage, which nursing action would have the highest priority?

A. Have patient turn every two hours.

B. Assess hemodynamic status and urine output hourly.

C. Maintain patency of the NG tube.

D. Medicate for pain every three hours.

34. Presence of muscle twitching and tremors can indicate which condition in a patient with acute pancreatitis?

   A. hypokalemia

   B. hypocalcemia

   C. dehydration

   D. acidosis

35. For the patient with pancreatitis, the nurse would question an order for which of the following pain medications?

   A. Demerol 25 mg IVP, every three hours

   B. Talwin 30 mg IM, every three hours

   C. codeine 30 mg IM, every four hours

   D. morphine Sulfate 10 mg IV, every three hours

36. The best position for the patient with acute pancreatitis to prevent respiratory problems would be

   A. supine

   B. prone

   C. Fowler's

   D. Sims'

37. An individual with chronic pancreatitis will generally seek medical attention when he or she

   A. notices blood in the stools

   B. is unable to tolerate food

   C. begins to retain fluid

   D. experiences acute attacks of pain

38. Laboratory findings consistent with chronic pancreatitis would include

   A. increased alkaline phosphate, decreased serum glucose

   B. increased serum glucose, increased pancreatic juices

   C. decreased alkaline phosphate, decreased pancreatic juices

   D. increased alkaline phosphate, decreased pancreatic juices

39. Because of the vitamin deficiencies associated with chronic pancreatitis, the nurse is aware that a patient with this condition is at risk for developing

   A. duodenal ulcer

   B. gastric bleeding

   C. pernicious anemia

   D. lactase deficiency

40. Which metabolic problem is associated with chronic pancreatitis?

   A. hyperglycemia

   B. hypoglycemia

   C. hypercalcemia

   D. hypokalemia

41. In the patient with chronic pancreatitis, it is not uncommon for the stools to appear

   A. black and liquid

   B. white and chalky

   C. tan, oily, foul-smelling

   D. frothy, bulky, foul-smelling

42. When a patient with pancreatic cancer has a jaundiced appearance, the nurse would suspect

   A. chronic pancreatitis

   B. biliary obstruction

   C. gastritis

   D. nutritional deficiency

43. The purpose of performing the Whipple procedure as a treatment for cancer of the pancreas is

   A. as a palliative approach to stop the disease

   B. to prevent a recurrence of the disease

   C. to allow enzymes to empty in the jejunum to allow normal digestion to take place

   D. to remove the pancreas and allow its functions to be taken over by the other accessory organs of digestion

44. A patient is scheduled for a Whipple procedure. Lab results indicate a prothrombin deficiency. What treatment would be indicated? Administration of

    A. antibiotics

    B. vitamin B_{12}

    C. KCl 40 mEq

    D. vitamin K

45. One of the major complications of the Whipple procedure is

    A. hemorrhage

    B. necrosis

    C. fistula formation

    D. all of the above

Nursing Care Plans

46. The nurse is caring for the patient with acute pancreatitis. Write a nursing care plan using the following diagnosis.

    Nursing diagnosis: Potential for fluid volume deficit

    Patient outcome:

    Interventions:

47. Write a nursing care plan for the individual with chronic pancreatitis who will need to comply with taking medications and following diet restrictions.

    Nursing diagnosis:

    Patient outcome:

    Interventions:

48. A major problem for the individual who has had a Whipple procedure will be a nutritional alteration. Write a care plan using this as your focus.

    Nursing diagnosis:

    Patient outcome:

    Interventions:

Case Studies

Case Study No. 1

Mr. T. is admitted to the hospital with acute pain in his side, nausea, and vomiting. After examination, the physician diagnoses acute pancreatitis.

49. After obtaining a patient history, the nurse identifies which of the following behaviors as related to the diagnosis?

    A.   smokes two packs of cigarettes per day

    B.   takes Tylenol 10 gr four times a day for arthritis

    C.   follows a low-sodium, low-cholesterol diet

    D.   takes Bactrim for urinary stasis

50. The initial diagnosis of pancreatitis would be confirmed if Mr. T. has a significant elevation in serum

    A.   glucose

    B.   amylase

    C.   creatinine

    D.   calcium

51. Because Mr. T. has a strong religious aversion to drinking, he becomes very upset when the physician asks him several times if he has a problem with alcohol intake. The nurse would explain to the family that the reason for these questions is

    A.   there is a strong link between alcohol use and this disease

    B.   use of alcohol will cause inaccurate results in the lab test

    C.   all patients admitted to the hospital are asked these questions

    D.   the physician is new and not very sensitive

52. During the initial assessment, the nurse notices that Mr. T. has muscle twitching in his forearms. The nurse should report this finding immediately because patients with this condition are at serious risk for

    A.   hypoglycemia

    B.   hypocalcemia

    C.   hyperkalemia

    D.   hyponatremia

53. During the acute period of his illness, Mr. T.'s diet will most likely be

    A.   NPO

    B.   clear liquids

    C.   bland, no stimulants

    D.   low fat, high carbohydrate

54. The nurse assesses Mr. T. and finds his abdomen has a small reddened area that is warm to touch. He has a temperature of 101.2° F. What is a likely cause of this finding? The patient has

    A.   developed an abscess

    B.   developed a fistula

    C.   internal bleeding

    D.   developed an ulcer

Case Study No. 2

Mr. B. is admitted with a diagnosis of chronic pancreatitis. He has a history of alcohol abuse and has been admitted twice in the past five years for the same problem. He is complaining of severe abdominal pain. He has lost 20 pounds in the last six months.

55. The nurse is reviewing the chart to determine Mr. B.'s nutrition status. Malnutrition would be a probable diagnosis if there is a significant low level in serum

    A.   glucose

    B.   total protein

    C.   potassium

    D.   calcium

56. What is the probable reason for the weight loss?

    A.   drinking causes him to forget to eat

    B.   malabsorption and vitamin deficiencies

    C.   hyperactivity of pancreas uses up the calories

    D.   increase in digestive enzymes

57. The nurse is aware that the goal of medical therapy is to decrease stimulation of pancreatic function. One of the drugs which would be useful is

    A. cimetidine

    B. morphine Sulfate

    C. Motrin

    D. Inderal

58. Once Mr. B. is stabilized he will be given information about his diet. An appropriate diet for the individual with chronic pancreatitis would be

    A. low-protein, high-fiber diet with five meals

    B. low-fat, bland diet with five meals

    C. high-calcium, soft diet with three meals

    D. low-residue, high-protein, high-fat diet

59. Mr. B. will also be taking pancreatic enzymes. How would the nurse teach him to monitor for the effectiveness of the therapy?

    A. monitor fluid intake

    B. do daily fingersticks for blood sugar

    C. observe stools for steatorrhea

    D. monitor urine for sediment

Case Study No. 3

Mrs. M., 56, is admitted for an open cholecystectomy. She has a history of cholelithiasis for several years and has been having attacks more frequently. She is 5' 6", and weighs 225 pounds. She currently has right quadrant pain.

60. Based on the patient's history, the nurse is aware that all of the following factors would predispose Mrs. M. to cholelithiasis EXCEPT

    A. age

    B. weight

    C. sex

    D. diet

61. In caring for Mrs. M., the nurse realizes that her diagnosis means that she has

    A. an infection in her gall bladder

    B. an obstruction in the bile duct

    C. presence of stones in the gall bladder

    D. all of the above

Following the surgery, Mrs. M. returns to the unit with an IV of dextrose/.45 normal saline at 100 cc/hour and a nasogastric tube to low wall suction. Her abdominal dressing is dry and intact and vital signs are stable.

62. When Mrs. M. complains of nausea and distention, what should the nurse do first?

    A. increase the IV rate

    B. give the patient an antiemetic

    C. medicate the patient for pain

    D. assess the NG tube for patency

63. Based on the above information, what would be an important nursing diagnosis at this time? Potential for

    A. alteration in fluid and electrolytes

    B. alteration in bowel elimination

    C. activity intolerance

    D. role disturbance

Learner Self-Evaluation

Do I fully understand the content? If no, then the areas I need to review are:

I need more information from my instructor on:

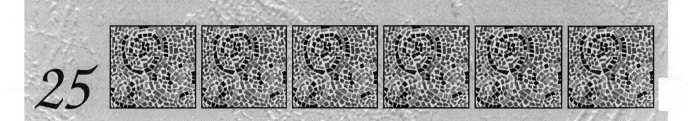

25

Knowledge Base for Patients with Hepatic Dysfunction

Objectives

1.0   Review the anatomy and physiology of the hepatic system.
    1.1   Identify the parts of the hepatic system.
    1.2   Demonstrate an understanding of the metabolic processes of the hepatic system.
    1.3   List five functions of the liver.
    1.4   Identify the underlying pathology associated with certain clinical manifestations of hepatic dysfunction.

2.0   Demonstrate an understanding of the assessment data related to hepatic dysfunction.
    2.1   List clinical manifestations associated with hepatic disorders.
    2.2   Match specific diagnostic tests with the description.
    2.3   Identify correct lab values for liver function tests.
    2.4   Identify results of specific diagnostic tests as they relate to the hepatic disorders.
    2.5   Plan the nursing care for the patient undergoing diagnostic studies.

3.0   Demonstrate an understanding of the interventions appropriate for patients with hepatic dysfunction.
    3.1   Identify the medical treatment and surgical procedures for patients with hepatic disorders.
    3.2   Plan the nursing care for the patient with hepatic encephalopathy.
    3.3   Write appropriate nursing interventions for the patient with hepatic dysfunction.

*L*earning Activities

Identification

1. Demonstrate your knowledge of anatomy by identifying the following parts of the hepatic system.

    A.   Right lobe of liver

    B.   Left lobe of liver

    C.   Inferior vena cava

    D.   Gall bladder

    E.   Hepatic ducts

    F.   Cystic duct

    G.   Common bile duct

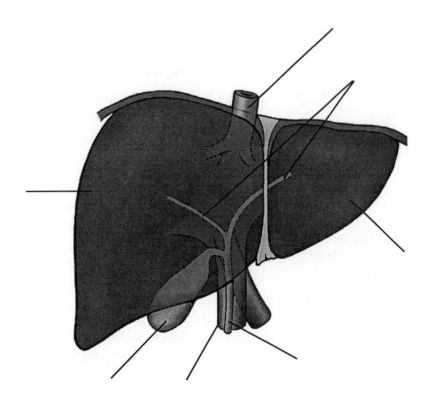

Short Answers

2.   List five functions of the liver.
1.

2.

3.

4.

5.

3.   The hepatic vein empties into the

     _____ .

4.   In carbohydrate metabolism, the liver has an
     important role in maintaining normal blood

     _____ .

5.   Five clinical manifestations associated with
     hepatic dysfunction are
1.

2.

3.

4.

5.

6.   _____ _____ are oxidized by the liver to
     produce energy when glucose is not avail-
     able to meet the body's needs.

7.   The end products of the digestion of proteins

     are _____ _____ .

8.   Another name for jaundice is

     _____ .

9.   Obstructive jaundice occurs when the flow of

     _____ is obstructed.

10.   An individual with ascites would need to

      restrict _____ and _____ intake.

Identification

Match each of these diagnostic tests with the
correct definition.

A.   Liver scan

B.   Abdominal ultrasound

C.   Esophagoscopy

D.   Peritoneoscopy

11.   _____   Permits the direct visualization of the
              liver

12.   _____   Determines the size, shape, position,
              and functioning of the liver

13.   _____   Can be used to identify esophageal
              varices

14.   _____   Uses sound waves to differentiate
              tissues within the abdominal cavity

Interpretation

Fill in the normal value for each of the following
blood studies, then indicate if the value will
increase (I) or decrease (D) with liver dysfunction.

	Value	Increase/ Decrease
15.	Urine urobilinogen ____ mg/24 hrs	_____
16.	Total serum protein ____ g/dL	_____
17.	Serum albumin ____ g/dL	_____
18.	Blood ammonia ____ mg/dL	_____
19.	Total cholesterol ____ mg/dL	_____
20.	Prothrombin time ____ sec	_____
21.	Alpha-fetoprotein ____ ng/mL	_____
22.	AST ____ U/L	_____

Knowledge Application

23. The functional units of the liver are the

    A. nephrotic capsules

    B. sinusoids

    C. hepatic lobules

    D. capsules of Glisson

24. The blood supply to the liver is transported via the

    A. hepatic artery

    B. hepatic portal vein

    C. inferior vena cava

    D. mesenteric artery

25. The process by which the liver converts glycogen to glucose to meet energy needs is known as

    A. glycogenesis

    B. glycogenolysis

    C. glucolysis

    D. glyconeogenesis

26. An important function of the liver that aids the body in the digestion of fats is production of

    A. cholesterol

    B. ketones

    C. bile

    D. amino acids

27. Ammonia, an end product of protein metabolism, is removed from the body by

    A. destruction in the liver

    B. filtration in the hemopoietic system

    C. destruction to amino acids and excretion in urine

    D. conversion to urea and excretion in urine

28. Which of the following clinical manifestations would indicate to the nurse that a patient has a deficiency in bile production?

    A. steatorrhea

    B. dermatitis

    C. glossitis

    D. osteomalacia

29. If a patient has a hepatic disorder and a deficiency in vitamin K, the nurse would assess for

    A. clotting disorders

    B. hypoglycemic reactions

    C. anemia

    D. fluid volume changes

30. A nurse is assessing a patient with jaundice. The nurse realizes that this is caused by

    A. rapid increase in byproducts of protein metabolism

    B. elevated levels of bilirubin

    C. increase in red blood cells

    D. excessive excretion of bile salts

31. In caring for the patient with jaundice, an appropriate nursing intervention would be to

    A. bathe in cool water, apply lotion

    B. massage skin every four hours

    C. monitor intake and output frequently

    D. encourage fluid intake

32. A patient is admitted with a diagnosis of intrahepatic obstruction. Which of the following problems is most likely related to this condition? A history of

    A. bowel obstruction

    B. congestive heart failure

    C. hepatitis

    D. diabetes

33. When assessing a patient with liver failure, what nursing assessment is used to detect portal hypertension?

   A.   heart sounds every shift

   B.   abdominal girth daily

   C.   for change in level of consciousness

   D.   patient weight weekly

34. A patient is admitted with ascites. The nurse may be administering _____ to help remove excessive sodium.

   A.   nifedipine

   B.   Catapres

   C.   digoxin

   D.   Aldactone

35. Assuming all these patients have ascites, which one would be most likely to have a paracentesis? A patient with

   A.   10-pound weight gain

   B.   irregular heart rhythm

   C.   respiratory difficulty

   D.   recent change in mental status

36. A patient has a LeVeen shunt inserted to control ascites. What is the best indication INITIALLY that the treatment is effective? Improved

   A.   cardiac output and urine output

   B.   breathing patterns

   C.   ability to ambulate

   D.   appetite

37. Which of the following is considered an adverse effect of a LeVeen shunt insertion?

   A.   weight loss of 10 pounds in one week

   B.   abdominal girth has decreased by one inch

   C.   hematuria and bleeding at IV site

   D.   nausea and vomiting

38. Following insertion of a LeVeen shunt, which intervention by the nurse will prevent fluid from being removed too rapidly from the peritoneal cavity?

   A.   ambulate the patient for 100 feet twice daily

   B.   restrict fluids to 1000 mL daily

   C.   place the patient in a sitting position

   D.   monitor abdominal girth daily

39. When checking a patient with liver failure, the nurse notices petechia and bruising on the forearms. This suggests

   A.   a clotting disorder exists

   B.   the LeVeen shunt has malfunctioned

   C.   a nutritional deficiency exists

   D.   a fluid imbalance is present

40. The nurse observes hematuria in a patient with a liver disorder. An appropriate nursing intervention would be to

   A.   instruct patient to avoid activities that can precipitate bleeding

   B.   apply pressure at all venipuncture sites for five minutes

   C.   have patient shave with an electric razor

   D.   all of the above

41. The nurse is aware that hepatic encephalopathy can occur in a patient with cirrhosis as a result of

   A.   excessive intake of fluids

   B.   excessive ingestion of protein and gastric bleeding

   C.   excessive restriction of proteins and fats

   D.   exposure to stressors

42. When a patient with a liver disorder exhibits restlessness, slurred speech, and tremors, the nurse would suspect

   A.   clotting disorder

   B.   portal hypertension

   C.   nutritional deficiency

   D.   hepatic encephalopathy

43. A patient with a hepatic disorder is on a diet to restrict ammonia production. The nurse instructs the patient to restrict

    A. fruit and fruit juice

    B. cheese and dairy products

    C. bread and cereal

    D. green and yellow vegetables

44. In caring for the patient with signs of hepatic encephalopathy, the nurse would probably administer

    A. Lasix or Dyazide

    B. Neosporin

    C. penicillin

    D. neomycin

45. The nurse is administering Lactulose to a patient. What is likely to occur as a result of this treatment?

    A. fluid diuresis

    B. hypokalemia

    C. diarrhea

    D. hematuria

46. In caring for a patient with hepatic encephalopathy, the nurse would expect to see an improvement in the condition when there is a decrease in the serum level of

    A. amylase

    B. ammonia

    C. potassium

    D. glucose

47. A nurse is assessing a patient with hepatic encephalopathy. Which assessment datum is a sign of impending coma?

    A. refusal to answer questions

    B. presence of asterixis (liver flap)

    C. presence of ecchymosis on abdomen

    D. increase in abdominal girth

48. A patient with alcoholism and a hepatic disorder is admitted with a nutritional deficiency. The reason for this condition is most likely

    A. inadequate nutrient intake

    B. excessive carbohydrate intake

    C. insufficient finances

    D. unilateral neglect

49. The chronic alcoholic is often at risk for developing malabsorption of certain vitamins because of

    A. insufficient fluid intake

    B. excessive intake of nonessential nutrients

    C. inflammation of the gastrointestinal tract

    D. lack of a balanced diet

50. The nurse is aware that the alcoholic patient often exhibits signs of impaired carbohydrate metabolism. Findings would include

    A. hyperglycemia

    B. hypoglycemia

    C. albuminuria

    D. proteinemia

51. A patient would likely be ordered to receive vitamin K if which of the following lab results is obtained?

    A. Prothrombin time is prolonged.

    B. Prothrombin time is decreased.

    C. Thromboplastin time is decreased.

    D. SGOT is elevated.

Nursing Care Plans

52. Write a nursing care plan for the patient who has had a paracentesis. Use the following nursing diagnosis.

    Nursing diagnosis: Fluid volume excess

    Patient outcome:

    Interventions:

53. Write a nursing care plan for the patient with advanced hepatic encephalopathy. Use the following diagnosis.

    Nursing Diagnosis: Potential for injury

    Patient outcome:

    Interventions:

54. Write a nursing care plan that will address the nutritional needs of the patient with cirrhosis and alcoholism who is being discharged and will be followed by a home-care nurse.

    Nursing diagnosis:

    Patient outcome:

    Interventions:

Case Studies

Case Study No. 1

Mr. H., 55, is admitted for diagnostic testing for possible liver disease. He has a history of drug- and alcohol abuse.

55. The nurse is reviewing the records. Liver damage would be indicated by an increase in serum

    A. AST or SGOT

    B. CK or CPK

    C. BUN and creatinine

    D. WBC, platelets

56. When assessing the patient, the nurse finds Mr. H. has rapid, shallow respirations and a large, firm abdomen. These findings would suggest the presence of

    A. jaundice

    B. dehydration

    C. ascites

    D. encephalopathy

57. Mr. H. is scheduled for a paracentesis. An important nursing intervention would include

    A.   positioning patient in prone position

    B.   having patient void immediately before procedure

    C.   administering preoperative medication

    D.   administering oxygen

58. After the procedure, which of the following symptoms would indicate a complication?

    A.   increase in pulse and decrease in blood pressure

    B.   discomfort in area of needle insertion

    C.   abdominal girth decreased by three inches

    D.   rise in blood pressure and pulse rate

The doctor diagnoses Mr. H. with portal hypertension and ascites. The patient will be discharged on medication and diet therapy.

59. The nurse would instruct the patient on the rationale for taking

    A.   diuretics

    B.   antibiotics

    C.   steroids

    D.   anticoagulants

60. The type of diet that is prescribed includes

    A.   low-sodium, high-protein food

    B.   high-sodium, high-carbohydrate food

    C.   low-sodium, moderate-protein food and avoidance of alcohol

    D.   high-protein, high-fat food and moderate alcohol intake

Case Study No. 2

Mr. B. is being treated for cirrhosis. He is exhibiting symptoms of hepatic encephalopathy. He has been admitted many times in the past with gastrointestinal bleeding and respiratory distress.

61. Assessment findings include rapid respirations, distant heart sounds, enlarged abdomen, altered thought process with confusion and tremors. The patient is at risk for

    A.   gastrointestinal bleeding

    B.   impending coma

    C.   fluid deficit

    D.   impaired tissue perfusion

62. The nurse would anticipate that this patient would exhibit an increase in serum levels of _____ as a result of his advanced cirrhosis.

    A.   albumin

    B.   globulin

    C.   total cholesterol

    D.   glucose

63. Medical management of Mr. B. will include preventing clotting disorders. The nurse would anticipate administering

    A.   vitamin B_{12}

    B.   vitamin C

    C.   vitamin K

    D.   potassium

64. In order to determine the source of Mr. B.'s bleeding, the nurse will prepare him for a(n)

    A.   MRI

    B.   CT scan

    C.   abdominal ultrasound

    D.   esophagoscopy

65. Mr. B. is receiving neomycin by mouth qid. The nurse is aware that the rationale for this treatment is

  A.   removal of byproducts of carbohydrate metabolism

  B.   reduction of the bacteria in the blood-stream

  C.   reduction in fluid retention in abdomen

  D.   reduction of ammonia-producing organisms in the intestine

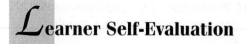

Learner Self-Evaluation

Do I fully understand the content? If no, then the areas I need to review are:

I need more information from my instructor on:

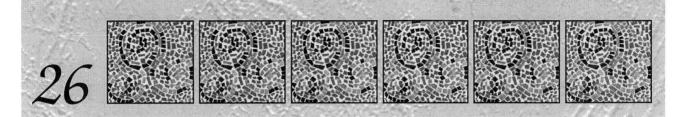

26

Nursing Care of Patients with Hepatic Disorders

Objectives

1.0 Demonstrate an understanding of the infectious and inflammatory disorders of the hepatic system.

    1.1 Identify the etiology, clinical manifestations and diagnostic procedures for infectious disorders.

    1.2 Identify and differentiate types of hepatitis.

    1.3 Identify ways to prevent hepatitis.

    1.4 Recognize the medical management of hepatitis.

    1.5 Write a nursing care plan for the patient with hepatitis.

2.0 Demonstrate an understanding of structural abnormalities of the hepatic system.

    2.1 Demonstrate an understanding of the etiology of several types of cirrhosis.

    2.2 Recognize the medical management of the patient with cirrhosis.

    2.3 Identify complications associated with cirrhosis.

    2.4 Identify nursing interventions appropriate for the patient with cirrhosis.

    2.5 Write a nursing care plan for the patient with cirrhosis.

3.0 Identify types of traumatic injuries that can affect the liver.

    3.1 Identify clinical manifestations associated with liver trauma.

    3.2 Identify medical management for the patient with liver trauma.

4.0 Demonstrate an understanding of the neoplasms that can affect the hepatic system.

    4.1 Identify clinical manifestations of hepatic tumors.

    4.2 Recognize the types of medical management for individuals with hepatic tumors.

    4.3 Recognize the surgical management of the patient with hepatic abnormalities.

*L*earning Activities

Short Answers

1. Acute viral hepatitis is characterized by

    inflammation and _____ of hepatic

    cells.

2. The _____ route is the major route of
    transmission of the hepatitis B virus (HBV).

3. Hepatitis C (HCV) is the leading cause of

    _____ hepatitis in the United States, Japan,

    and Europe.

4. The icteric phase of hepatitis begins with the

    appearance of _____.

5. The administration of immune serum

    globulin (ISG) can provide _____

    immunity for hepatitis A (HAV).

6. Chronic hepatitis C is one of the most

    common indications for _____

    _____.

7. Cirrhosis is a chronic disease that follows

    hepatocellular _____.

8. In all types of cirrhosis, abstinence from

    _____ is important.

9. _____ is the procedure of choice for
    long-term control of actively bleeding
    esophageal varices.

10. Candidates for liver transplant must be in

    the _____ stage of hepatic disease.

True/False

11. _____ Hepatitis B (HBV) is found in sweat,
    tears, semen, and saliva.

12. _____ Hepatitis E (HEV) is transmitted by
    needle sticks.

13. _____ Vaccines for HAV have been found to
    be effective.

14. _____ Hepatitis B vaccine is recommended for
    all health-care workers.

15. _____ Previously healthy individuals who
    develop hepatitis usually recover
    completely.

16. _____ In chronic hepatitis, there is liver cell
    necrosis and portal tract obstruction.

17. _____ Chronic active hepatitis can progress to
    cirrhosis.

18. _____ Individuals who develop fulminant
    hepatitis will recover completely.

19. _____ Primary biliary cirrhosis is the most
    common form of cirrhosis.

20. _____ Bleeding from esophageal varices is
    life-threatening.

Knowledge Application

21. The type of hepatitis that is related to poor
    sanitation and can be spread by contami-
    nated food is
    A.   HAV
    B.   HBV
    C.   HCV
    D.   HGV

22. The type of hepatitis that is related to an
    increase in IV drug use and sexual activity
    with multiple partners is
    A.   HAV
    B.   HBV
    C.   HDV
    D.   all of the above

23. The best way to characterize the process of hepatitis is

    A. liver cell necrosis, inflammation, cell regeneration

    B. liver cell necrosis, degeneration, chronicity

    C. liver cell hypoxia, obstruction

    D. liver cell destruction, scarring, infiltration

24. A nurse has been exposed to HBV. The incubation for this disease can be as long as

    A. 20 days

    B. 45 days

    C. 90 days

    D. 160 days

25. Clinical manifestations associated with the preicteric phase of hepatitis include

    A. anorexia, jaundice

    B. fatigue, nausea, anorexia

    C. right upper quadrant pain, fatigue

    D. vomiting, diarrhea, dark urine, dark stool

26. The nurse should explain to a patient with hepatitis with obstruction of bile flow that he or she will have

    A. light-colored urine

    B. dark, tarry stools

    C. dark-colored urine

    D. pale skin

27. A patient is admitted with acute viral hepatitis. The nurse would expect to see a rise in serum _____.

    A. PT, PTT

    B. AST, ESR

    C. potassium

    D. BUN, creatinine

28. Assessment findings that would demonstrate to the nurse that the patient with hepatitis is in the recovery phase would include

    A. weight returns to normal, ascites disappear

    B. jaundice disappears, normal energy levels return

    C. normal heart and breath sounds, active bowel sounds

    D. stool and urine normal in color, appetite improves

29. When an individual with hepatitis has an obstruction in bile flow, it is due to

    A. hepatocyte inflammation

    B. liver cell necrosis

    C. leukopenia

    D. biliary obstruction

30. A health-care institute is testing its staff for presence of hepatitis markers. The best explanation of what the presence of which markers in the serum indicates is

    A. exposure to a hepatitis virus with antibody formation

    B. active hepatitis current in system

    C. past infection with hepatitis virus

    D. immunity to the HAV

31. If one of the nurses is found to have the hepatitis marker HBeAg in her serum, it would indicate

    A. current infection of HAV

    B. current infection of HBV

    C. past infection of HBV

    D. present infection of HCV

32. Medical management for the patient with acute viral hepatitis would include

    A. hospitalization, antibiotic therapy

    B. bed rest, hydration, antibiotics

    C. rest, avoid fatigue, well-balanced diet

    D. bed rest, low-calorie diet, force fluids

33. Once an individual has had an episode of hepatitis, the nurse would be sure to include which of the following instructions?

   A.   avoid all foods high in protein

   B.   avoid alcohol

   C.   don't donate blood

   D.   stop smoking

34. The administration of HBV immunoglobin is indicated in which of the following instances?

   A.   A nurse has received a needlestick injury.

   B.   A person is positive for HBsAg.

   C.   A person is splashed in the face with HBsAg material.

   D.   A patient is traveling to an area where HBV is endemic.

35. There is an increase in the number of cases of both HAV and HBV in health-care institutes. Nurses are at the highest risk of developing HBV in which area?

   A.   emergency room

   B.   intensive care unit

   C.   dialysis unit

   D.   cardiac unit

36. The administration of HBV vaccine would be recommended for which of the following individuals?

   A.   hemodialysis patient

   B.   homosexually active males

   C.   sexual contacts of HBV carriers

   D.   all of the above

37. When a patient is admitted with a possible liver abscess, which test would be most helpful during diagnosis?

   A.   chest x-ray

   B.   ultrasonogram

   C.   V-Q scan

   D.   MRI scan

38. Which nursing action has the highest priority when caring for the patient with multiple liver abscesses?

   A.   maintain strict bed rest

   B.   administer antibiotics on time

   C.   maintain fluid restrictions

   D.   administer pain medications as needed

39. A patient is admitted to the hospital with toxic hepatitis. On review of the chart, the nurse identifies which information as having a possible relationship to the current problem?

   A.   recent travel to Haiti

   B.   recent discharge from the army

   C.   employed by dry-cleaning company

   D.   ingestion of two glasses of wine daily

40. In caring for the patient with toxic hepatitis, the nurse's responsibility would include

   A.   prevention of reexposure to hepatotoxin

   B.   administration of analgesics frequently

   C.   prevention of skin breakdown

   D.   administering antibiotics

41. Elderly individuals are at risk for the development of toxic hepatitis because of

   A.   poor dietary habits

   B.   decrease in level of activity

   C.   increased susceptibility to infection

   D.   use of multiple medications

42. The type of cirrhosis that has been linked to alcohol consumption is known as

   A.   primary biliary cirrhosis

   B.   necrotic cirrhosis

   C.   Laennec's cirrhosis

   D.   secondary obstructive cirrhosis

43. One of the first manifestations of liver damage that results from alcoholism is

    A. fatty cirrhosis

    B. muscle wasting

    C. alcoholic hepatitis

    D. biliary obstruction

44. When working with individuals with cirrhosis, the nurse is aware that regardless of the cause of the problem, the end result will be

    A. fatty nodules and liver abscess formation

    B. biliary tract obstruction

    C. destruction and regeneration of liver cells

    D. destruction of hepatocytes and impaired liver function

45. The nurse should consider which nursing diagnosis a priority when caring for a patient with newly diagnosed Laennec's cirrhosis?

    A. Ineffective breathing patterns

    B. Ineffective coping strategies related to chronic disease

    C. Alteration in nutrition: more than body requirements

    D. Knowledge deficit related to disease cause and prognosis

46. The nurse's responsibility in preventing complications associated with cirrhosis includes monitoring for

    A. signs of bleeding

    B. fluid and electrolyte imbalance

    C. signs of skin breakdown

    D. signs of malnutrition

47. Medical management of a patient who has esophageal varices would include the administration of

    A. corticosteroids

    B. antibiotic therapy

    C. vasopressin

    D. streptokinase

48. The physician orders oral neomycin every four hours for a patient with cirrhosis. The nurse explains to the patient that the purpose of this therapy is to

    A. reduce edema and abdominal swelling

    B. remove intestinal contents and block ammonia formation

    C. prevent esophageal and rectal bleeding

    D. prevent infection from spreading throughout system

49. The nurse carefully observes the patient with cirrhosis for signs of portal systemic encephalopathy. A change in which of the following may be a precursor to encephalopathy?

    A. blood pressure and pulse

    B. level of consciousness

    C. urine output

    D. level of mobility

50. A patient is admitted to the emergency room following a car accident. Which of the following signs would indicate liver trauma?

    A. restlessness, signs of shock, absent bowel sounds

    B. anxiety, rise in blood pressure and heart rate

    C. vomiting, sharp abdominal pain

    D. agitation, altered level of consciousness

51. Management of a suspected liver laceration in an unstable patient would involve

    A. monitoring vital signs every hour

    B. surgical intervention

    C. administering blood products

    D. stabilizing and transferring to a trauma unit

52. A patient is admitted with a possible neoplasm of the liver. The nurse is aware that a definitive diagnosis can be made by

    A. scanning techniques

    B. results of lab work

    C. liver biopsy

    D. abdominal x-ray

53. A patient with liver cancer is to receive chemotherapy via a hepatic catheter. An important nursing responsibility would be to

    A.   prepare patient for a lengthy hospitalization

    B.   instruct patient to perform wet-to-dry dressing changes

    C.   provide dietary instructions and limitations

    D.   instruct patient in aseptic care of the catheter and pump

54. A primary nursing responsibility when caring for the patient who has received a liver transplant involves

    A.   frequent vital signs and neuro checks

    B.   monitoring for signs of infection or rejection

    C.   monitoring continuous feedings

    D.   preventing ventilator malfunction

55. The nurse is caring for a patient who has received a liver transplant. Which of the following is a positive sign indicating liver function?

    A.   thick, green bile drainage from the T-tube

    B.   decrease in abdominal girth

    C.   increased output with decreased edema

    D.   stable vital signs, normal urine and stools

56. When assessing the patient who has had a liver transplant, the nurse finds the patient has a low-grade fever and joint pain. This can indicate

    A.   infection

    B.   rejection

    C.   suppression

    D.   either A or B

57. Because the patient who has received a liver transplant must take large doses of steroids and immunosuppressants, the nurse would monitor for signs of

    A.   infection

    B.   rejection

    C.   hemorrhage

    D.   obstruction

Nursing Care Plans

58. Write a nursing care plan for the patient with HAV. Use the following diagnosis.

    Nursing diagnosis: High risk for altered health maintenance related to insufficient knowledge of disease process and mode of transmission

    Patient outcome:

    Interventions:

59. Write a nursing care plan for the patient with cirrhosis and encephalopathy. Use the following nursing diagnosis.

    Nursing diagnosis: Potential for injury related to altered thought process

    Patient outcome:

    Interventions:

60. Plan the care of the person who has undergone a liver transplant and is ready for discharge. Focus on the discharge planning.

Nursing diagnosis:

Patient outcome:

Interventions:

Case Studies

Case Study No. 1

Ms. A. is admitted with fatigue, anorexia, and jaundice. She is homeless and was brought to the hospital by police. A tentative diagnosis of hepatitis is made.

61. Because of the symptoms that Ms. A. currently has, the nurse would expect to see an increase in serum

    A. WBC

    B. BUN

    C. ammonia

    D. bilirubin

62. A diagnosis of HAV is made. This is confirmed by the presence of which hepatitis marker?

    A. HAV-Ab/IgM

    B. HAV-Ab/IgG

    C. HBeAg

    D. anti-HCV

63. Which of the following information provided by Ms. A. is a clue as to how she contracted the disease?

    A. "I sleep in the shelters."

    B. "I don't have warm clothes."

    C. "I eat out of garbage cans."

    D. "I have a friend who uses drugs."

64. An important nursing intervention for the acute phase of Ms. A.'s illness would be to

    A. provide rest periods frequently throughout day

    B. increase fluid intake, especially water

    C. measure abdominal girth daily

    D. increase activity as tolerated

65. The nurse is aware that the virus that causes HAV will be excreted from Ms. A.'s system mainly through

    A. skin

    B. feces

    C. urine

    D. saliva

Case Study No. 2

Mr. B. is admitted with cirrhosis. He states he drinks heavily and has been admitted several times for bleeding. He has jaundice and a protruding abdomen. He is complaining of right upper quadrant pain.

66. During the initial assessment, the nurse gathers enough data to indicate that Mr. B. may have portal hypertension. Assuming all these findings are present, which one would lead to that conclusion?

    A. jaundiced appearance

    B. low-grade fever

    C. ascites and edema

    D. palpable liver

67. Mr. B. begins to hemorrhage. The physician inserts a Sengstaken-Blakemore tube to control the bleeding. The rationale for this treatment is

   A.   the suction removes the bleeding

   B.   it provides a route to administer medications

   C.   the inflated balloon exerts pressure on the bleeding site

   D.   it provides a route for rapid blood administration

68. To prevent any complications associated with the use of the Sengstaken-Blakemore tube, the nurse will carefully assess

   A.   cardiac function

   B.   respiratory status

   C.   fluid status

   D.   neurologic status

69. The physician is able to stop the bleeding and stabilize the patient. He decides that Mr. B. may benefit from sclerotherapy. The nursing care would include

   A.   preparing the patient for endoscopy procedure

   B.   preparing the patient for surgery

   C.   administering vasopressors

   D.   administering antibiotics

70. Mr. B. is complaining of dry, itchy skin. The nurse is aware that this is a result of which problem associated with cirrhosis?

   A.   elevated protime

   B.   elevated bilirubin

   C.   decreased sodium and potassium

   D.   impaired synthesis of vitamin K

Mr. B. is discharged, but is readmitted in five days with another episode of bleeding.

71. The physician orders vasopressin (Pitressin). The purpose of this medication is to

   A.   increase the portal venous pressure

   B.   lower the portal venous pressure

   C.   stimulate clotting factors

   D.   prevent further necrosis

72. Unfortunately, Mr. B. does not respond well to medical therapy or sclerotherapy. Another treatment option would involve

   A.   liver transplant

   B.   portocaval shunt

   C.   insertion of Levin tube

   D.   transjugular intrahepatic shunt

73. Upon discharge, the family is aware that this procedure may have controlled the bleeding but

   A.   it does not improve long-term survival

   B.   he will still need a transplant

   C.   he will need further sclerotherapy

   D.   he may develop liver cancer

_L_earner Self-Evaluation

Do I fully understand the content? If no, then the areas I need to review are:

I need more information from my instructor on:

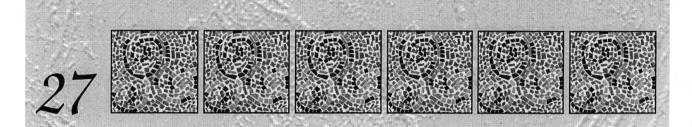

Knowledge Base for Patients with Endocrine Dysfunction

Objectives

1.0 Review the functions of the endocrine system.

    1.1 Identify the major endocrine glands on a diagram.

    1.2 Identify specific hormones secreted by the specific glands.

    1.3 Match specific hormones with their primary hormonal functions.

2.0 Demonstrate an understanding of specific manifestations of endocrine dysfunctions.

    2.1 Identify assessment data that are characteristic of endocrine dysfunction.

    2.2 Demonstrate application of the nursing process when caring for a patient with an endocrine dysfunction.

$\mathcal{L}$earning Activities

Identification

1. On the diagram, identify the major endocrine glands.

   A. Pituitary gland

   B. Hypothalamus

   C. Thyroid

   D. Parathyroid

   E. Adrenal gland

   F. Pancreatic islets

   G. Ovaries

   H. Testes

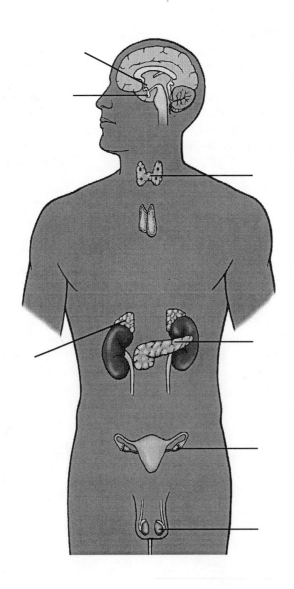

Short Answers

2. Hormones can affect a _____ or can have a general effect on the entire body.

3. One way that the concentration of hormones in the blood is maintained is by

   _____.

4. The pituitary gland is also known as

   _____.

5. Secretion of insulin in the pancreas occurs in

   the _____.

6. Interactions between hormones and their target organs are controlled by the

   _____ system and the

   _____ system.

7. When the blood level of a substance affected by a hormone falls, hormone production is

   _____.

8. Dysfunction of the hypothalamus will result

   in _____ dysfunction.

9. The primary glucocorticoid secreted by the

   adrenal cortex is _____.

10. The adrenal _____ is the primary source of epinephrine in the body.

Basic Knowledge

Next to each of the following endocrine glands, list the principal hormone it secretes.

Hormone

11. Thymus _____

12. Pineal _____

13. Hypothalamus _____

14. Pituitary _____

15. Thyroid _____

16. Adrenals _____

17. Pancreatic islets _____

Identification

Match each of the hormones with its primary function.

    A. Insulin

    B. Glucagon

    C. Estrogen

    D. Testosterone

    E. Somatotropin

    F. Thyroxine

    G. Calcitonin

    H. Adrenalin

    I. Aldosterone

    J. Antidiuretic hormone

18. _____ Promotes sodium and water retention and potassium excretion

19. _____ Regulates energy production, growth, and development

20. _____ Stimulates closure of the epiphysial plates at puberty

21. _____ Stimulates the stress response

22. _____ Regulates osmolality of extracellular fluids

23. _____ Regulates metabolism of fat, protein, and carbohydrates

24. _____ Increases the rate that calcium is deposited in the bones

25. _____ Necessary for the maturation of the reproductive system

26. _____ Stimulates growth of cells, bones, and muscles

27. _____ Raises blood glucose levels by promoting hepatic glycogenolysis

True/False

28. _____ A cell will not respond to a hormone unless it has receptor sites for that hormone.

29. _____ The functions of the adrenal cortex are nonessential.

30. _____ Dysfunction of one endocrine gland often affects the function of another.

31. _____ Hypersecretion from an endocrine gland is often the result of a tumor.

32. _____ Secondary glandular dysfunction is usually permanent.

Knowledge Application

33. The nurse would monitor for signs of glucose intolerance when a patient has
    A. acromegaly
    B. Cushing's disease
    C. pheochromocytoma
    D. Graves' disease

34. An individual with abnormal production of _____ is at risk for developing osteoporosis.
    A. adrenalin
    B. aldosterone
    C. calcitonin
    D. cortisol

35. A deficiency in the production of which hormone will lead to symptoms of diabetes insipidus?
    A. insulin
    B. glucagon
    C. estrogen
    D. antidiuretic hormone

36. A deficiency in the production of which hormone will lead to symptoms of diabetes mellitus?
    A. glucagon
    B. insulin
    C. prolactin
    D. epinephrine

37. When a patient has an alteration in serum calcium and phosphorus levels, the nurse would suspect an alteration in function of this gland.
    A. thyroid
    B. parathyroid
    C. pancreas
    D. adrenal

38. When an individual has a low dietary intake of iodine and protein, they are at risk for dysfunction of which of the following glands?
    A. thyroid
    B. parathyroids
    C. adrenal
    D. pituitary

39. When an individual is subjected to a very stressful experience, he or she would have increased amounts of _____ secreted.
    A. epinephrine
    B. insulin
    C. estrogen
    D. thyroxine

40. One of the most noticeable age-related changes in the endocrine system is
    A. decrease in the ability to respond to stress
    B. increase in the number of endocrine disorders
    C. change in glucose production
    D. erratic production of hormones

41. The primary function of thyroxine is to
    A. regulate cell metabolism and energy production
    B. cause release of corticosteroids
    C. regulate water reabsorption
    D. regulate blood glucose levels

Case Study

A patient is admitted with a suspected endocrine abnormality. Symptoms include alteration in blood sugar, weakness, and irritability.

42. Diagnostic testing to determine the cause of the problem will mainly include

    A.   x-ray

    B.   laboratory studies

    C.   ultrasound

    D.   MRI

43. Based on the initial symptoms, the nurse would suspect an alteration in the function of which gland?

    A.   adrenal

    B.   thyroid

    C.   pancreas

    D.   parathyroids

44. If this condition is a primary endocrine gland dysfunction it implies that

    A.   the gland is secreting too much or too little hormone due to a defect in the gland itself

    B.   the gland is secreting abnormal amounts of hormone in response to changes in the pituitary gland

    C.   there is idiopathic hyperplasia of the affected gland

    D.   the primary gland is causing dysfunction of the secondary gland

45. While collecting the history from the patient, it would be important to

    A.   determine if the patient knows the reason for admission

    B.   have someone familiar with the patient present

    C.   determine if symptoms developed gradually or rapidly

    D.   determine if the patient has characteristic symptoms

    E.   all of the above

46. Emotional support and teaching are probably the most important nursing functions to help the individual because

    A.   the disease is usually life-threatening

    B.   it is almost impossible to comply with the many restrictions they will have

    C.   the individual will need to make adjustments in lifestyle and take lifelong medications

    D.   the disease will require a change of profession and much less activity

*L*earner Self-Evaluation

Do I fully understand the content? If no, then the areas I need to review are:

I need more information from my instructor on:

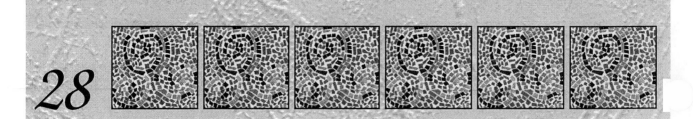

28

Nursing Care of Patients with Diabetes Mellitus

Objectives

1.0 Demonstrate an understanding of the pathophysiology of diabetes mellitus.
   1.1 Demonstrate an understanding of the hormonal regulation of blood glucose levels.
   1.2 Identify clinical manifestations of diabetes mellitus.
   1.3 Identify characteristics of type I and type II diabetes.
   1.4 Identify how the diagnosis of diabetes mellitus is made.

2.0 Demonstrate an understanding of the medical management of diabetes mellitus.
   2.1 Identify medications used in the treatment of diabetes mellitus.
   2.2 Identify ways to manage the diabetic during illness.
   2.3 Identify alternative treatments and care settings for individuals with diabetes.

3.0 Demonstrate an understanding of the complications that can occur in the patient with diabetes.
   3.1 Identify acute and chronic complications of diabetes mellitus.
   3.2 Identify nursing interventions used to treat complications of diabetes mellitus.
   3.3 Write a nursing care plan for the patient with diabetes mellitus.

Learning Activities

Short Answers

1. Diabetes mellitus is characterized by persistent _____.

2. The effects of insulin on carbohydrate metabolism are to _____ glucose metabolism, _____ blood glucose concentration, and _____ glycogen stores.

3. Insulin promotes fatty acid synthesis by converting _____ into fatty acids.

4. The process of converting glycogen back to glucose, called glycogenolysis, is done by the

   _____.

5. It has been proven that close control of

   _____ _____ levels will delay or prevent development of long-term complications of diabetes.

6. The level at which glucose enters the kidney tubules and spills into the urine is known as

   the _____ _____.

7. The most widely used concentration of

   insulin is _____.

8. The goal of insulin therapy is to

   _____ normal insulin production.

9. Symptoms of hyperglycemic hyperosmolar nonketotic syndrome (HHNKS) include

   profound _____ and _____.

10. The _____ phenomenon is characterized by an increase in fasting blood glucose levels between 5 AM and 9 AM.

True/False

11. _____ Gestational diabetes usually disappears after delivery.

12. _____ Opened bottles of insulin may be stored at room temperature.

13. _____ Patients with type II diabetes mellitus often do not have classic symptoms.

14. _____ The sulfonylureas should be considered oral insulin.

15. _____ Hypoglycemic reactions cannot occur when taking sulfonylureas.

16. _____ The diabetic patient must assume responsibility for management of his or her condition.

17. _____ The diabetic diet is the cornerstone of treatment for the diabetic patient.

18. _____ It is very important to exercise if blood glucose is higher than 250 mg/dL.

19. _____ Humulin insulin comes from cadaver pancreases.

20. _____ Diabetics should stop taking insulin if they become ill.

21. _____ Glucose tolerance declines with increasing age.

Knowledge Application

22. All of the following are counterregulatory hormones and will oppose the action of insulin EXCEPT

   A. glucagon

   B. cortisol

   C. growth hormone

   D. antidiuretic hormone

23. When a patient with hyperglycemia is admitted, the nurse would assess carefully for signs of

   A. dehydration, electrolyte depletion

   B. fluid retention, high potassium levels

   C. cardiac arrhythmias

   D. infection, pain

24. If the fasting blood glucose level is over _____ mg/dL on more than one occasion, the diagnosis of diabetes can be made.

   A. 80

   B. 100

   C. 140

   D. 180

25. When the patient with diabetes has insufficient insulin to metabolize carbohydrates there will be a(n)

    A.   decrease in breakdown of fats

    B.   increase in the production of ketones

    C.   decrease in breakdown of ketones

    D.   development of respiratory alkalosis

26. The major characteristic of type II diabetes is

    A.   impaired receptor sites

    B.   excess of insulin

    C.   lack of insulin

    D.   insulin resistance

27. The main difference between type I and type II diabetes is that the type I diabetic

    A.   must follow a diabetic diet

    B.   must take daily insulin

    C.   has more complications

    D.   has a history of obesity

28. The diagnosis of diabetes is based on

    A.   glucose tolerance test, hormone testing

    B.   presence of symptoms, fasting glucose levels

    C.   symptoms of polyuria, polydipsia, polyphagia

    D.   family history, current complaint

29. An appropriate diet for a diabetic should include _____ carbohydrates, _____ fat, and _____ protein.

    A.   30%, 30%, 40%

    B.   40%, 20%, 40%

    C.   55%, 30%, 15%

    D.   55%, 15%, 30%

30. It is important for the nurse to instruct the patient with diabetes about the value of exercise since it

    A.   acts as a hypoglycemic

    B.   can help normalize blood sugar

    C.   can eliminate the need for insulin

    D.   helps prevent infections

31. When an elderly patient with type II diabetes develops influenza, he or she is at risk for developing

    A.   hypoglycemia

    B.   diabetic ketoacidosis

    C.   HHNKS

    D.   systemic infection

32. The initial therapy for the newly diagnosed elderly patient with diabetes whose blood glucose levels are below 250 mg/dL would be

    A.   diet therapy

    B.   oral hypoglycemics

    C.   insulin therapy

    D.   insulin and exercise program

33. It would be important for the nurse to instruct the diabetic patient that if he or she becomes ill, to

    A.   monitor blood sugar levels every four to six hours

    B.   stop taking insulin until symptoms subside

    C.   come to the hospital immediately

    D.   follow any diet that makes him or her feel better

34. When a diabetic patient is admitted for surgery, the methods of administering the daily insulin would be to

    A.   give the normal dose of insulin

    B.   give ⅓ to ½ the usual dose of long-acting insulin

    C.   make the patient NPO and withhold insulin

    D.   give regular insulin every two hours

35. When a patient has diabetic neuropathy, it is very important for the nurse to monitor for

    A.   neurologic changes

    B.   changes in skin on lower extremities

    C.   signs of nausea, vomiting, diarrhea

    D.   signs of infection

36. The rationale for the measurement of glycosylated hemoglobin in the individual with diabetes is

    A. to be sure the patient is taking insulin

    B. to assess if the patient is following the diet

    C. to assess blood glucose levels over the previous three months

    D. so that the patient doesn't have to do the daily blood glucose testing

37. Emergency treatment for the patient admitted with diabetic ketoacidosis would include

    A. rapid administration of D_5W and insulin

    B. replacement of fluid, electrolytes, and dextrose

    C. administration of .45% saline and insulin via pump

    D. the use of .9% saline, sodium bicarbonate, and potassium

38. What is the reason that the patient should be instructed to bring insulin to room temperature before injecting?

    A. It will hurt if it is cold.

    B. Cold temperatures can affect the rate of absorption.

    C. To prevent hypoglycemia.

    D. It is harder to draw up when it is cold.

39. If a diabetic patient exhibits symptoms of shaking, sweating, weakness, hunger, and drowsiness, the nurse should administer

    A. 4 oz. fruit juice or regular soda

    B. 8 oz. of juice with two lumps of sugar

    C. 1 ampule of 50% dextrose

    D. regular insulin as ordered

40. When a patient is to be discharged with an insulin pump, he or she needs to be instructed on possible complications. These can include (check all that apply)

    A. hypoglycemia

    B. ketoacidosis

    C. infection at site

    D. pump failure

41. Which of the following patients would be the best candidate for a pancreas transplant?

    A. insulin-dependent male, age 20

    B. patient who is poorly controlled with insulin and has frequent episodes of hypo- and hyperglycemia

    C. patient who is unable to learn how to administer insulin or follow diet

    D. female, age 70, who can no longer take oral hypoglycemics

42. The nurse would monitor the patient with a pancreas transplant for early signs of rejection including

    A. hypoglycemia

    B. hyperglycemia

    C. fever, weakness

    D. nausea, vomiting

43. If a patient with diabetes has a hyperglycemic reaction, typical symptoms include

    A. diaphoresis, hunger, confusion

    B. blurred vision, thirst, nausea, vomiting

    C. cool, clammy skin; dizziness; drowsiness

    D. any of the above

44. The individual most likely to develop HHNKS is

    A. elderly hospitalized patient with type II diabetes

    B. newly diagnosed middle-aged female with type II diabetes

    C. hospitalized young adult with type I diabetes

    D. young adult athlete with type I diabetes

45. For the patient with diabetic nephropathy, an important nursing measure is

    A.   maintaining normal blood pressure

    B.   providing dietary instruction

    C.   contacting a support group

    D.   administration of insulin

46. The _____ _____ is characterized by periods of hypoglycemia followed by rebound hyperglycemia.

    A.   dawn phenomenon

    B.   degenerative effect

    C.   Somogyi phenomenon

    D.   ketosis effect

47. The main treatment for diabetic retinopathy is

    A.   medication

    B.   corrective lens

    C.   laser treatment

    D.   surgical correction

48. When a patient with peripheral neuropathy develops muscle weakness and sensory loss, the nursing goal would be to

    A.   prevent pain

    B.   prevent injury

    C.   treat symptoms

    D.   educate patient

49. When a diabetic patient has symptoms that include hyperglycemia, proteinuria, hypertension, and edema, this suggests diabetic

    A.   nephropathy

    B.   retinopathy

    C.   neuropathy

    D.   ketosis

50. To prevent rejection following a pancreas transplant, the patient must take

    A.   insulin

    B.   oral hypoglycemics

    C.   immunosuppressive medications

    D.   prophylactic antibiotics

51. If the nurse administers 35 units of Humulin NPH insulin at 7:30 AM, it would be important for the patient to receive a snack at

    A.   11 AM

    B.   1 PM

    C.   4 PM

    D.   8 PM

52. To help determine if a patient with symptoms of hyperglycemia has DKA or HHNKS, which laboratory finding would the nurse check?

    A.   blood sugar

    B.   potassium

    C.   white blood count

    D.   ketones

Nursing Care Plans

53. Write a care plan for the patient with diabetes mellitus. Focus on the discharge planning for the newly diagnosed diabetic.

    Nursing diagnosis: High risk for altered health maintenance related to insufficient knowledge of diabetic self-management

    Patient outcome:

    Interventions:

54. Write a care plan for the hospitalized patient with macrovascular disease secondary to diabetes. Write an appropriate nursing diagnosis and care plan.

    Nursing diagnosis:

    Patient outcome:

    Interventions:

Case Studies

Case Study No. 1

A young adult male is admitted to the hospital with a severe respiratory infection. Lab results show a blood glucose of 450 mg/dL. Further testing establishes that the patient has diabetes type I. The patient denies any history or symptoms of the disease.

55. Why would this patient develop diabetes at this time?

    A. The acute infection precipitated the event.

    B. He used up all his insulin.

    C. He is in the high-risk age group.

    D. He must have parents with the disease.

56. The treatment of choice for this patient will include (Check all that apply.)

    A. _____ diet

    B. _____ insulin

    C. _____ exercise

    D. _____ oral hypoglycemics

    E. _____ pancreatic transplant

57. The nurse would instruct the patient to watch for signs of hypoglycemia when he is taking insulin. Causes of this condition include all EXCEPT

    A. too much insulin

    B. too much food

    C. too much activity

    D. ingestion of alcohol

58. Because of the long-term complications that often occur with type I diabetes, the nurse would instruct the patient to

    A. have a yearly eye exam

    B. join a health club

    C. check his feet daily

    D. have a yearly exam by a cardiologist

Case Study No. 2

A 50-year-old male was found to have a blood glucose of 288 mg/dL during a spot check at a local health fair. He is very surprised by this.

59. Which of the characteristic findings might the nurse expect to find in the history? (Check all that apply.)

    A. _____ obesity

    B. _____ inactivity

    C. _____ family history

    D. _____ recent infection

60. What is the most likely diagnosis for this patient?

    A. type I diabetes

    B. type II diabetes

    C. gestational diabetes

    D. impaired glucose tolerance

61. The treatment of choice for this patient will probably involve

    A. insulin and diet

    B. exercise and diet

    C. oral hypoglycemics and diet

    D. insulin and antibiotics

62. This individual is most at risk for developing which of the following complications?

    A.   diabetic retinopathy

    B.   diabetic foot ulcer

    C.   hypoglycemia

    D.   diabetic ketoacidosis

Case Study No. 3

A 75-year-old female is admitted to the hospital from a nursing home. She has a history of type II diabetes, arthritis, and cerebrovascular accident. Currently she is dehydrated and having diarrhea. Laboratory findings show a blood sugar of 880 mg/dL and an osmolality of 400 mOsm/kg.

63. Based on the above information, the nurse would suspect that this individual has

    A.   hyperglycemia

    B.   diabetic ketoacidosis

    C.   HHNKS

    D.   sepsis

64. Appropriate treatment would involve

    A.   fluid replacement, correction of electrolyte deficiency, regular insulin

    B.   giving NPH insulin and .9% saline for dehydration

    C.   insulin drip, 10% dextrose in saline

    D.   electrolyte replacement, sodium bicarbonate

65. On the second day, the nurse finds the patient talking incoherently. She is shaky, diaphoretic, tachycardiac, and very anxious. These symptoms suggest

    A.   hyperglycemia

    B.   hypoglycemia

    C.   dehydration

    D.   stroke

66. An appropriate nursing intervention at this time would be to

    A.   stop insulin infusion, check blood glucose

    B.   call the physician

    C.   draw blood gases

    D.   increase IV fluids, give patient simple sugar

Learner Self-Evaluation

Do I fully understand the content? If no, then the areas I need to review are:

I need more information from my instructor on:

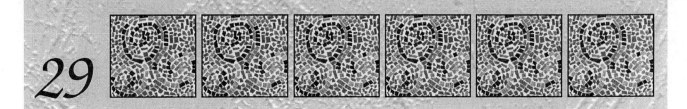

29

Nursing Care of Patients with Other Endocrine Disorders

*O*bjectives

1.0 Demonstrate an understanding of the pathophysiology of the endocrine system.
    1.1 Demonstrate an understanding of the role of hormonal regulation in other endocrine disorders.
    1.2 Identify clinical manifestations of endocrine disorders.

2.0 Demonstrate an understanding of adrenal, pituitary, thyroid, and parathyroid disorders of the endocrine system.
    2.1 Identify the etiology and clinical manifestations of common endocrine disorders.
    2.2 Identify diagnostic procedures and medical and surgical management of common endocrine disorders.

2.3 Demonstrate an understanding of the nursing interventions used in caring for the patient with a common endocrine disorder.
2.4 Plan the nursing care for patients with common endocrine disorders.
2.5 Identify the special considerations for the elderly patient with an endocrine disorder.

*L*earning Activities

Short Answers

1. The _____ gland is a vital link between the hypothalamus and the endocrine system.

2. Addison's disease most often results from destruction of the adrenal gland by an

    _____ process.

3. Cushing's syndrome is a disorder characterized by oversecretion of _____ hormones.

4. Catecholamine-producing tumors that occur in the adrenal medulla are known as

    _____.

5. Adequate daily intake of _____ and

    _____ is necessary for the synthesis of
    thyroid hormones.

6. The production and secretion of thyroxine is

    controlled by the secretion of _____.

7. The thyroid secretes _____, which
    lowers serum calcium.

8. The most common form of chronic thyroidi-

    tis is known as _____.

9. The primary function of the parathyroid

    gland is to regulate _____ and

    _____ levels.

10. Serum calcium levels will _____ as parathy-
    roid hormone is secreted.

Identification

Match the following adrenal hormones with their
action(s).

    A. Mineralocorticoids

    B. Glucocorticoids

    C. Androgens

11. _____ Promote sodium retention and potas-
    sium excretion

12. _____ Influence development of secondary
    sex characteristics

13. _____ Stimulate gluconeogenesis by the liver

14. _____ Aldosterone is an example of these

15. _____ Secretion is controlled by ACTH
    secretion

16. _____ Cortisol is the primary example of these

True/False

17. _____ The posterior lobe of the pituitary
    gland is neural in origin.

18. _____ Secretion of all anterior pituitary
    hormones is monitored by the hypo-
    thalamus.

19. _____ Following treatment for acromegaly,
    the symptoms will be reversed.

20. _____ Epinephrine secretion has a major effect
    on the cardiovascular system.

21. _____ The incidence of hypothyroidism
    increases with age.

22. _____ Treatment for hypothyroidism lasts six
    to nine months.

23. _____ Hyperthyroidism may be precipitated
    by stress.

24. _____ Acute hypocalcemic tetany is a medical
    emergency.

25. _____ Vitamin D is necessary for calcium
    absorption.

26. _____ Calcium supplements are given after a
    parathyroidectomy.

Knowledge Application

27. The most common manifestation of a pitu-
    itary tumor is

    A. frequent headaches

    B. visual disturbances

    C. dizziness

    D. vomiting

28. When a patient has had surgical removal of a pituitary neoplasm, the nurse would monitor carefully any early sign of increasing intracranial pressure (ICP), such as:

    A. lethargy

    B. narrow pulse pressure

    C. tachycardia

    D. agitation

29. Following surgery for a pituitary adenoma the nurse would monitor for signs of the most common complication, which is

    A. fluid retention

    B. diabetes insipidus

    C. seizures

    D. panhypopituitarism

30. Which of the following would indicate a potential complication following transsphenoidal microsurgery for a pituitary adenoma?

    A. urine output less than 40 mL/hour

    B. urine output greater than 100 mL/hour

    C. headache postoperatively

    D. nausea and anorexia

31. Individuals with excess secretion of somatotropin are at high risk for development of

    A. renal failure

    B. cardiac disease

    C. diabetes mellitus

    D. infections

32. The most accurate way to test for an excess of growth hormone is by

    A. CT scan

    B. laboratory testing

    C. MRI

    D. radioimmunoassay

33. The treatment of choice for the individual with severe symptoms of acromegaly due to a trauma is

    A. external irradiation

    B. treatment with Parlodel

    C. transsphenoidal microsurgery

    D. chemotherapy

34. Discharge instructions for the patient with a deficiency in pituitary hormone would include information on

    A. lifelong hormone replacement

    B. proposed surgery

    C. diabetes insipidus

    D. diet therapy

35. Regulation of secretion of ADH is controlled by receptors in the hypothalamus, which respond to changes in fluid _____.

    A. electrolytes

    B. osmolality

    C. vasopressin

    D. levels

36. In the patient with diabetes insipidus, the nurse would monitor carefully for signs of

    A. hypoglycemia and hypokalemia

    B. dehydration and sodium depletion

    C. hyperglycemia

    D. vascular overload

37. Short-term medical treatment of diabetes insipidus includes the administration of

    A. vasopressin

    B. desmopressin acetate

    C. lypressin

    D. Parlodel

38. Discharge instruction for the patient with diabetes insipidus who will be taking DDAVP would include

    A. administration of injection

    B. information on diet low in potassium

    C. instruction to measure weight daily

    D. information on fluid restriction

39. A patient who develops the syndrome of inappropriate antidiuretic hormone would be treated by

    A. insulin, saline, electrolytes

    B. antibiotics, analgesics

    C. fluid replacement, potassium

    D. fluid restriction, diuretics

40. The result of aldosterone deficiency in the individual with Addison's disease will be

    A. retention of sodium and potassium

    B. retention of sodium, chloride, and water

    C. excretion of sodium, increased potassium retention

    D. excretion of sodium, water, potassium, chloride

41. If the symptoms of Addison's disease were to continue without intervention, the end result would be

    A. septic shock

    B. inability to fight infection

    C. renal failure

    D. circulatory collapse and hypovolemic shock

42. Discharge instructions for the individual with Addison's disease would include how to prevent precipitating a crisis by avoiding

    A. stress

    B. dehydration

    C. illness

    D. all of the above

43. In making a diagnosis of primary Addison's disease, the nurse would expect to see which laboratory results?

    A. low levels of cortisol

    B. elevated levels of ACTH

    C. low levels of ACTH and cortisol

    D. low levels of androgens, low sodium and potassium

44. The medical management for the adult with Addison's disease would include administration of

    A. mineralocorticoids

    B. hydrocortisone, Florinef

    C. ACTH

    D. cortisone, androgen

45. When caring for the patient in Addisonian crisis, the most important nursing goal would be aimed at

    A. preventing infection

    B. preventing rise in ICP

    C. lowering blood pressure

    D. reestablishing fluid and electrolyte balance

46. The primary cause of Cushing's syndrome is

    A. hyperplasia of the adrenal cortices

    B. oversecretion by the hypothalamus

    C. tumor of the adrenal cortex

    D. high doses of steroids

47. Assessment of the patient with Cushing's syndrome involves observation for typical symptoms such as

    A. thin skin with hyperpigmentation

    B. truncal obesity, thin extremities, moon face

    C. weight gain, obesity, edema

    D. any of the above

48. To confirm a medical diagnosis of Cushing's syndrome, the nurse would expect which laboratory findings?

    A. decrease in cortisol and hydrocorticosteroid levels

    B. high cortisol level, hypoglycemia, hypernatremia

    C. high plasma cortisol and urinary ketosteroid levels

    D. elevation of plasma ACTH level

49. Unregulated hypersecretion of aldosterone will result in

    A. decreased fluid volume, hypotension

    B. increased sodium retention, excess potassium excretion

    C. hypotension, retention of potassium and sodium

    D. excessive secretion of sodium, potassium, fluids

50. The treatment of choice for the patient with primary aldosterone-secreting adenoma would be

    A. steroidal blocking agents

    B. antihypertensives, antibiotics

    C. unilateral adrenalectomy

    D. diet control, steroids

51. When a patient with primary aldosteronism exhibits a positive Chvostek's sign, the nurse would monitor for signs of

    A. tetany

    B. respiratory distress

    C. cardiac irregularities

    D. hyporeflexia

52. The symptoms associated with pheochromocytoma are due to

    A. overstimulation of sympathetic nervous system

    B. decreased production of catecholamines

    C. overproduction of corticosteroids

    D. oversecretion of pituitary and adrenal hormones

53. The most significant clinical feature of pheochromocytoma is

    A. nausea, vomiting

    B. hypertension

    C. hypotension, tachycardia

    D. headaches, bradycardia

54. Following an adrenalectomy, it would be important for the nurse to monitor for complications such as

    A. hyperreflexia

    B. pulmonary edema

    C. hypertensive crisis

    D. hypovolemic shock

55. One of the earliest clinical manifestations seen with chronic thyroiditis is

    A. pain

    B. goiter

    C. redness

    D. hoarseness

56. A patient with tertiary hypothyroidism will have a low level of

   A.   TSH

   B.   T4

   C.   T3

   D.   TRH

57. Early symptoms of hypothyroidism would include

   A.   mental deterioration

   B.   puffy appearance to tissue

   C.   dull sparse hair, loss of hair

   D.   fatigue, lethargy, increased somnolence

58. Chronic headaches in a patient with hypothyroidism are significant because they may indicate

   A.   decreased metabolism

   B.   cerebral hypoxia

   C.   brain damage

   D.   paresthesia

59. Medical treatment of primary hypothyroidism includes

   A.   surgery

   B.   radiation therapy

   C.   thyroid replacement

   D.   iodine replacement

60. Which of the following medications would be contraindicated for a patient receiving thyroid replacement therapy?

   A.   estrogen

   B.   antibiotics

   C.   aspirin

   D.   Feosol

61. A patient who will be taking thyroid replacement therapy should be taught to monitor for side effects such as

   A.   palpitations, tachycardia

   B.   chest pain, headache

   C.   nausea, diarrhea, anorexia

   D.   menstrual irregularities

   E.   any of the above

62. Elderly patients starting thyroid replacement therapy should increase the dose gradually in order to avoid

   A.   cardiovascular side effects

   B.   rapid slowdown of metabolic rate

   C.   nausea and vomiting

   D.   psychotic reactions

63. When a patient with Graves' disease develops exophthalmos, this is due to

   A.   increased volume of the orbital contents

   B.   inflammation of the extraocular muscles

   C.   pretibial edema

   D.   unknown etiology

64. When assessing a patient with Graves' disease, the nurse would monitor for clinical manifestations such as (Check all that apply.)

   A.   _____   nervousness

   B.   _____   insomnia

   C.   _____   tachycardia

   D.   _____   impaired coordination

   E.   _____   fatigue

   F.   _____   warm, moist skin

65. A patient who is taking antithyroid drugs should not stop them abruptly because it may precipitate

   A.   respiratory distress

   B.   hypothyroidism

   C.   exophthalmos

   D.   thyroid crisis

66. The drug of choice to treat hyperthyroidism is

   A.   levothyroxine

   B.   methimazole

   C.   prednisone

   D.   propylthiouracil

67. Teaching the patient who is to have radioactive iodine therapy would include providing information about

   A.   thyroid replacement therapy

   B.   type of anesthesia

   C.   precautions to follow

   D.   postoperative care

68. After a subtotal thyroidectomy, the nurse would monitor the patient for complications such as (Check all that apply.)

   A.   _____   infection

   B.   _____   hemorrhage

   C.   _____   tetany

   D.   _____   vocal cord paralysis

   E.   _____   hypotension

69. Early manifestations of acute hypocalcemia would include

   A.   difficulty breathing, stridor

   B.   cardiac arrhythmias, hypertension

   C.   irritability, muscle cramps

   D.   change in level of consciousness

70. The nurse is assessing a patient for signs of low serum calcium by tapping the facial nerve. This is known as

   A.   Chvostek's sign

   B.   Trousseau's sign

   C.   Homans' sign

71. The nurse monitors serum calcium levels carefully, knowing that when the serum calcium drops below 7 mg/dL, the patient is at risk for

   A.   respiratory arrest

   B.   cardiac tamponade

   C.   convulsions

   D.   hyperthermia

72. Dietary recommendations for a patient with chronic hypoparathyroidism would include

   A.   high calcium, high phosphorus, low sodium

   B.   high calcium, low phosphorus, vitamin D supplement

   C.   high calcium, high potassium, high sodium

73. A condition that could precipitate secondary hyperparathyroidism in a patient is

   A.   diabetes

   B.   hypothyroidism

   C.   acromegaly

   D.   congestive heart failure

74. The majority of patients with hyperparathyroidism are known to develop

   A.   renal calculi

   B.   vitamin D deficiency

   C.   anemia

   D.   osteoporosis

75. The medical management of the patient with primary hyperparathyroidism includes

   A.   vitamin C and D supplements, phosphate salts

   B.   diuretics, antihypertensives

   C.   limited fluids, increase calcium, decrease phosphate

   D.   increase fluids, decrease calcium, increase phosphate

76. Which of the following medications might be administered to help promote phosphorus excretion?

   A. calcium

   B. Amphojel

   C. Feosol

   D. Lasix

77. The nurse would recommend that a patient with high calcium levels include _____ in his or her diet.

   A. dairy products

   B. red meats

   C. cranberry or tomato juice

   D. complex carbohydrates

Nursing Care Plans

78. Write a nursing care plan for the patient who has had surgical removal of a pituitary adenoma. Use the following nursing diagnosis.

   Nursing diagnosis: Altered tissue perfusion, cerebral, related to increased intracranial pressure secondary to surgical trauma

   Patient outcome:

   Interventions:

79. Write a nursing care plan for the patient in Addisonian crisis. Use the following nursing diagnosis.

   Nursing diagnosis: Fluid volume deficit related to extracellular sodium and water loss secondary to vomiting, diarrhea, and adrenocorticoid insufficiency

   Patient outcome:

   Interventions:

80. Write a nursing care plan for the patient with Cushing's syndrome who needs discharge instructions. Use the following nursing diagnosis.

   Nursing diagnosis: High risk for infection related to impaired immune response and tissue repair

   Patient outcome:

   Interventions:

81. Write a nursing care plan for a patient with hypothyroidism who will be taking thyroid replacements after discharge. Use the following diagnosis.

Nursing diagnosis: High risk for altered health maintenance related to insufficient knowledge of self-management

Patient outcome:

Interventions:

82. Write a nursing care plan for a patient with hyperthyroidism. Use the following nursing diagnosis.

Nursing diagnosis: High risk for altered tissue perfusion, systemic, related to dehydration, hyperthermia, and decreased cardiac output

Patient outcome:

Interventions:

Case Studies

Case Study No. 1

Mr. M. has just returned to the unit following surgery to remove a pituitary adenoma.

83. Since this patient has had a hypophysectomy, how should he be positioned?

A. prone

B. supine

C. high-Fowler's

D. elevated 30 degrees

84. Which of the following nursing interventions would be contraindicated for this patient?

A. avoid activities that cause exertion

B. cough and deep breathe 10 times each hour

C. medicate promptly if nauseated

D. report urine output of > 100 cc to physician

85. Why will the nurse assess for signs of nuchal rigidity or headaches?

A. the patient may be septic

B. the patient may have meningitis

C. this is a sign of decreased ICP

D. these signs may precede a seizure

86. Discharge instructions for this patient would include

A. take antibiotics for two weeks

B. rinse frequently with mouthwash

C. use foam toothette and dental floss daily

D. continue to do coughing and deep breathing exercises q.i.d.

Case Study No. 2

An elderly patient has been diagnosed as having primary thyroid dysfunction as a result of thyroiditis.

87. During the initial interview, the nurse would assess for clinical manifestations of the disease such as (Check all that apply.)

    A. _____ low blood pressure, low heart rate

    B. _____ impaired wound healing

    C. _____ pale, cool skin

    D. _____ anorexia and diarrhea

    E. _____ heat intolerance

    F. _____ slowed speech, forgetfulness

88. This disorder can be very serious in the elderly because it can lead to myxedema coma. Which of the following might be a precipitating factor?

    A. exposure to temperature extremes

    B. use of central nervous system depressants

    C. use of caffeine, alcohol

    D. immobility

89. Which medication would be the drug of choice to treat this patient?

    A. desiccated thyroid

    B. Cytomel

    C. levothyroxine

    D. iodine

90. To avoid an overdose of medication the nurse would instruct the patient to monitor

    A. pulse

    B. weight

    C. urine output

    D. diet

91. Because the nurse is aware of potential side effects of this drug, it would be important to ask about a history of

    A. renal disease

    B. pulmonary fibrosis

    C. gastric reflux

    D. coronary artery disease

Case Study No. 3

Mrs. B. is admitted for thyroid surgery for Graves' disease after other methods of treatment were unsuccessful.

92. Before surgery, the patient states she has been taking

    A. Synthroid

    B. Cytomel

    C. ampicillin

    D. propylthiouracil

93. A subtotal thyroidectomy is performed. Six hours after surgery, she complains of numbness of her toes. The nurse notices muscle twitching. This suggests

    A. hyperthyroidism

    B. hypothyroidism

    C. tetany

    D. cerebral hypoxia

94. After receiving appropriate medical orders, the nurse would administer

    A. potassium

    B. calcium

    C. Dilantin

    D. morphine

95. Mrs. B. is having difficulty breathing and is becoming anxious. An appropriate nursing intervention is to

    A. assess vital signs

    B. release the dressing and check for bleeding

    C. obtain tracheostomy set

    D. all of the above

96. Mrs. B. is stabilized and the rest of the hospitalization is uneventful. Check statements that the nurse would include in the discharge teaching.

    A. _____ need to continue antithyroid medications

    B. _____ need to monitor blood level of thyroid hormone

    C. _____ possible need to take hypothyroid medication

    D. _____ side effects of therapy

Case Study No. 4

A patient is admitted to the hospital with a diagnosis of possible Addisonian crisis.

97. During the initial assessment, the nurse would observe for symptoms of the disease including

    A. respiratory distress, edema

    B. hyporeflexia, hypertension, bradycardia

    C. hypotension, hypoglycemia, hyponatremia

    D. hyporeflexia, hypotension

98. Treatment should be initiated quickly and the nurse would anticipate administration of

    A. fluids and steroids

    B. insulin and dextrose

    C. ventilatory support

    D. surgical intervention

99. It would be important for the nurse to observe for complications such as

    A. infection, septic shock

    B. hypovolemic shock, dysrhythmias

    C. fluid overload, pulmonary edema

    D. thrombophlebitis, pulmonary emboli

100. Which statement by the patient would signify an event that may have precipitated this crisis?

    A.   "I started a new diet."

    B.   "I recently lost my job."

    C.   "I am taking a new medication."

    D.   "I have a new baby."

101. One of the ways that an individual with Addison's disease can prevent a crisis from occurring would be to

    A.   reduce level of activity

    B.   follow dietary restrictions

    C.   stop medications during illness

    D.   increase medication during stressful times or illness

*L*earner Self-Evaluation

Do I fully understand the content? If no, then the areas I need to review are:

I need more information from my instructor on:

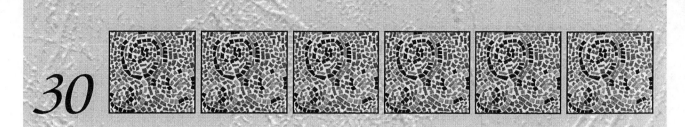

30

Knowledge Base for Patients with Urinary Dysfunction

*O*bjectives

1.0 Review the anatomy and physiology of the urinary system.
    1.1 Identify the parts of the kidney.
    1.2 List the functions of the renal system.
    1.3 Explain the physiology of the urinary system.
    1.4 Explain the physiology of micturition.

2.0 Demonstrate an understanding of the assessment data related to the urinary system.
    2.1 Identify clinical manifestations of urinary tract dysfunctions.
    2.2 Match diagnostic tests used to diagnose abnormalities of the urinary system with the best definition.
    2.3 Plan nursing care for the patient having a cystoscopy.

3.0 Demonstrate an understanding of the interventions used to treat adults with urinary tract dysfunction.
    3.1 Identify the medical treatment and some surgical interventions used for patients with urinary tract dysfunction.
    3.2 Plan teaching measures for the patient who is performing self-catheterization.
    3.3 Plan nursing measures for the patient who has a problem with urinary incontinence.

$\mathcal{L}$earning Activities

Identification

1.   Label the following diagram.

    A.   Cortex

    B.   Major calyx

    C.   Medulla

    D.   Glomeruli

    E.   Renal artery

    F.   Renal pelvis

    G.   Ureter

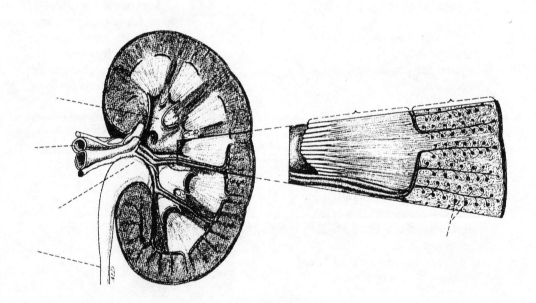

Short Answers

2. The _____ is the functional *tissue* of the kidney.

3. The _____ is the functional *unit* of the kidney.

4. List five main functions of the renal system.
   1.

   2.

   3.

   4.

   5.

5. List three factors responsible for the glomerular filtration rate in the kidney.
   1.

   2.

   3.

6. _____ is an end product of a substance in skeletal muscle.

7. The kidneys regulate blood pressure through regulation of plasma volume and the ____ _____ system.

8. The kidneys regulate fluid and electrolyte balance by adjustments in _____, _____, and _____.

9. Three factors that contribute to normal micturition are
   1.

   2.

   3.

10. Incontinence is a _____, not a disease.

11. An indwelling Foley catheter greatly increases a patient's risk of developing

    _____ _____.

12. When caring for an indwelling catheter, the nurse is responsible for preventing complications. List five nursing interventions that should be implemented.
    1.

    2.

    3.

    4.

    5.

Identification

Match these signs of dysfunctional voiding with the appropriate definition.

   A.   Frequency

   B.   Urgency

   C.   Dysuria

   D.   Nocturia

   E.   Hesitancy

13. _____ Nighttime urinary frequency
14. _____ Excessive need to urinate
15. _____ Sudden and strong desire to urinate
16. _____ Painful or difficult urination
17. _____ Delay in the start of urination

Match the following diagnostic tests with the definition.

   A.   KUB x-ray

   B.   Voiding urogram

   C.   Cystogram

   D.   Ultrasound

   E.   Magnetic resonance imaging (MRI)

   F.   Cystometrogram

   G.   Urodynamics

18. _____ Series of diagnostic tests to evaluate voiding disorders.

19. _____ Study based on the reaction to a magnetic field of protons and electrons in living tissue.

20. _____ Radiologic study where patient is catheterized, contrast dye is instilled, and films are taken.

21. _____ Radiographic film of the major organs of the urinary tract.

22. _____ Measures bladder pressure during the filling and storage phases of micturition.

23. _____ Transducer is passed over the kidney to evaluate for abnormalities.

24. _____ Radiographic study using contrast dye, which is observed as it passes through the urinary tract.

Knowledge Application

25. Which part of the renal system is responsible for most of the process of reabsorption?

   A.   glomerulus

   B.   proximal tubule

   C.   loop of Henle

   D.   distal tubule

26. The kidneys receive _____% of the total cardiac output.

   A.   10

   B.   25

   C.   40

   D.   60

27. The normal creatinine clearance in an adult with normal kidneys would be

   A.   40–60 mL/min

   B.   60–80 mL/min

   C.   80–100 mL/min

   D.   100–120 mL/min

28. The normal response of the kidney when acidosis occurs is to

   A.   secret excess hydrogen ions

   B.   reabsorb excessive hydrogen

   C.   retain potassium

   D.   excrete chloride

29. When an individual is dehydrated, the body will respond by

   A.   increasing release of antidiuretic hormone

   B.   decreasing release of antidiuretic hormone

   C.   retaining sodium

   D.   excreting potassium

30. The production of _____ in the renal parenchyma is necessary for red blood cell production.

   A.   creatinine

   B.   erythropoietin

   C.   calcitonin

   D.   hemoglobin

31. Which of the following would not be a cause of urinary frequency?

   A.   anxiety

   B.   increased volume of urine

   C.   decreased volume of urine

   D.   inflammation of the bladder

32. Which of the following would lead to nocturia in an elderly patient?

    A. fluid retention during the day

    B. consumption of two cups of coffee at 2 PM

    C. consumption of four cups of water daily

    D. medication for angina

33. Which statement best explains the process of bladder emptying?

    A. It occurs by parasympathetic facilitation and sympathetic inhibition.

    B. It occurs by sympathetic facilitation and parasympathetic inhibition.

34. A definition of urinary retention would be

    A. voiding frequently during the day

    B. residual urine of > 50 mL

    C. residual urine of > 100 mL

    D. voiding less than 200 mL daily

35. The primary reason that the patient will seek a urologic consultation is usually

    A. bleeding with urination

    B. inability to urinate

    C. pain within the urinary tract

    D. inability to control urination

36. Symptoms of hesitancy, intermittent stream, and dribbling in a 55-year-old male suggest

    A. urinary infection

    B. enlarged prostate

    C. neurologic disorder

    D. renal failure

37. Reflex incontinence is associated with

    A. urinary retention

    B. neurologic disorder

    C. trauma

    D. bladder infection

38. The presence of blood in the urine is a situation that requires evaluation. Which of the following is NOT a cause of hematuria?

    A. presence of a tumor

    B. urinary infection

    C. benign prostatic hypertrophy

    D. hydronephrosis

39. Urinary output of 100–400 mL in a 24-hour period is defined as

    A. anuria

    B. oliguria

    C. nonuria

    D. polyuria

40. Two tests most commonly used to measure glomerular filtration are

    A. PSP and WBC

    B. WBC and BUN

    C. BUN and creatinine

    D. creatinine and CPK

41. As the nurse caring for a patient having a workup for possible renal disease, what is the most important information to obtain?

    A. history of cardiac dysfunction

    B. family history of diabetes and hypertension

    C. allergy to contrast dye

    D. presence of gastrointestinal problems

42. An excretory urogram would be contraindicated for an individual with a history of

    A. diabetes

    B. heart disease

    C. renal failure

    D. hypertension

43. A patient has just returned from an intravenous pyelogram. Which nursing intervention would you implement following the test?

    A. assess vital signs every 10 minutes for 2 hours

    B. maintain patient on bed rest for 48 hours

    C. encourage fluid intake and monitor output

    D. maintain patency of the urinary drainage system

44. Which of the following diagnostic tests are most informative in terms of the urologic evaluation?

    A. KUB

    B. cystoscopy and IVP

    C. ultrasound and CT scan

    D. BUN and IVP

45. Which of the following conditions can be diagnosed using cystoscopic examination?

    A. recurrent urinary infections

    B. congenital defects

    C. prostatism

    D. all of the above

46. You are doing discharge instruction for a patient who has had a cystoscopy this morning. You explain that

    A. urine may be slightly blood-tinged for 24–48 hours

    B. urine should be clear after the first urination

    C. burning with urination is common after this test

    D. fluids should be limited for the first 24 hours

47. Ms. M. calls the clinic at 10 AM. She reports that since her cystoscopy test yesterday at 11 AM, she has not been able to urinate. You would have her

    A. drink fluids and call back at 6 PM

    B. come to the clinic as soon as possible

    C. go downtown to the emergency room

    D. call back when she has urinated

48. A patient who is predisposed to urinary calculus formation would be on which type of diet?

    A. low sodium

    B. fluid restriction

    C. low calcium

    D. low protein

49. An individual with chronic renal failure is being discharged. The nurse is reinforcing information on which diet?

    A. low sodium, low potassium, low protein, high carbohydrate

    B. low sodium, high potassium, high protein, high carbohydrate

    C. high sodium, low potassium, low protein, high carbohydrate

    D. high sodium, high potassium, low protein, low carbohydrate

50. What diagnostic procedure would you expect the physician to perform on the patient who has been having hematuria and is suspected to have adenocarcinoma of the bladder?

    A. voiding cystogram

    B. intravenous pyelogram

    C. cystoscopy with biopsy

    D. CT scan of abdomen

51. A bladder biopsy would be contraindicated when a patient is currently taking which of the following medications?

    A. Coumadin

    B. Indocin

    C. Lasix

    D. ampicillin

52. Mr. C. has just returned to the unit following a closed renal biopsy. The nurse is aware that the most common complication of this procedure is

    A. infection

    B. bleeding

    C. obstruction

    D. incontinence

53. The nurse would suspect a problem if Mr. C. exhibits which of the following symptoms?

    A. sudden drop in blood pressure

    B. presence of pink-tinged urine

    C. tenderness in flank area

    D. anxiety after procedure

54. Which of the following symptoms would probably result in a delay of urodynamic testing?

    A. temperature of 98.9° F

    B. presence of sugar in the urine

    C. presence of bacteria in the urine

    D. blood pressure of 150/90, pulse of 92

55. When would a patient be a candidate for a suprapubic catheter rather than an indwelling catheter? When

    A. he or she has recurrent bladder infections

    B. there is a urethral obstruction

    C. there is hydronephrosis of the kidney

    D. a kidney stone is present

56. An appropriate nursing intervention implemented when caring for the patient with a suprapubic catheter is

    A. change catheter every week

    B. irrigate to maintain patency

    C. limit fluid intake

    D. change dressing twice daily

57. What is the purpose of the Crédè procedure? To

    A. aid in the passage of urine from the bladder

    B. avoid having to catheterize the patient

    C. prevent recurrent bladder infections

    D. minimize trauma to the urethra

58. Management of the patient with a urinary tract disorder may involve diet therapy. The nurse would teach the patient all of the following EXCEPT

    A. increase intake of acidotic foods

    B. increase fluids to 3000 cc per day

    C. increase intake of dairy products

    D. decrease intake of caffeine and alcohol

59. A nurse is teaching a patient with a urinary dysfunction to perform Kegel exercises. The purpose for these exercises is to

    A. regain voluntary bladder control

    B. control involuntary loss of urine

    C. prevent hematuria

    D. prevent recurrent bladder infections.

True/False

60. _____ Painless hematuria should be considered a serious symptom.

61. _____ Incontinence is related to the aging process.

62. _____ Both men and women can use external catheters.

63. _____ When obtaining a culture from an indwelling catheter, disconnect catheter and take 5 mL of urine for analysis.

64. _____ Weekly changing of indwelling catheters will help reduce the bacteria count.

Nursing Care Plans

65. You are the home-care nurse working with an elderly female with diabetes and total urinary incontinence. Write a nursing care plan to help her cope with this problem.

    Nursing diagnosis:

    Patient outcome:

    Interventions:

66. Write a nursing care plan for the surgical patient with urinary retention. Use the following nursing diagnosis.

    Nursing diagnosis: Urinary retention related to postoperative complications

    Patient outcome:

    Interventions:

67. Write a nursing care plan for the patient in a subacute care facility with an indwelling Foley catheter. Use the following nursing diagnosis.

    Nursing diagnosis: Alteration in pattern of urinary elimination related to irritation of the mucosa due to catheterization

    Patient outcome:

    Interventions:

Case Studies

Case Study No. 1

Ms. N. is seen in the emergency room of her local hospital. She is complaining of a sudden onset of severe colicky pain that radiates from the left side to the groin.

68. The nurse would ask the patient if she has a history of

    A. kidney stones

    B. bladder infections

    C. diabetes

    D. incontinence

69. Ms. N. says that she had a small kidney stone several years ago. Based on this information, what is the most likely cause of her current problem?

    A. urinary tract infection

    B. urinary tract obstruction

    C. severe menstrual cramps

    D. pelvic inflammatory disease

70. Ms. N. has a urine culture and sensitivity test. The nurse explains that the purpose of this test is to

    A. rule out an obstruction

    B. determine the presence of a neoplasm

    C. identify any bacteria

    D. determine if she has diabetes

71. A diagnostic procedure that will probably be ordered for this patient is

    A. intravenous pyelogram

    B. sonogram

    C. Doppler studies

    D. angiogram

72. Following this procedure, what is an important nursing intervention?

    A. increase fluid intake

    B. limit fluid intake

    C. keep patient on bed rest for 24 hours

    D. maintain patency of drainage catheter

73. Ms. N. is able to pass her kidney stone during the hospitalization. She is discharged on a low-calcium diet. Which food should she avoid?

    A. green leafy vegetables

    B. rice and pasta

    C. fish

    D. soft drinks

Case Study No. 2

Ms. W. has a neurogenic bladder condition and upon discharge from the hospital will be doing self-catheterization. She will need discharge instructions.

74. The first step in your teaching plan would be to

    A. emphasize that this is a sterile procedure

    B. review the female anatomy with Ms. W.

    C. gather all the appropriate equipment

    D. provide a sedative before she begins the procedure

75. To instruct Ms. W. in this procedure, the nurse would tell her to

    A. look for meatus in a mirror, insert catheter straight in two inches

    B. locate meatus, clean with Betadine, insert catheter four inches

    C. palpate meatus, insert catheter in an upward direction for three inches

    D. view meatus, clean with soap and antiseptic solution, insert catheter six inches

76. To further instruct Ms. W. in the care of the catheter, the nurse would tell her to

    A. clean after use, soak once a week to remove exudate, and discard after 4–6 weeks of use

    B. use a clean, sterile catheter each time

    C. sterilize with alcohol after each use and discard after using three times

    D. clean as recommended by physician after using catheter for 24 hours, discard after one week

*L*earner Self-Evaluation

Do I fully understand the content? If no, then the areas I need to review are:

I need more information from my instructor on:

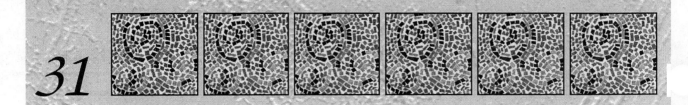

31

Nursing Care of Patients with Urinary Disorders

*O*bjectives

1.0　Demonstrate an understanding of the infections and inflammations of the urinary tract.

   1.1　Identify several inflammatory disorders of the urinary tract.

   1.2　Recognize the clinical manifestations of several inflammatory disorders of the urinary tract.

   1.3　Plan the nursing care for the patient with glomerulonephritis.

   1.4　Plan the nursing care for the patient with cystitis.

2.0　Demonstrate an understanding of renal failure.

   2.1　Identify the effects of acute and chronic renal failure.

   2.2　Demonstrate an understanding of the pathology involved in chronic renal failure.

   2.3　Review the medical management of the patient with renal failure.

   2.4　Demonstrate an understanding of treatment options for the patient with renal failure.

   2.5　Plan the nursing care for the patient with renal failure.

3.0　Demonstrate an understanding of obstructive disorders of the renal system.

   3.1　Identify the clinical manifestations of the patient with an obstructive disorder.

   3.2　Plan the nursing care for the patient with renal calculi.

3.3　Review the medical and surgical treatment options for the patient with an obstructive disorder.

3.4　Plan appropriate nursing interventions for the patient with an obstructive disorder.

4.0　Demonstrate an understanding of the types of traumatic injuries that can affect the renal system.

   4.1　Identify the clinical manifestations of renal trauma.

   4.2　Review the medical and surgical treatments used for patients with traumatic injuries.

   4.3　Plan nursing interventions for the patient with a traumatic injury.

5.0　Demonstrate an understanding of the neoplasms that can affect the renal system.

   5.1　Identify the clinical manifestations of several types of renal neoplasms.

   5.2　Review the surgical interventions used in the treatment of renal neoplasms.

   5.3　Plan the nursing care for the patient with a neoplasm of the renal system.

Learning Activities

Short Answers

1. The most common urologic disorders are

   _____ and _____.

2. An individual with azotemia who is symp-

   tomatic is said to have _____.

3. Individuals with uncomplicated, acute

   cystitis are usually treated with _____.

4. Urinary tract _____ is a blockage of the
   normal glomerular filtrate flow anywhere
   along the urinary tract.

5. A pathologic narrowing of the urethra is

   called a _____.

6. Traumatic injuries to the genitourinary tract

   are usually the result of _____ or

   _____ injuries.

Identification

Demonstrate your basic knowledge by matching
these terms with the correct definition.

   A.   Pyelonephritis

   B.   Cystitis

   C.   Urethritis

   D.   Glomerulonephritis

   E.   Acute renal failure

   F.   Chronic renal failure

   G.   Azotemia

7. _____ Chronic, progressive, irreversible loss
   of renal function

8. _____ Infection of the bladder

9. _____ Sudden, potentially reversible loss of
   kidney function

10. _____ Infection of the upper urinary tract

11. _____ Inflammation of the urethra

12. _____ Buildup of nitrogenous waste products
    in the blood

13. _____ Inflammation of the kidney affecting
    the capillary loops in the glomeruli

Knowledge Application

14. When reviewing the laboratory results for a
    patient, the nurse is aware that a urinary
    tract infection is present if there are more
    than _____ organisms per mm^3
    in the clean-catch specimen.

    A.   10,000

    B.   30,000

    C.   50,000

    D.   100,000

15. In females the most common way that
    cystitis occurs is it develops

    A.   secondary to a strep infection

    B.   after exposure to a bacteria or virus

    C.   after bacteria from the rectum or vagina
         ascend to the bladder

    D.   as a result of an existing problem in the
         urinary tract

16. Discharge planning for the patient who has
    had cystitis should include which of the
    following information?

    A.   take antibiotics for six more weeks

    B.   maintain restricted activity

    C.   refrain from sexual activity

    D.   proper hygienic methods

17. Which of the following nursing interventions would help alleviate bladder spasm for the patient with cystitis?

  A. administer antispasmodics or analgesics as ordered

  B. encourage fluid intake

  C. encourage the patient to urinate frequently

  D. all of the above

18. The most common cause of pyelonephritis is

  A. invasion of bacteria into bladder

  B. reflux of infected urine

  C. contamination from GI tract

  D. sepsis

19. A medical diagnosis of pyelonephritis is confirmed by which of the following tests?

  A. urine culture, WBC, KUB

  B. urinalysis, CBC, WBC

  C. urine culture, IVP, BUN

  D. CT of abdomen

20. Mr. H. has been diagnosed with acute pyelonephritis. There is an order to obtain a urine specimen for culture and sensitivity. When should the specimen be obtained?

  A. immediately upon admission

  B. immediately after starting his antibiotic

  C. as soon as he urinates 100 cc

  D. within the first 24 hours of admission

21. Mr. H. has been treated with antibiotics for the past week. He continues to have a persistent fever and edema over the area of his right kidney. What is a possible explanation for his symptoms? He may

  A. be resistant to antibiotic therapy

  B. have developed an abscess

  C. have developed a neoplasm

  D. have a hematoma

22. What type of diet would probably be ordered for a patient with acute glomerulonephritis who is edematous?

  A. low fat, low protein

  B. low salt, high protein

  C. low protein, low salt

  D. high fat, high calories

23. Which of the following statements is MOST accurate about the cause of glomerulonephritis? It

  A. is caused by staphylococcus

  B. develops secondary to streptococcus infection

  C. is caused by an immunologic reaction

  D. usually leads to renal failure

24. In a large portion of the individuals who develop urinary calculi, what is the causative factor?

  A. fluid restrictions

  B. dietary habits

  C. geographic location

  D. heredity

25. When caring for the patient admitted with a calculus in the urinary tract, the primary nursing goal is

  A. alleviation of pain

  B. maintain fluid balance

  C. promote mobility

  D. prevent respiratory complications

26. The treatment of choice for large renal or ureteral calculi that do not pass spontaneously is

  A. surgical removal of stone

  B. pain control and fluid therapy

  C. extracorporeal lithotripsy

  D. renal angioplasty

27. A patient with a kidney stone is being managed conservatively. Knowing the usual medical treatment, what information would the nurse give to this patient?

    A. stay on complete bed rest

    B. strain all urine

    C. avoid pain medication because it masks symptoms

    D. limit fluid to 1000 cc daily

28. Following extracorporeal lithotripsy, the nurse should consider which goal as primary?

    A. control of pain

    B. maintain patency of urinary system

    C. maintain electrolyte status

    D. prevent infection of suture line

29. Diagnosis of a stricture of the urinary system is most likely to be made by

    A. angiogram

    B. excretory urogram

    C. KUB

    D. CAT scan

30. If untreated, the nurse is aware that obstructive disorders of the urinary system will eventually lead to

    A. renal neoplasm

    B. tubular osmosis

    C. hydronephrosis

    D. renal calculi

31. The treatment goals for the person with ureteropelvic obstruction are aimed at

    A. restoring renal function

    B. providing relief of symptoms

    C. eliminating infection

    D. correcting anatomic abnormalities

    E. all the above

32. Renal failure will occur when there is functional loss of what portion of the kidney's nephrons?

    A. 20%

    B. 40%

    C. 60%

    D. 75%

33. Prerenal failure is thought to be caused by

    A. hypovolemia

    B. low cardiac output

    C. renal artery obstruction

    D. all of the above

34. For the patient in acute renal failure, which of the following laboratory findings is most serious?

    A. Hgb 10.8

    B. BUN 28

    C. creatine 1.8

    D. potassium 6.2

35. The management of patients with acute renal failure is primarily directed toward decreasing _____.

    A. sodium and chloride levels

    B. BUN and creatinine levels

    C. Hgb and Hct Levels

    D. CO_2 levels

36. Which assessment data indicates the presence of acute renal failure?

    A. urine excretion of 500 cc/day, hypertension, nausea

    B. urine excretion of 200 cc/day, edema, mental changes

    C. urine excretion of 600 cc/day, BUN 30, creatinine 1.8

    D. urine excretion of 500 cc/day, fever, flank pain

37. The nursing assessment of a renal patient reveals a fever, nausea, pleuritic pain, and an audible friction rub. The nurse suspects the patient has developed

   A.   chronic renal failure

   B.   uremia

   C.   pericarditis

   D.   pneumonia

38. The nurse's responsibility in caring for the patient with renal failure would be centered around controlling

   A.   fluid and electrolyte balances

   B.   pain and anxiety

   C.   altered level of consciousness

   D.   altered breathing patterns

39. In the individual with chronic renal failure, which symptoms would always be present?

   A.   oliguria, hypokalemia, alkalosis

   B.   polycythemia, hypovolemia, acidosis

   C.   uremia, anemia, acidosis

   D.   dehydration, anemia, hypercalcemia

40. Which condition in a patient with chronic renal failure would be a reason to institute dialysis?

   A.   severe dehydration

   B.   uremia

   C.   hypokalemia

   D.   hypertension

41. The type of dialysis that involves dialyzing for 40 hours/week with 3–7 dialysis runs is _____. It involves a cycling machine and the abdomen is dry between runs.

   A.   hemodialysis

   B.   intermittent peritoneal dialysis

   C.   continuous ambulatory dialysis

   D.   continuous cycle peritoneal dialysis

42. Why would peritoneal dialysis be the treatment of choice over hemodialysis? It

   A.   provides for less chance of infection

   B.   provides for more patient independence

   C.   allows for more rapid removal of waste products

   D.   is appropriate for all patients

43. A patient is scheduled for peritoneal dialysis. Presence of which condition would contraindicate this procedure?

   A.   cardiac disease

   B.   diabetes

   C.   neurologic impairment

   D.   inflammatory bowel disease

44. What is the most appropriate action for the nurse to take if during the peritoneal dialysis procedure the patient becomes short of breath and diaphoretic?

   A.   call for respiratory treatment

   B.   stop procedure for this time

   C.   continue infusion but notify physician

   D.   elevate the bed, assess respiratory status

45. What is the main difference between hemodialysis and peritoneal dialysis?

   A.   Peritoneal dialysis is more effective.

   B.   Hemodialysis requires vascular access.

   C.   Hemodialysis takes longer to complete.

   D.   Peritoneal dialysis has fewer complications.

46. Which of the following statements is FALSE?

   A.   Hemodialysis is a treatment for both acute and chronic renal failure.

   B.   Hemodialysis can be done at home.

   C.   Peritoneal dialysis can be done at home.

   D.   Peritoneal dialysis is a clean procedure.

47. When checking the patient who returns from dialysis, the nurse notices periods of confusion and altered perception. This is most likely due to

    A. rapid removal of fluid volume

    B. rapid removal of creatinine

    C. sudden rise in blood pressure

    D. sudden onset of infection

48. In the patient who has had a renal transplant the most common infection that can result in graft loss is

    A. CMV

    B. HIV

    C. fungal

    D. herpes

49. The management of a patient who has had a renal transplant involves administering immunosuppressive agents to prevent what complication?

    A. rejection of the transplanted organ

    B. systemic infection

    C. fungal infection

    D. clotting of graft

50. For the patient who is receiving immunosuppressive agents, the nurse would be concerned if he or she finds which symptom during assessment?

    A. weight loss of two pounds

    B. temperature of 98.8° F

    C. productive cough

    D. hyperactive bowel sounds

51. In a patient who had acute renal failure in the past, which of the following conditions will increase the risk for developing further renal problems?

    A. cholecystitis

    B. abdominal aneurysm

    C. angina

    D. rheumatic fever

52. Which clinical manifestation is a sign of an obstruction of a urethral stricture?

    A. hematuria and burning with urination

    B. hesitancy, urinary retention

    C. flank pain, dysuria

    D. frequency, pain with intercourse

53. The most common therapy for a urethral stricture would involve

    A. extracorporeal lithotripsy

    B. balloon angioplasty

    C. mechanical dilatation

    D. intravenous pyelogram

54. Which of the following patients would be at the greatest risk for the development of an extrinsic urethral obstruction? A patient

    A. receiving chemotherapy for lung cancer

    B. who is undergoing popliteal revascularization

    C. who is receiving pelvic radiation therapy

    D. with diabetes on insulin therapy

55. Urethral trauma is generally treated by

    A. drug therapy

    B. bed rest and fluids

    C. surgical repair

    D. antibiotics

56. Mr. F. is admitted following a crushing injury. Presence of which of the following symptoms might indicate a ruptured bladder?

    A. flank pain, hematuria, frequency

    B. lower abdominal pain, inability to void

    C. abdominal rigidity; sharp, knifelike pain

    D. bladder spasm, urinary retention

57. Since Mr. F. has not yet urinated, it would be important to implement which of the following interventions first?

   A. catheterize the patient

   B. assess the type of injury sustained

   C. encourage fluid intake

   D. medicate for pain

58. In the patient who has a urethral tear without extravasation the nurse would expect that treatment would involve

   A. insertion of a Foley catheter for 7–10 days

   B. surgical repair as soon as possible

   C. surgical repair after bleeding has ceased

   D. analgesic and anti-inflammatory medications

59. In caring for the patient who has had a radical nephrectomy, the nurse should set which goal as the priority during the immediate postoperative period?

   A. maintaining stable fluid and electrolyte status

   B. maintaining effective breathing patterns

   C. maintaining adequate nutrition

   D. preventing problems related to immobility

60. The most common symptom in the patient with bladder cancer is

   A. pain

   B. incontinence

   C. hematuria

   D. urinary retention

61. Which of the following therapies is used MOST often in the treatment for papillary (superficial) bladder cancer?

   A. transurethral resection

   B. intravesical chemotherapy

   C. laser therapy

   D. radical surgery

62. Which form of therapy has been successful in curing some patients with nonpapillary (muscle invasive) bladder cancer?

   A. transurethral resection

   B. intravesical chemotherapy

   C. intravesical immunotherapy

   D. partial cystectomy

63. Which of the following patients would be a candidate for external radiation therapy to treat a malignant bladder tumor?

   A. young adult with papillary bladder cancer

   B. middle-aged female with nonpapillary bladder neck tumor

   C. elderly female with invasive bladder cancer

   D. any of the above

64. Which of the following statements is FALSE?

   A. Metastasis of a renal cell carcinoma occurs in about 25% of cases.

   B. Chemotherapy is the treatment of choice for renal cell carcinoma.

   C. Malignant bladder tumors are the most frequent tumors within the urinary system.

   D. The most common symptom of bladder cancer is painless hematuria.

Nursing Care Plans

65. Write a nursing care plan for the patient with cystitis. Use the following nursing diagnosis.

Nursing diagnosis: Urinary elimination, alteration in patterns related to inflammation

Patient outcome:

Interventions:

66. Write a nursing care plan for the patient with chronic renal failure. Use the following nursing diagnosis.

Nursing diagnosis: Alteration in renal tissue perfusion related to chronic renal failure

Patient outcome:

Interventions:

67. An important part of the nursing care for the patient who is to undergo CAPD is preventing complications related to the procedure. Write a nursing care plan for this patient.

Nursing diagnosis:

Patient outcome:

Interventions:

Case Studies

Case Study No. 1

Ms. R. is admitted with a sore throat, fever, flank pain, and peripheral edema. The diagnosis is possible glomerulonephritis.

68. The nurse reviews Ms. R.'s lab results. Which of the following findings would tend to confirm this diagnosis?

A. presence of protein and blood in the urine, high BUN

B. elevated white count, low hemoglobin

C. presence of *E. coli* in the urine

D. high sedimentation rate, low platelet count

69. A renal biopsy is performed and the diagnosis is confirmed. Ms. R. wonders is this is a serious condition. You would explain that

    A. this is a mild inflammation that is easily treated

    B. this can be a serious condition that needs aggressive treatment

    C. this is a chronic condition that often leads to end-stage renal disease

    D. everyone you have seen with the condition does well with treatment

70. Following the renal biopsy, you would monitor carefully for

    A. signs of bleeding

    B. signs of infection

    C. signs of respiratory distress

    D. hypertension

71. What is the reason that Ms. R. is on bed rest? To

    A. prevent further damage to the renal tubules

    B. prevent the spread of infection

    C. conserve energy

    D. prevent injury from falls

Case Study No. 2

Mr. P. has chronic renal failure and has now been told he has end-stage renal failure. A decision is made to start hemodialysis. He is admitted for the placement of an AV graft (GoreTex) in the right forearm.

72. When an individual is classified as having ESRD, this means that over _____% of renal function is lost.

    A. 50

    B. 70

    C. 85

    D. 95

73. Mr. P. asks the nurse to explain to him what this procedure involves. The nurse would explain that

    A. a vein and artery are surgically joined together

    B. a bridge is made between an artery and vein using a synthetic material

    C. a graft of Teflon is implanted outside the femoral artery

74. Mr. P. returns to the unit after the graft insertion. How should the nurse assess for patency of the graft?

    A. perform circulation check every hour

    B. check vital signs every 30 minutes

    C. assess graft for presence of thrill and bruit

    D. keep compression dressing in place for 24 hours

The physician also inserts a subclavian dialysis catheter and sends Mr. P. for his first dialysis treatment.

75. Mr. P. asks why they can't use his new graft. You reply

    A. "It takes time to mature."

    B. "It would rupture."

    C. "I don't know."

    D. "Ask the doctor."

76. Following dialysis, Mr. P. is groggy and irritable. The nursing priority should be to

    A. assess blood pressure

    B. listen to breath sounds

    C. monitor urine output

    D. all of the above

77. Mr. P. wonders if he can have a kidney transplant from his brother. You tell him that the two major factors in donor and recipient determination are

    A. age and blood type of donor

    B. blood type and histocompatibility

    C. blood type and sex of donor

    D. blood cross-match and donor desire to participate

Case Study No. 3

Mr. B. was injured when he hit a tree on his motorcycle. In addition to a concussion and fractured ribs, he received a laceration of the right kidney. After stabilization, he was taken to surgery for repair of the laceration.

78. Which information would it be important for the floor nurse to obtain from the recovery room nurse?

    A.   vital signs

    B.   level of consciousness

    C.   presence of drainage tubes

    D.   all of the above

79. Mr. B. has a nephrostomy tube (stent) as well as an indwelling catheter. Which information is true about this type of drainage?

    A.   Most of the urinary drainage occurs through the stent.

    B.   Most of the urinary drainage occurs through the catheter.

    C.   All drainage occurs through the stent.

    D.   All drainage occurs through the catheter.

80. As part of his discharge instruction, it would be important for Mr. B. to know how to

    A.   handle the urinary drainage system

    B.   change his abdominal dressing

    C.   irrigate the catheter

    D.   prevent problems related to immobility

Case Study No. 4

Mrs. W., age 50, is admitted with bladder cancer that has not responded to conservative methods of treatment. She is scheduled for a radical cystectomy. The physician is planning on constructing an ileal reservoir.

81. What is the best way to explain this procedure to Mrs. W.?

    A.   The bladder is removed and the urethra is brought to the abdominal wall.

    B.   A section of ileum is resected and the ureters are implanted into it, and the end of the colon forms a stoma.

    C.   The ureters are resected into the distal ileum and urine drains out the rectum.

    D.   The bladder is removed and the ureters attached to the transverse colon which forms the stoma.

82. Following surgery, the nurse would watch for which of the following?

    A.   Fluid intake and output is balanced.

    B.   Urinary output is 30 mL or more per hour.

    C.   Vital signs are within normal range for patient.

    D.   All of the above

83. After surgery, Mrs. W. does well for the first 48 hours, but today she is withdrawn. She turns away when you assess her urinary drainage system. Which nursing diagnosis might be applicable at this time?

    A.   Alteration in respiratory functioning

    B.   Alteration in fluid and electrolytes

    C.   Alteration in body image

    D.   Alteration in nutrition

84. Which would be an appropriate referral for the primary nurse to implement?

    A.   consultation with the enterostomal therapist

    B.   referral to social services for home care

    C.   referral for a psychiatric evaluation

    D.   referral to the physician about condition

85. The nurse would realize that teaching had been effective when Mrs. W. says which of the following?

     A.   "I'm glad everything is back to normal."

     B.   "I didn't realize how the diversion would really look."

     C.   "I didn't realize that I couldn't have sex again."

     D.   "I'm just glad to be alive."

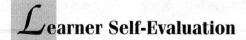

Learner Self-Evaluation

Do I fully understand the content? If no, then the areas I need to review are:

I need more information from my instructor on:

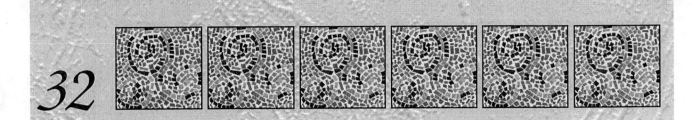

32

Knowledge Base for Patients with Immune Dysfunction

Objectives

1.0 Review the anatomy and physiology of the immune system.
    1.1 Identify the parts of the immune system.
    1.2 Match the types of white cells with their functions.
    1.3 Identify the function of T-cells and B-cells.

2.0 Demonstrate an understanding of the specific immune responses that occur in the body.
    2.1 List the three stages of the immune response.
    2.2 Identify types of specific and nonspecific immune responses.
    2.3 Demonstrate an understanding of types of immunity.

3.0 Demonstrate an understanding of assessment data related to adults with immune dysfunction.
    3.1 Identify clinical manifestations of immune dysfunction.
    3.2 Review diagnostic procedures used to identify immune dysfunctions.

3.3 Match the specific allergy test with its characteristics.
3.4 Plan the nursing care of the patient having a bone marrow aspiration.
3.5 Write a discharge plan for an individual with a bone marrow transplant.

4.0 Demonstrate an understanding of the interventions used to manage adults with immune dysfunction.
    4.1 Identify types of medical treatment currently used.
    4.2 Demonstrate an understanding of the reasons certain treatments are used.
    4.3 Plan the nursing care for an adult with an immune dysfunction.

Learning Activities

Short Answers

1. List the three primary functions of the immune system.
   1.

   2.

   3.

2. The generative (primary) lymphoid organs in

   humans are the _____ and

   _____.

3. The T-cells are produced in the _____ and

   are responsible for the _____ response.

4. The B-cells are produced in the _____
   and are responsible for producing

   _____.

5. The major serum antibody is _____ ,
   which comprises about 70% of the total
   circulating antibodies.

6. The first antibody produced in response to

   an antigen is _____.

7. In the body, a goal of phagocytosis is the

   removal of _____.

8. Describe the three stages of the inflammatory
   response.
   1.

   2.

   3.

9. A critical factor in the success of any bone
   marrow transplant is a compatible

   _____.

10. Immunofluorescence is a technique that
    allows for identification of specific

    _____.

Identification

Match each kind of leukocyte type with its specific function.

   A.   Neutrophil

   B.   Eosinophil

   C.   Monocyte

   D.   Lymphocyte

11. _____ Ingests large numbers of microorganisms through phagocytosis.

12. _____ Responsible for the specific immune response.

13. _____ One of the first lines of defense during infection.

14. _____ Responds primarily to allergic reactions.

The body evokes either specific or nonspecific responses to an invader. Put an S (specific) or an N (nonspecific) next to each of the following defense mechanisms.

15. Physical barrier   _____

16. Interferon   _____

17. Inflammation   _____

18. Antigen   _____

19. Phagocytosis   _____

Match each type of allergy test with its description.

A.   Scratch test

B.   Prick test

C.   Intradermal

D.   Radioallergosorbent (RAST) test

20. _____   A drop of antigen is placed on the skin, then skin is pricked with a small-gauge needle.

21. _____   Done on the back or forearms, tests antigens one at a time.

22. _____   Determines the presence of allergen-specific IgE antibodies in blood.

23. _____   A small amount of antigen is injected under the skin.

True/False

24. _____   Live vaccines can be given safely to pregnant women.

25. _____   Multiple antigens can be administered simultaneously.

26. _____   The arm is the preferred injection site for vaccines in adults.

27. _____   Vaccines should not be given to adults who are allergic to eggs.

28. _____   Corticosteroids are a type of immuno-suppressant agent.

29. _____   Cytotoxic drugs kill immunologically competent cells.

30. _____   There is a gradual decrease in immuno-logic competency with aging.

Knowledge Application

31.   The function(s) of the lymph nodes include

A.   filtration of foreign material from lymph

B.   providing a place where immunologically active cells and antigens interact

C.   drainage of regions of the body

D.   all of the above

32.   An example of a chemical barrier within the body would be

A.   lysozyme

B.   sweat

C.   urine

D.   interferon

33.   Neoplastic diseases can lead an individual to become more susceptible to infections. This is usually a result of

A.   anemia

B.   neutropenia

C.   thrombocytopenia

D.   all of the above

34.   Choose the statement that best describes the inflammatory response.

A.   it is an attempt to maintain homeostasis and repair injured tissue

B.   it is an abnormal response to a threat of invasion

C.   it is a specific response by the body to protect against any threat of invasion

35.   If an individual has abnormal phagocytosis, the nurse would see which of the following in the patient's history?

A.   presence of neoplastic disease

B.   recurrent bacterial infections

C.   recurrent viral infections

D.   recurrent colds and fevers

36.   A substance that produces an immune response when introduced into a host is known as a(n)

A.   antigen

B.   phagocyte

C.   antibody

D.   lymphocyte

37. What type of immune process is found in the newborn infant?

   A.   maternal

   B.   natural

   C.   active

   D.   acquired

38. Immunity to a disease can develop as the result of exposure to an antigen. This is called _____ immunity.

   A.   natural

   B.   acquired

   C.   systemic

   D.   lifelong

39. What does the term *artificial exposure* refer to? Immunity received

   A.   from the mother

   B.   from exposure to virus

   C.   after receiving vaccine

   D.   after exposure to bacteria

40. When the nurse takes a health history on a patient, what information should be gathered related to the immune system? (Check all that apply.)

   A.   _____ infections

   B.   _____ cancer

   C.   _____ childhood disease

   D.   _____ immunizations

41. One main use of immunosuppressive therapy is to

   A.   treat viral infections that don't otherwise respond

   B.   treat adults with allergies

   C.   help with the success of organ transplants

   D.   treat surgical complication

42. A specific type of induced immunosuppression would be

   A.   allergy desensitization

   B.   administration of an antibody from one individual to another

   C.   administration of RhoGAM

   D.   all of the above

43. Which of the following statements is NOT true about cytotoxic drugs? They

   A.   can kill any cell that is replicating

   B.   may affect both the T-cells and the B-cells

   C.   have few side effects

   D.   have been used to treat rheumatoid arthritis

44. A patient is having a bone marrow aspiration. She wants to know what site will be used. Which is the most common?

   A.   hip

   B.   iliac crest

   C.   scapula

45. When bone marrow is harvested from a matched donor and infused into the recipient, this is known as

   A.   allogeneic transplant

   B.   matched transplant

   C.   syngeneic transplant

   D.   autologous transplant

46. Following a bone marrow transplant, new marrow begins to mature and function in

   A.   2–6 days

   B.   10–20 days

   C.   1–4 weeks

   D.   1–2 months

47. After bone marrow transplant, how long does it take for the body to regain the normal immune function?

   A.   1–3 months

   B.   3–6 months

   C.   6–12 months

   D.   12–18 months

48. For the individual who has had a bone marrow transplant, which of the following gifts would not be allowed?

   A.   flowers

   B.   candy

   C.   cards

   D.   puzzle

49. What is the biggest threat to the individual who has had a bone marrow transplant?

   A.   nutritional deficiency

   B.   interstitial bleeding

   C.   graft versus host disease

   D.   infection

50. Which of the following statements is most accurate in terms of the clinical manifestation of an infection in an 80-year-old female?

   A.   Fever is always present.

   B.   White blood cell count is always elevated.

   C.   Behavior changes are often present.

   D.   Pain and inflammation are often present.

Nursing Care Plan

51. Write a nursing care plan for the individual who is having a bone marrow aspiration.

   Nursing diagnosis: Knowledge deficit related to procedure

   Patient outcome:

   Interventions:

52. Write a nursing care plan for the patient who is being discharged following a bone marrow transplant. Focus on patient education.

   Nursing diagnosis:

   Patient outcome:

   Interventions:

Case Studies

Case Study No. 1

The nurse is assigned to care for Ms. K., a 19-year-old with leukemia. She is scheduled for a bone marrow transplant. The following questions refer to this situation.

53. Ms. K.'s mother wants to know why the physician wants to insert a Hickman catheter. Your response would be

    A. "It will prevent Ms. K. from getting infections."

    B. "It is always inserted for this procedure."

    C. "It makes it easier to administer drugs and draw blood."

    D. "It prevents any complications from occurring."

54. Ms. K.'s mother cannot understand why Ms. K. is going to receive chemotherapy before the transplant. "Isn't one procedure enough?" she asks. As the nurse, you explain to her that chemotherapy is done to

    A. prevent transplant rejection

    B. suppress the patient's immune system

    C. prevent side effects of the procedure

    D. prevent graft versus host disease

55. Following the procedure, the patient is in the recovery period. What is an appropriate nursing role at this time?

    A. Review behaviors that might indicate a knowledge deficit.

    B. Place the patient in a room with another teenager to allow her to verbalize her concerns.

    C. Encourage family and friends to visit.

56. Because the nurse knows that pancytopenia can persist for several weeks, Ms. K. should

    A. increase her activity slowly

    B. eat a high-protein diet

    C. remain on protective isolation

    D. have frequent visits with friends

57. Because Ms. K.'s platelet count is still low, the nurse would monitor for signs of

    A. infection

    B. bleeding

    C. stress

    D. anemia

58. Because mucositis is often a problem following chemotherapy and transplantation, the nurse would recommend

    A. small, frequent meals

    B. frequent rest periods

    C. deep-breathing exercises every two hours

    D. frequent mouth care with dilute peroxide

Case Study No. 2

Mrs. P. is admitted to your unit. She is 80 years old and was brought to the hospital by her husband because of fatigue, apathy, and confusion. She has a history of diabetes and angina.

59. As a nurse, you often work with geriatric patients and recognize that these symptoms may indicate that the patient may have

    A. organic brain syndrome

    B. a nutritional deficit

    C. low blood sugar

    D. an infection

60. Assessment findings reveal that she has poor cough effort, low urine output, and poor intake. It would be important to check the

    A. CBC

    B. chest x-ray

    C. urinalysis

    D. all of the above

61. Part of your nursing care of this patient will include monitoring for signs of

    A.   decreased metabolic rate

    B.   hypoglycemia

    C.   adequate oxygenation

    D.   sepsis

62. Discharge instructions for Mrs. P. would include which of the following information?

    A.   stay in bed as much as possible

    B.   avoid excessive contact with children

    C.   limit fluids during the day

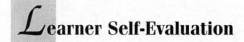

*L*earner Self-Evaluation

Do I fully understand the content? If no, then the areas I need to review are:

I need more information from my instructor on:

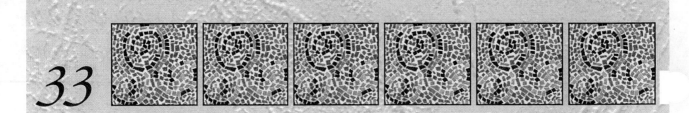

Nursing Care of Patients with HIV/AIDS and Other Immune Disorders

33

Objectives

1.0 Demonstrate an understanding of the etiology and pathology of the disorders of the immune system.
   1.1 Identify clinical manifestations of an immunodeficiency.
   1.2 Review the etiology and pathophysiology of several immune disorders.

2.0 Demonstrate application of the nursing process when caring for the patient with HIV/AIDS.
   2.1 Describe the etiology and transmission of HIV/AIDS.
   2.2 List the clinical manifestations of HIV/AIDS.
   2.3 Describe treatment options available for the patient with HIV/AIDS.
   2.4 Plan the nursing care for the patient being treated for HIV/AIDS.

3.0 Demonstrate an understanding of the nursing process when caring for the patient with a hypersensitivity reaction.
   3.1 Identify several of the hypersensitive disorders.
   3.2 Recognize the medical management for the adult with a hypersensitivity reaction.
   3.3 Plan the nursing care for the patient who has a hypersensitive reaction.

4.0 Demonstrate application of the nursing process when caring for the adult with a dysfunction of the immune system.
   4.1 Demonstrate an understanding of the needs of the adult with systemic lupus erythematosus (SLE).
   4.2 Identify the clinical manifestations and management goals for the patient with SLE.

Learning Activities

Short Answers

1. In immunodeficiency disorders, the immune system fails to _____.

2. Stem cell deficiency is an example of a _____ deficiency.

3. AIDS is the result of infection with _____.

4. A vascular neoplasm that causes dermatologic manifestations and occurs in about 25% of the patients with AIDS is known as _____.

5. The most frequent pulmonary manifestation of AIDS is pneumonia caused by the proto-

zoa _____.

6. List four syndromes associated with AIDS.
1.

2.

3.

4.

7. List the clinical manifestations of HIV infection. Include the four stages.
1.

2.

3.

4.

8. _____ is a sudden life-threatening reaction to an antigen.

9. The most useful drugs used in the treatment

of hay fever are _____.

10. A form of immunotherapy in which the patient is injected with extracts of the pollen he or she is allergic to is known as

_____.

11. _____ is an impaired hypersensitive reaction to an antigen that the patient has been exposed to previously.

12. _____ is a condition in which the body is reacting against itself.

13. Presence of the _____

_____ in the serum is an

important diagnostic finding with systemic lupus erythematosus (SLE).

True/False

14. _____ The more sexual partners a person has, the greater the risk of acquiring HIV.

15. _____ Transmission of HIV often occurs through contaminated blood.

16. _____ Women can pass the HIV virus to their infants.

17. _____ Health-care workers are at an increased risk of being infected by HIV.

18. _____ AIDS can be easily diagnosed by laboratory testing for HIV antibodies.

19. _____ Use of latex barriers by health-care workers will lessen the chance of exposure.

20. _____ Chronic fatigue syndrome often starts as the flu.

21. _____ Scleroderma is a potentially fatal disease.

22. _____ Scleroderma is an autoimmune collagen disease.

23. _____ Symptoms with systemic lupus follow a typical pattern.

24. _____ There is an increase in infection among the elderly.

25. _____ Elderly patients exhibit classical symptoms of infection.

Match the following types of hypersensitivity reactions with the correct description.

A. Type I
B. Type II
C. Type III
D. Type IV

26. _____ Occurs within minutes of the antigen-antibody reaction

27. _____ Delayed reaction caused by the release of lymphokines by T-cells

28. _____ Cytotoxic reaction that causes cell damage

29. _____ Occurs when soluble antigens react with antibodies

30. _____ Hay fever is an example of this type

31. _____ A transplant reaction is an example of this type

Knowledge Application

32. Identify the primary symptom(s) of an immunodeficient disease.

    A.   failure to thrive

    B.   chronic infection

    C.   weakness and malaise

    D.   chronic pain

33. Stem cell deficiency is characterized by absence of

    A.   T-cell function

    B.   B-cell function

    C.   both T-cell and B-cell function

    D.   thymic development

34. AN individual who has had _____ may be at risk for developing a secondary immunodeficiency.

    A.   tuberculosis

    B.   cytomegalovirus

    C.   acquired immunodeficiency syndrome (AIDS)

    D.   malignancies

    E.   all of the above

35. Education of the patient with an immunodeficiency would include teaching all of the following EXCEPT?

    A.   need to avoid crowds

    B.   ways to avoid infection

    C.   importance of good hygiene

    D.   need to take prophylactic medication

    E.   signs and symptoms of infections

36. What happens within the body when HIV infects the helper T-cells?

    A.   RNA is transformed into viral DNA, which destroys the helper T-cells if activated by exposure to antigens.

    B.   DNA is transformed into RNA, which destroys the B-cells and T-cells and destroys the immune system.

    C.   RNA is transformed into DNA, which when transformed, enters the leukocytes that subsequently multiply rapidly and immaturely.

    D.   HIV infects the entire immune system and renders the individual helpless when exposed to any bacteria or virus.

37. The nurse is aware that HIV is transmitted by

    A.   saliva and droplet infection

    B.   sexual contact that involves exchange of body fluids

    C.   contaminated food products

    D.   prolonged exposure to an AIDS victim

38. When an individual infected with HIV develops an acute infection, the nurse might expect to see symptoms such as

    A.   fever, sweats, malaise, anorexia, vomiting

    B.   maculopapular rash on chest

    C.   lymphadenopathy, enlarged spleen

    D.   any of the above

39. Current medical management for AIDS consists primarily of

    A.   palliative treatment since there is no cure

    B.   early treatment of infections, symptomatic management

    C.   antiretroviral therapy and protease inhibitors

    D.   bone marrow transplants

40. The nurse admits a patient who has a diagnosis of AIDS. During the physical assessment, she notices white patches in the buccal cavity. This finding suggests

    A. Kaposi's sarcoma

    B. *Candida albicans*

    C. *Pneumocystis carinii*

    D. *Shigella*

41. Mr. M., a 25-year-old patient with AIDS, is admitted with a serious fluid and electrolyte imbalance. When gathering information, it would be important to ask about history of

    A. excessive exercise patterns

    B. adherence to prescribed medications

    C. changes in bowel patterns

    D. changes in fluid intake

42. The nurse is assisting Mr. M. with his hygienic needs. One important reason for offering a back rub is to help him

    A. combat the sense of isolation

    B. to prevent formation of skin lesions

    C. bathe since he can't reach his back

    D. acknowledge his feelings

43. A patient with AIDS develops fever, dyspnea, tachypnea, and dry cough. These symptoms suggest the patient has

    A. *Entamoeba histolytica*

    B. *Shigella*

    C. *P. carinii* pneumonia

    D. tuberculosis

44. Because the nurse recognizes that most individuals with AIDS will be managed in home-care settings, what information should be available for persons with AIDS?

    A. referrals to social service, support groups

    B. public assistance programs

    C. complementary therapies such as vitamins, herbs

    D. legal and financial aid sources

    E. all of the above

45. The group of medications that have been found to be most helpful in treating allergic rhinitis is

    A. systemic corticosteroids

    B. antibiotics

    C. antihistamines

    D. antivirals

46. When an individual cannot control the symptoms of allergic rhinitis with environment control and medications, the patient may be a candidate for

    A. dustproofing the environment

    B. psychologic counseling

    C. protective isolation

    D. desensitization

47. A patient is admitted with a diagnosis of hypersensitivity pneumonitis. The nurse would expect to find symptoms such as

    A. shortness of breath

    B. fever, chills

    C. malaise

    D. all of the above

48. The nurse is aware that hypersensitivity pneumonitis results from

    A. autoimmune response

    B. arthus reaction

    C. antigen-antibody response

    D. any of the above

49. All of the following are common characteristics of autoimmune disease EXCEPT it

    A. occurs more often in men than women

    B. tends to run in families

    C. improves with immunosuppressive therapy

    D. may involve all of the body systems

50. SLE is an autoimmune disease. From the list below, star those factors that may trigger this disease.

   A.   use of sex hormones

   B.   ultraviolet radiation

   C.   viral infection

   D.   pregnancy

   E.   fatigue

   F.   stress

51. A patient is newly diagnosed with SLE and is asking the nurse to explain this disease. The nurse replies

   A.   "There is a basic imbalance in the immune system with depressed T-cell activity and increase in antibody production."

   B.   "This is a chronic systemic disease with very typical signs and symptoms."

   C.   "This is an acute disease that will go into remission once treatment is begun."

   D.   "This is a serious disease that may progress rapidly."

52. Providing which of the following information would meet the educational needs of the patient with SLE?

   A.   explain medical treatments that can cure the disease

   B.   teach how to avoid factors that cause exacerbation

   C.   teach which drugs are given prophylactically

   D.   explain that this disease won't interrupt lifestyle

53. The management goals for the patient with SLE are to

   A.   induce remission

   B.   control pain and inflammation

   C.   control inflammation and relieve symptoms

   D.   cure the disease with medication

54. If a patient with scleroderma were to exhibit malnutrition and weight loss, the probable cause would be

   A.   renal failure

   B.   CREST syndrome

   C.   esophageal stricture

   D.   pericarditis

55. An autoimmune disorder characterized by the increased destruction of red blood cells is

   A.   aplastic anemia

   B.   thrombocytopenia

   C.   hemolytic anemia

   D.   hemophilia

56. The following statements about chronic fatigue syndrome are all true EXCEPT

   A.   the etiology is uncertain

   B.   it occurs in Caucasians and blacks

   C.   it occurs mainly in young adults

   D.   it is characterized by unrelenting fatigue

57. Which of the following are reasons for the increase in infection rates with aging? (Check all that apply.)

   A.   _____ weakening of respiratory muscles

   B.   _____ calcification of heart valves

   C.   _____ increase in gastric motility

   D.   _____ increase in renal function

   E.   _____ chronic illnesses

Nursing Care Plans

58. Write a nursing care plan for an adult with AIDS. Use the following diagnosis.

     Nursing diagnosis: Knowledge deficit related to etiology, transmission, clinical course, and treatment protocols

     Patient outcome:

     Interventions:

59. Plan the nursing care for a patient who is diagnosed with SLE to help cope with the disease. Use the following diagnosis.

     Nursing diagnosis: Alteration in comfort related to inflammatory effects

     Patient outcome:

     Interventions:

60. Plan the nursing care for the patient with chronic fatigue syndrome who is being followed by a home-health nurse. Use the following diagnosis.

     Nursing diagnosis: Fatigue related to chronic fatigue syndrome

     Patient outcome:

     Interventions:

Case Studies

Case Study No. 1

Mr. B., a 35-year-old patient, has had AIDS for eight months. He has tried many types of treatments. He is admitted for treatment of secondary infections and general debilitation.

61. During assessment the nurse finds he is 5' 10" and weighs 125 lbs. He is pale and has poor skin turgor. He has white patches in his mouth. What other information will add to this assessment data?

     A.   dietary history

     B.   list of medications he is taking

     C.   number of past hospitalizations

     D.   list of contacts

62. Mr. B. states he has had severe diarrhea during the last month. The nurse would carefully assess for signs of

   A.   fluid and electrolyte imbalance

   B.   malnutrition

   C.   skin breakdown

   D.   all of the above

63. To help manage Mr. B.'s nutritional status, the nurse would suggest

   A.   drugs to increase appetite, dietary supplements

   B.   insertion of a feeding tube

   C.   injections of antiemetics prior to meals

   D.   prophylactic anti-infectives

64. A primary nursing diagnosis is Knowledge deficit related to treatment and self-care. Which action by the patient indicates the nurse's intervention has been effective? He

   A.   describes correct use of prescribed analgesic

   B.   states symptoms that require immediate medical attention

   C.   can chew soft foods with minimal discomfort

   D.   does not get short of breath with activity

65. It would be important to provide a nonjudgmental atmosphere to help Mr. B. cope with his feelings. An appropriate intervention would be to help the patient

   A.   deal with death and dying

   B.   manage home care

   C.   understand his medical care

   D.   all of the above

Case Study No. 2

Ms. S. is brought into the ER. She is dyspneic and diaphoretic. Her husband states she was stung by a bee. The physician administers epinephrine.

66. The nurse should consider which action of primary importance when performing the nursing assessment?

   A.   calm the patient and reassure her that she will be fine

   B.   document her reaction and response to treatment

   C.   assess for signs of allergic reaction to epinephrine

   D.   insist that her husband wait outside

67. Ms. S. is breathing much easier now. She asks you if this will ever happen again. What would be an appropriate response?

   A.   "I don't know, ask your doctor."

   B.   "No, these type of reactions generally don't recur."

   C.   "Yes, another sting could cause a similar reaction."

68. The nurse should plan to explain to Ms. S. that she should

   A.   avoid areas where bees are prevalent

   B.   carry a bee sting kit and know how to use it

   C.   wear a medic alert band

   D.   all of the above

Case Study No. 3

A 23-year-old college student is admitted to the hospital with a diagnosis of scleroderma. She has been treated by her family physician until this episode.

69. Which of the following statements best describes this disorder?

   A.   It occurs mainly in men.

   B.   It is an autoimmune collagen disorder.

   C.   It is an allergic reaction to antigens.

   D.   It is caused by a bacteria.

70. Specific characteristics that the nurse would ask about would include

    A. fibrosis in the skin

    B. edema in joints

    C. thickening of dermis

    D. vasospasmodic episodes

    E. any of the above

71. The patient is having difficulty breathing and swallowing. This may be a result of

    A. pulmonary fibrosis, esophageal stricture

    B. pericarditis, heart failure

    C. formation of plaque

    D. Raynaud's syndrome

72. Because of the systemic nature of this disease, an important laboratory finding for the nurse to review would be

    A. CBC, WBC

    B. BUN, creatinine

    C. CPK, AST

    D. ABGs

73. The nurse would expect medical treatment to involve

    A. antibiotics

    B. prednisone

    C. vasodilators

    D. vasoconstrictors

*L*earner Self-Evaluation

Do I fully understand the content? If no, then the areas I need to review are:

I need more information from my instructor on:

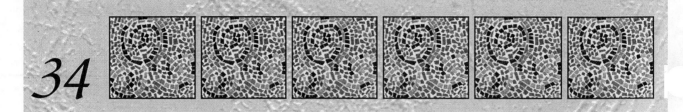

Nursing Care of Patients with Oncologic Disorders

Objectives

1.0 Demonstrate an understanding of the etiology and clinical manifestations of oncologic disorders.
 1.1 Identify current terminology.
 1.2 Identify signs and symptoms associated with cancer.

2.0 Demonstrate an understanding of the diagnostic testing and assessment data used to identify an oncologic disorder.
 2.1 Identify risk factors related to cancer formation.
 2.2 Identify diagnostic procedures used when an oncologic disorder is suspected.

3.0 Demonstrate application of the nursing process when caring for the patient receiving radiation therapy.
 3.1 Compare internal and external radiation therapy.
 3.2 Describe indications for radiation therapy.
 3.3 Identify the side effects related to radiation therapy.
 3.4 Plan the nursing care for the adult receiving radiation therapy.

4.0 Demonstrate application of the nursing process when caring for the patient receiving chemotherapy.
 4.1 Describe the types and actions of various chemotherapeutic agents.
 4.2 Identify types of delivery systems for chemotherapeutic agents.
 4.3 Identify the side effects related to chemotherapy.

5.0 Demonstrate an understanding of the diverse needs of the patient being treated for cancer.
 5.1 Describe methods to meet the nutritional needs of the patient with an oncologic disorder.
 5.2 Demonstrate an understanding of the needs of the patient who has pain secondary to cancer.
 5.3 Plan the nursing care for patients being treated for cancer.
 5.4 Identify the needs of patients being treated in alternative care settings within the community.
 5.5 Identify special considerations for the elderly patient with cancer.

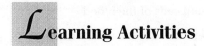

*L*earning Activities

Short Answers

1. List the seven warning signs of cancer.
    1.

    2.

    3.

    4.

    5.

    6.

    7.

2. List three risk factors associated with lung cancer.
    1.

    2.

    3.

3. List three risk factors associated with cervical cancer.
    1.

    2.

    3.

4. The process of transforming normal cells into malignant cells is known as _____.

5. The method of identifying the extent of the disease in the person who has cancer is known as _____.

6. Explain what is meant by a "cancer-prone" personality.

7. Proteins and hormones that are produced by certain types of cancers are known as

    _____.

8. A biopsy may be done to _____ or _____ a suspicious mass.

9. Loss of taste sensation secondary to radiation therapy is known as _____.

10. _____ drugs disrupt cell development and reproduction.

11. The incidence of cancer has been found to

    _____ with age.

Developing Understanding

Understanding how cancer is thought to develop is important. Explain how each of these factors may contribute to carcinogenesis.

12. Genetic factors

13. Environmental factors

14. Smoking

15. Diet

16. Immunologic defects

17. Psychosocial factors

18. Aging

Identification

Match these terms with the best definition.

   A.   Benign neoplasm

   B.   Carcinomas

   C.   Malignant neoplasm

   D.   Sarcoma

   E.   Leukemia

   F.   Neoplasm

19. _____ Malignant cells of connective tissue

20. _____ Cells which resemble the tissue of origin

21. _____ Malignant cells of the blood

22. _____ Undifferentiated cells unlike tissue of origin

23. _____ Malignant cells in epithelial tissue

24. _____ Group of cells with abnormal growth pattern

Knowledge Application

25. Cancer cells differ from normal cells in that they are anaplastic, which means

   A.   they are primitive, undifferentiated cells

   B.   they replicate slowly

   C.   they closely resemble the original cells

   D.   all of the above

26. Malignant tumors can spread through a direct or indirect process, known as

   A.   tissue invasion

   B.   metastasis

   C.   replication

   D.   duplication

27. Indirect spread of a tumor can be by invasion of (Check all that apply.)

   A.   _____ muscle cells

   B.   _____ vascular system

   C.   _____ lymphatic system

   D.   _____ immune system

   E.   _____ neuron fibers

28. Research has found that there is a correlation between heavy consumption of alcohol and the development of

   A.   esophageal, liver cancer

   B.   rectal, stomach cancer

   C.   breast, cervical cancer

   D.   brain, lung cancer

29. Research has shown that there is a relationship between _____ and onset of illness.

    A. diet

    B. smoking

    C. stress

    D. alcohol use

30. An example of a blood test used to diagnose cancer is the test for carcinoembryonic antigen. With what type of cancer has it been most often associated?

    A. cervical

    B. gastrointestinal

    C. brain

    D. bone

31. Which of the following statements is NOT true about magnetic resonance imaging? The patient is

    A. seen in a three-dimensional image

    B. not exposed to radiation

    C. checked first with a metal detector

    D. made NPO after midnight

32. The type of diagnostic test that uses high-frequency sound waves directed over a specific body part is called

    A. tomography

    B. ultrasonography

    C. mammography

    D. radionuclide scanning

33. The radiographic procedure that produces a detailed three-dimensional image that can be analyzed by a computer is called

    A. radionuclide scanning

    B. magnetic resonance imaging

    C. computed axial tomography

    D. ultrasonography

34. Mrs. J. is scheduled for a Pap smear and biopsy to rule out a neoplasm. From the list below, pick the most appropriate nursing diagnosis at this time.

    A. Anxiety related to uncertain outcome of tests

    B. Alteration in comfort related to diagnostic procedure

    C. Alteration in elimination related to diagnostic procedure

35. In assessing Mrs. J., who has now been diagnosed as having cancer, which of the following is important to ask?

    A. "Have you talked with your family about the diagnosis?"

    B. "What do you usually do when you have a problem?"

    C. "What kind of medical plan do you have?"

    D. all of the above are appropriate

36. The type of biopsy that removes all of the tumor is called

    A. needle biopsy

    B. incisional biopsy

    C. excisional biopsy

    D. irradiation biopsy

37. Which statement by the nurse would best describe the rationale for radiation therapy? "The purpose is to

    A. remove the neoplasm."

    B. damage and kill cancer cells."

    C. prevent metastasis."

    D. all of the above

38. When radiation is used in the early stages of cancer, the goal is to cure the neoplasm.

    A. true

    B. false

39. The rationale for giving radiation therapy over a period of several weeks is so that

    A. normal cells can have time for cellular repair

    B. costs will be decreased

    C. alopecia will be prevented

    D. radiation burns will not occur

40. The nurse is caring for a patient who has an internal radiation implant for uterine cancer. Pick the nursing measures that should be implemented.

    A. Call for a private room.

    B. Have the same nurse care for the patient.

    C. Cover the patient with a lead apron.

    D. Spend only 30 minutes in the room at a time.

41. Which of the following is NOT a relevant part of the assessment of the patient receiving radiation therapy of the esophagus?

    A. changes in skin color

    B. mouth ulcerations

    C. pain in chest

    D. ability to ambulate

42. The physician had ordered steroids for a patient who will have a series of radiation treatments for a brain tumor. The rationale for this medication is to

    A. prevent infection

    B. prevent skin excoriation

    C. stimulate the appetite

    D. prevent cerebral edema

43. Which of the following explanations would the nurse give to a patient to explain how chemotherapeutic drugs work?

    A. "They destroy only the abnormal cells."

    B. "They work quickly and have few side effects."

    C. "They prevent a recurrence of the cancer."

    D. "They disrupt the development and reproduction of cells."

44. Which of the following is a major advantage of chemotherapy? It

    A. has few side effects

    B. is less expensive

    C. is systemic

    D. prevents a return of the neoplasm

45. Which of the following statements is NOT true about the plant alkaloids. They

    A. inhibit DNA and protein synthesis

    B. come from the periwinkle plant

    C. are active during the mitosis phase

    D. are most effective against tumors with increased metabolic rates

46. The type of chemotherapeutic drugs that interfere with normal biochemical processes are

    A. antimetabolites

    B. plant alkaloids

    C. hormones

    D. steroids

47. The type of chemotherapeutic drugs that would most likely be given to the individual with prostate cancer would be

    A. plant alkaloid

    B. steroid

    C. hormonal therapy

    D. antimetabolite

48. Because chemotherapeutic agents are cytotoxic, special precautions are needed. Which of the following precautions are not necessary?

    A. wear protective gloves, gown, and mask when preparing agents

    B. use laminar airflow hood during large volume preparation

    C. wash skin with Betadine if agent is spilled

    D. wear gloves to administer

49. In preparing for the delivery of chemo-therapy, a variety of routes may be used. Which method involves the surgical place-ment of a catheter near the right atrium?

    A. central venous catheter

    B. intra-arterial catheter

    C. intrapleural catheter

    D. intravascular

50. Following surgery for liver cancer, Mr. M. is having a method of chemotherapy known as adjuvant therapy. This is done

    A. for the cure, control, or palliation of the tumor

    B. to stop further cell division of meta-static cells

    C. to prevent a recurrence of the tumor

    D. because he is not a candidate for radiation therapy

51. The reasons that patients undergoing chemo-therapy are at risk for side effects is because

    A. having cancer causes debilitation

    B. chemotherapy destroys normal cells

    C. the drugs are very potent

    D. chemotherapy causes toxic reactions

52. Since one of the side effects of chemotherapy is irritation of the gastrointestinal tract, the nurse might treat this problem with any of the following EXCEPT

    A. administer antiemetic drugs as ordered

    B. use relaxation therapy with the patient

    C. administer antihistamines as ordered

    D. administer anxiolytic drugs as ordered

    E. administer a small feeding prior to chemotherapy

53. During the administration of a chemothera-peutic drug the nurse finds that the medica-tion has infiltrated. What is an appropriate nursing action?

    A. stop the infusion and give the recom-mended antidote

    B. slow the infusion and call the physician

    C. change the infusion site and continue the medication

    D. wait and see if problems occur before taking action

54. Ms. B. has received chemotherapy for the past six weeks. Today she states that she feels uncoordinated, is weak, and has ringing in her ears. These symptoms suggest

    A. cardiotoxicity

    B. neurotoxicity

    C. pulmonary toxicity

    D. tissue extravasation

55. Chemotherapy can cause a variety of side effects. What should the nurse monitor to prevent an infection in a patient?

    A. signs of leukopenia

    B. signs of anemia

    C. energy levels

    D. stomatitis

56. If the patient undergoing chemotherapy has a low platelet count, the nurse would moni-tor for

    A. infection

    B. fluid and electrolyte imbalance

    C. bleeding

    D. hypoxia

57. The type of treatment for cancer with a chemical or biologic agent intended to assist the immune system to destroy cancer cells is known as

    A. chemotherapy

    B. hormonal therapy

    C. immunotherapy

    D. radiation therapy

58. Which of the following is NOT an example of a chemotherapeutic agent?

    A. vincristine

    B. dobutamine

    C. doxorubicin

    D. nitrogen mustard

59. Cancer presents a variety of psychosocial problems. From the list below, pick those that occur most frequently.

    A. anxiety and fear

    B. threat to self-concept

    C. alteration in breathing patterns

    D. potential for injury

    E. isolation and alienation

    F. family stress

60. Isolation is often a problem with individuals who have cancer. Which of these would be an appropriate nursing intervention?

    A. call the local minister

    B. offer suggestion of a referral to the cancer society

    C. offer tapes on pain control

    D. provide a book on hospice care

61. What is one of the reasons that patients with advanced cancer have pain?

    A. tissue damage and tissue infiltration

    B. bleeding into the tissue

    C. severe infection

    D. all of the above

62. Chemicals produced by the body in response to pain are known as

    A. narcotics

    B. neurotransmitters

    C. stimulants

    D. depressants

63. Pharmacologic agents that control pain by acting on the central nervous system are

    A. psychotropic agents

    B. narcotic agents

    C. anti-inflammatory agents

    D. nonnarcotic agents

64. A type of cutaneous therapy that stimulates the peripheral nervous system in an attempt to override the pain stimulus is called

    A. acupuncture

    B. skin massage

    C. transcutaneal electrical stimulation (TENS)

    D. cold application

Nursing Care Plans

65. Write a nursing care plan for the individual who is newly diagnosed with cancer. Use the following diagnosis.

    Nursing diagnosis: Knowledge deficit related to cause, prognosis, type of malignancy, and treatment methods

    Patient outcome:

    Interventions:

66. Plan the nursing care for the patient who is undergoing external radiation therapy. Use the following diagnosis.

    Nursing diagnosis: High risk for altered health maintenance related to lack of knowledge of side effects of treatment

    Patient outcome:

    Interventions:

Coping Strategies

When providing support to the cancer patient, the nurse needs to know the prognosis to help the patient deal successfully with the problems. Therefore, it is important to know if the treatment focus is to cure the disease, control symptoms, or only provide comfort. List two interventions that would be appropriate for each of the treatment foci.

67. Cure: How will the nurse help the patient cope with anxiety and fear?
    1.

    2.

68. Control: How will the nurse help the patient cope with problems related to sexuality?
    1.

    2.

69. Comfort: How will the nurse help the patient deal with loss of life and helplessness?
    1.

    2.

Working in the Home

Currently most of the treatment for cancer will be done in a clinic or outpatient facility with the patient returning home. The office nurse, the nurse practitioner, or the home-health nurse will be involved in teaching and monitoring for complications. Assume you are working with cancer patients in the community.

70. List three complications associated with chemotherapy that would be part of your teaching.
    1.

    2.

    3.

71. List two ways to cope with these complications.
    1.

    2.

72. List three complications associated with radiation therapy that would be part of your teaching.
    1.

    2.

    3.

73. List two ways to cope with these complications.
    1.

    2.

Food for Thought

Would the person with cancer of a specific organ (for example, liver or pancreas) be a candidate for transplant? Why or why not?

How are decisions made about who receives a bone marrow transplant?

What are the long-term survival rates associated with cancers?

Case Studies

Case Study No. 1

Mr. D. is 75 years old. He has had surgery for esophageal cancer to be followed by radiation therapy upon discharge.

74. The diagnosis of esophageal cancer is usually made by

    A.   endoscopy

    B.   chest x-ray

    C.   CT scan

    D.   angiogram

In Mr. D.'s situation, he is not a candidate for surgery because the cancer has already metastasized.

75. Why is cancer often not diagnosed until it has already spread?

    A.   Symptoms are often vague.

    B.   Patient does not seek treatment early.

    C.   Patient fears the results of tests.

    D.   all of the above

76. All of the following are side effects of radiation therapy EXCEPT

    A.   alopecia

    B.   erythema

    C.   esophagitis

    D.   weakness

77. Mr. D. develops a sore throat and esophagitis. What is the most relevant nursing diagnosis at this time?

    A.   Alteration in skin integrity

    B.   Potential for infection

    C.   Potential for alteration in elimination

    D.   Alteration in nutrition

78. At this time is would be important for the nurse to teach Mr. D. how to

    A.   perform good oral hygiene

    B.   perform coughing and deep breathing

    C.   control pain and discomfort

    D.   apply lotions and compresses

Case Study No. 2

The nurse is caring for a 66-year-old female, Mrs. A., who has a lymphoma. Part of your care for Mrs. A. involves giving a dose of vincristine. The following questions refer to this situation.

79. In order to be certified in the administration of chemotherapy, the nurse must have special training. Which of the following is NOT included in the training?

    A.   starting the intravenous solution with vincristine

    B.   awareness of the possibility of tissue extravasation

    C.   appropriate ways to treat nausea

    D.   understanding of emergency procedures

80. After a course of chemotherapy, Mrs. A. is to have several radiation therapy treatments. The purpose of radiation therapy in this case would be

    A.   adjuvant therapy

    B.   palliative therapy

    C.   primary curative therapy

81. The nurse is explaining to Mrs. A. what to expect during her first treatment. Which of the following statements is inaccurate?

    A. "You will be required to lie still."

    B. "You will have a radiologist with you."

    C. "You will not be radioactive after the treatment."

    D. "You will hear a noise from the machine."

82. As a result of the treatment, Mrs. A. develops dermatitis. All of the following are appropriate nursing measures, EXCEPT to apply

    A. moisturizer

    B. water-soluble lubricant

    C. warm compresses

    D. soap

Case Study No. 3

A patient is admitted to the hospital for further chemotherapy to treat lung cancer. Her tumor was resected two months ago, followed by four weeks of radiation therapy. As the primary nurse, you talk about the intended chemotherapy.

83. Which statement by the patient would indicate that the information given was effective?

    A. "Please review the purpose of chemotherapy."

    B. "Leave me alone; I'm not worried."

    C. "My husband doesn't need to know about this."

    D. "I've read that cancer is always fatal."

84. Following the first chemotherapy treatment, she complains of severe nausea and begins to vomit. A medication that has some effect on minimizing nausea is

    A. Demerol

    B. Valium

    C. Phenergan

    D. Haldol

85. A common complication of chemotherapy is mucositis. The nurse is aware that the reason for this is

    A. chemotherapy attacks cells that grow rapidly

    B. the drug is taken by this route

    C. unknown

    D. the drug is very irritating to tissue

86. To help prevent this problem, the nurse would

    A. offer a soft diet

    B. provide good oral hygiene

    C. provide pain medication

    D. provide diversional therapy

87. The patient also begins to have severe episodes of diarrhea. The most appropriate interventions would include

    A. nutritional interventions

    B. drugs such as Lomotil

    C. fluid replacement

    D. all of the above

88. When the patient is discharged, she is told that a common side effect of the medication she received is photosensitivity. Because of this she should avoid

    A. crowds

    B. exposure to sunlight

    C. any over-the-counter medications

    D. milk in her diet

*L*earner Self-Evaluation

Do I fully understand the content? If no, then the
areas I need to review are:

I need more information from my instructor on:

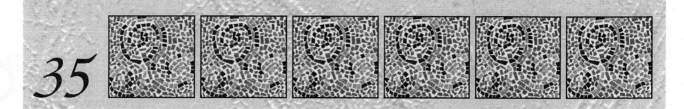

35

Knowledge Base for Patients with Integumentary Dysfunction

Objectives

1.0 Review the anatomy and physiology of the skin.
    1.1 Identify the layers of the skin.
    1.2 Match the skin structure with its function.

2.0 Demonstrate an understanding of the assessment data related to skin dysfunction.
    2.1 Identify the clinical manifestations of various skin diseases.
    2.2 Identify specific types of skin lesions.
    2.3 Identify basic diagnostic procedures.
    2.4 Apply the nursing process in caring for a patient who is having a skin biopsy.

3.0 Demonstrate an understanding of interventions used to treat alteration in skin function.
    3.1 Identify the pharmacologic treatments used.
    3.2 Identify the surgical procedures and techniques used for patients with skin dysfunction.
    3.3 Identify complications of surgical procedures used to treat skin dysfunctions.
    3.4 Identify nursing interventions applicable to patients with skin dysfunction.

Learning Activities

Identification

1. On the following figure, identify the following.

    A. Epidermis

    B. Dermis

    C. Subcutaneous layer

    D. Hair shaft

    E. Sweat gland

    F. Hair follicle

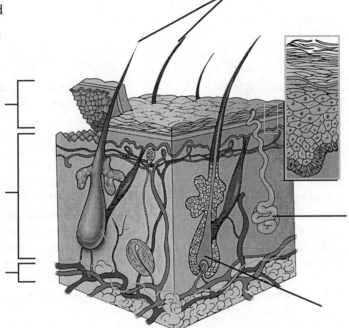

Match the skin structure with the appropriate function.

    A. Epidermis

    B. Dermis

    C. Subcutaneous fat tissue

    D. Sweat glands

    E. Melanocyte

    F. Blood vessels

    G. Sebaceous glands

2. _____ Provide skin pigment and color

3. _____ Outer layer of skin, protective barrier

4. _____ Provide nourishment

5. _____ Provides support and elasticity

6. _____ Provides insulation from cold and trauma

7. _____ Helps with temperature regulation

8. _____ Give bulk to the skin

9. _____ Oil-producing glands

Short Answers

10. A wart or mole is an example of a

    _____.

11. A skin abscess is often caused by a

_____ infection.

12. Pustules are common in _____.

13. A wheal is also known as a

_____.

14. Crusts are often seen with conditions such as

_____.

15. Loss of subcutaneous tissue can result in

_____.

16. The most common symptom in dermatology

is _____.

17. _____ agents can be applied
to the scalp to debride the scales of psoriasis.

18. List four areas that could show changes
when an individual has a skin dysfunction.
1.

2.

3.

4.

Identification

Match these common skin dysfunctions with the
best definition.

    A.   Macule

    B.   Papule

    C.   Cyst

    D.   Abscess

    E.   Wheal

    F.   Vesicle

19. _____ Circumscribed walled-off cavity filled
with pus and serosanguineous fluid

20. _____ Flat nonpalpable lesion characterized
by change in skin color

21. _____ Transient, irregularly shaped elevation
of the skin

22. _____ Raised, palpable, firm lesion less than 1
cm in diameter

23. _____ Lesion with a cavity that contains free
fluid

24. _____ Elevated, encapsulated mass in dermis
or subcutaneous layer; has fluid,
semifluid, or solid content

The ability of the nurse to assess alterations is an
important skill. Write the name of the skin lesion
depicted in each of the following illustrations.

Name

25.

26.

27.

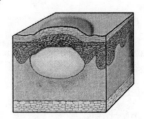

Name

28.

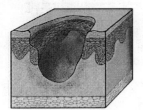

29.

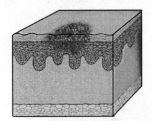

True/False

30. _____ A cream is an oil-in-water emulsion

31. _____ An ointment is a water-in-oil emulsion

32. _____ A lotion is a liquid suspension

33. _____ Systemic effects can result from the use of topical steroids

34. _____ Hydrocortisone cream ½% has no side effects

35. _____ Hexachlorophene can be used on any open skin lesion

36. _____ Occlusive dressings are used to enhance penetration of medications

37. _____ Occlusive dressings increase the risk of skin irritation and toxic side effects

Knowledge Application

38. The potassium hydroxide mount is an office procedure used to diagnose

    A.   viral infections

    B.   fungal infections

    C.   bacterial infections

    D.   scabies

39. A Tzanck smear is done to diagnose

    A.   herpes vial infections

    B.   fungal infections

    C.   staphylococcal infections

    D.   syphilis infection

40. A darkfield microscope examination is done to diagnose

    A.   fungal infections

    B.   viral herpes

    C.   active syphilis infection

    D.   scabies

41. The type of skin biopsy that would be done when malignant melanoma is suspected is

    A.   shave biopsy

    B.   punch biopsy

    C.   needle biopsy

    D.   excision biopsy

42. The nurse is aware that coal tar agents are usually used to treat a patient with

    A.   psoriasis

    B.   scabies

    C.   poison ivy

    D.   fungal infection

43. A topical skin preparation used for its antiproliferative and anti-inflammatory effect is

    A.   anthralin

    B.   corticosteroid

    C.   Hibiclens

    D.   Betadine

44. A topical agent known to be effective against fungal infections is

    A.   nystatin

    B.   acyclovir

    C.   Retinoid

    D.   hydrocortisone

45. The antiviral drug that is the treatment of choice for herpes simplex is

    A. hydrocortisone

    B. tetracycline

    C. Retin A

    D. acyclovir

46. AN antimetabolite medication useful in the treatment of psoriasis is

    A. fluorouracil

    B. Leukeran

    C. methotrexate

    D. Acyclovir

47. The most common procedure used for the removal of early basal cell cancer is

    A. curettage and desiccation

    B. punch biopsy

    C. scraping

    D. radiation treatment

48. A patient is undergoing outpatient ultraviolet radiation for treatment of eczema. The nurse would implement all of the following interventions EXCEPT

    A. have patient wear protective goggles

    B. have patient wear paper gown

    C. have patient stand nude in treatment area

    D. cover any sunburn-sensitive areas

49. The type of procedure that uses liquid nitrogen application to destroy lesions such as warts is known as

    A. radiation treatment

    B. cryosurgery

    C. nitrogen scraping

    D. dermabrasion

50. The nurse is aware that the carbon dioxide laser works by

    A. chemical irritation to the tissue

    B. freezing of tissue and subsequent destruction

    C. vaporizing of tissue by causing cells to swell and burst

    D. causing death to tissue by direct penetration of beam

51. The type of graft when skin is transplanted from one person to another is called

    A. autograft

    B. homograft

    C. heterograft

    D. dermograft

52. The most common donor site for a split-thickness skin graft is the

    A. upper arm

    B. scapula

    C. anterior thigh

    D. abdomen

53. The nurse caring for a patient with a skin graft is aware that the first dressing change is done in approximately

    A. 24 hours

    B. 48 hours

    C. 72 hours

    D. 1 week

54. The nurse would teach the patient how to care for the donor site. Instructions would include all of the following EXCEPT

    A. maintaining immobility of site

    B. preventing pressure on the site

    C. changing dressing every four hours

    D. keeping site free from contamination

55. A complication that the nurse would observe for following liposuction would be

    A.   fat embolism

    B.   hypotension

    C.   cardiac arrhythmia

    D.   infection

Nursing Care Plan

56. Write a care plan for the patient with a skin graft. Use the following nursing diagnosis.

    Nursing diagnosis: High risk for infection related to multiple routes of possible invasion by microorganisms caused by breaks in the skin

    Patient outcome:

    Interventions:

Case Studies

Case Study No. 1

A patient is admitted with psoriasis. It has been a problem for several months and she is seeking relief.

57. The nurse examines the skin, and finds that it is irregular and thick with flaky exfoliation. A word that may be used to describe this condition is

    A.   crusty

    B.   ulceration

    C.   atrophy

    D.   scaly

58. One type of medication found to be useful in the management of this condition is

    A.   hydrocortisone

    B.   anthralin

    C.   tetracycline

    D.   penicillin

59. The physician orders a hydrating therapeutic bath for this patient. The proper procedure would be to

    A.   have the patient soak in hot water for one hour, rinse, and pat dry

    B.   place in a whirlpool to which oils have been added

    C.   place in warm water for 30 minutes, wash with soft cloth to gently debride the scales

    D.   place in cool water, then brush away rough skin vigorously with a brush

60. The patient has signs of psoriasis on her scalp. What type of agent would the nurse expect the physician to order to help in debriding the lesions?

    A.   keratolytic agents

    B.   steroidal agents

    C.   antibiotic agents

    D.   coal tar products

61. AN example of this type of agent would be

    A.   hydrocortisone

    B.   tetracycline ointment

    C.   salicylic acid in oil base

    D.   acyclovir

Case Study No. 2

A nurse working in a clinical setting is caring for a patient who is having a basal cell cancer on the upper back removed by curettage and desiccation.

62.   Following the treatment, information that the nurse would tell the patient is

    A.   healing takes place in 1–3 weeks; the crust forms and sloughs in 7–10 days

    B.   healing takes 3–5 days; the crust drops off in 2–3 days

    C.   healing may take as long as six months; infection is a big problem

    D.   scabs drop off in 3 days; healing is complete in 1 week

63.   The patient asks if this type of cancer is going to be fatal. The nurse would reply

    A.   "You need to discuss that with your physician."

    B.   "The cure rate of early basal cell cancer with this procedure is excellent."

    C.   "The outcome with any type of cancer is very uncertain."

    D.   "Don't worry about that now."

Unfortunately, the cancer recurs. Micrographic surgery is recommended.

64.   The patient is worried and asks how the physician will know if all the cancer is removed. The nurse replies

    A.   "The physician takes out all the abnormal tissue that he can see."

    B.   "The lesion is removed and tissue is examined; if malignant cells are present more is removed until you are free from abnormal cells."

    C.   "An area twice the size of the cancer is removed so that the physician is sure that all the abnormal cells have been removed."

65.   The area that is removed is large enough to require use of a skin flap. The best definition of what a skin flap involves is

    A.   tissue is raised from one area of the body and transferred to an adjacent area

    B.   tissue is cut out from area that is highly vascular

    C.   a flap of skin is taken from the leg and placed on the back

    D.   a piece of skin is cut from the leg with a razor then laid on the area where the cancer was

66.   The donor site will heal by

    A.   scar formation

    B.   revascularization

    C.   re-epithelialization

    D.   forming a crust

Case Study No. 3

67.   Mr. P. had a skin graft to his upper arm following a burn. The nurse is instructing him on home management. Write four discharge instructions for Mr. P. to help protect the graft.

1.

2.

3.

4.

*L*earner Self-Evaluation

Do I fully understand the content? If no, then the
areas I need to review are:

I need more information from my instructor on:

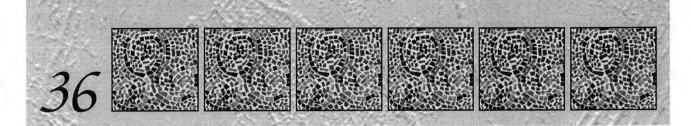

36

Nursing Care of Patients with Integumentary Disorders

*O*bjectives

1.0 Demonstrate an understanding of the infectious and inflammatory integumentary disorders.
   1.1 Match several types of skin disorders with the correct definition.
   1.2 Identify the clinical manifestations of several infections and inflammations of the skin.
   1.3 Demonstrate an understanding of the types of treatment options available for patients with skin disorders.
   1.4 Demonstrate an understanding of the teaching needs of the patient with a skin disorder.

2.0 Demonstrate an understanding of structural disorders of the integumentary system.
   2.1 Identify the clinical manifestations of several structural disorders of the skin.
   2.2 Demonstrate an understanding of the types of treatment options available for patients with structural disorders of the skin.

3.0 Demonstrate an understanding of the needs of patients with pressure ulcers.
   3.1 Demonstrate an understanding of the types of treatment options available for patients with pressure ulcers.
   3.2 Identify nursing interventions commonly applicable to patients with pressure ulcers.
   3.3 Identify the special needs of the elderly with pressure ulcers.

4.0 Demonstrate an understanding of the needs of the patient with skin cancer.
   4.1 Identify characteristics of neoplasms of the skin.
   4.2 Plan the nursing care for a patient with a neoplasm.

*L*earning Activities

Identification

Match the following common infectious or inflammatory skin disorders with the best definition.

A.   Pyoderma

B.   Folliculitis

C.   Furuncle

D.   Carbuncle

E.   Cellulitis

F.   Dermatophyte infections

G.   Eczematous dermatitis

H.   Acne

I.   Pemphigus vulgaris

1.   _____ Skin disorder that affects the sebaceous glands

2.   _____ Superficial fungal infection of skin (ringworm)

3.   _____ Bacterial skin infections

4.   _____ Pus-filled mass in dermis, drains purulent exudate

5.   _____ Autoimmune disease characterized by flaccid, easily ruptured bullae

6.   _____ Deep folliculitis, usually caused by *Staphylococcus aureus*, also known as a boil

7.   _____ Deep infection of the skin and subcutaneous tissue

8.   _____ Superficial inflammation of the skin characterized by itching, erythema, and edema

9.   _____ Superficial infection of the hair follicle

Short Answers

10.   Most pathogenic organisms that cause skin

infections reach the skin by an _____

route.

11.   Bacterial skin infections are most commonly

caused by _____ or _____.

12.   Fungal infections are classified as

_____ or _____ infec-

tions.

13.   Warts are caused by

_____.

14.   The varicella-zoster virus enters the

_____ nerves.

15.   Contact dermatitis is a common inflamma-

tory skin ailment caused by an _____

agent.

16.   Two factors that contribute to the develop-

ment of pressure ulcers are _____

and _____.

17.   Basal cell epitheliomas develop in areas of

the skin exposed to _____.

True/False

18.   _____ *Candida albicans* is normally present on the skin.

19.   _____ Warts cannot be transmitted by touch.

20.   _____ Herpes simplex virus is not contagious.

21.   _____ Drug reactions are the most common cause of generalized erythematous eruptions.

22.   _____ Acne is the most common skin disorder seen by dermatologists.

23.   _____ Psoriasis is a chronic hereditary disorder.

24.   _____ Pressure ulcers occur most often among the frail elderly.

25.   _____ Pressure ulcers can be easily treated.

Knowledge Application

26. A patient is seen in a clinic where a furuncle is diagnosed. The treatment might include all of the following EXCEPT

    A. applying hot compresses four times daily

    B. squeezing gently

    C. local antibiotics

    D. surgical excision

    E. systemic antibiotics

27. When caring for a patient with cellulitis, the nurse would expect to implement which of the following orders?

    A. administer oral and topical antibiotics

    B. warm compresses, oatmeal bath

    C. bed rest, parenteral antibiotics

    D. assist with surgical debridement, antibiotics

28. Medical management for the patient who has a severe tinea infection of the scalp would include

    A. topical antifungal agents, daily cleansing with soap and water

    B. cleansing, wet soaks, systemic antifungal agents

    C. oral antifungal agents, daily scrubbing with coal tar agents

    D. surgical debridement followed by wet-to-dry compresses

29. Presence of _____ in a skin culture would confirm the presence of a fungal infection in a patient.

    A. Streptococcus

    B. Staphylococcus

    C. Candidiasis

    D. *Escherichia coli*

30. Which of these factors would predispose a patient to the development of candidiasis?

    A. pregnancy

    B. diabetes

    C. antibiotic therapy

    D. steroid therapy

    E. any of the above

31. The nurse is aware that certain patients have increased risk for developing candidiasis. Which of the following individuals would be most likely to develop candidiasis?

    A. teenager with poor nutrition

    B. elderly male with leukemia

    C. young woman pregnant with first child

    D. middle-aged male with prostate cancer

32. The most common method of treating warts is

    A. laser surgery

    B. cytotoxic agents

    C. cryosurgery

    D. surgical incision

33. A patient is admitted to the hospital with pneumonia and shingles. The nurse is aware that shingles is caused by

    A. reactivation of herpes simplex

    B. activation of varicella-zoster in individuals who have had varicella

    C. exposure to individuals with genital herpes

    D. compromised immune system

34. A patient with shingles is complaining of severe pain and itching. Treatment might involve administration of

    A. antibiotics and analgesics

    B. antifungals and steroids

    C. analgesics and antipruritics

    D. antibiotics and steroids

35. One of the roles of the nurse in treating the individual with contact dermatitis would be

   A.   assisting the person to identify the cause

   B.   administering topical antivirals

   C.   applying wet-to-dry dressing

   D.   giving systemic antibiotics and steroids

36. During assessment of a patient, the nurse notices generalized, macular/papular, bright red eruptions over the trunk area. This is most likely related to

   A.   contract dermatitis

   B.   food allergy

   C.   drug allergy

   D.   any of the above

37. While working on the oncology unit, the nurse accidentally spills some of the chemotherapeutic medication on her hands. A possible result might be

   A.   contact dermatitis

   B.   seborrheic dermatitis

   C.   dermatophyte infection

   D.   stasis dermatitis

38. If the nurse did develop a reaction, which of the following clinical manifestations would occur?

   A.   pustules, macules

   B.   skin erosion followed by abscess

   C.   vesicles, fluid-filled papules

   D.   erythema following linear tracks

39. When checking a patient with peripheral vascular disease, the nurse notices edema, brown pigmentation, and thickened skin on the extremities. This would suggest

   A.   allergic dermatitis

   B.   seborrheic dermatitis

   C.   stasis dermatitis

   D.   contact impetigo

40. A nurse is about to administer the second dose of gentamicin to a patient. The patient complains of pruritus and the nurse notices a generalized macular/papular rash on the body. An appropriate nursing action is to

   A.   administer the medication then call the physician

   B.   hold the medication and call the physician

   C.   administer an antipyretic then administer medication

   D.   administer medication and recheck patient in one hour

41. A type of antibacterial and keratolytic agent that is used in the treatment of acne vulgaris is

   A.   tretinoin

   B.   isotretinoin

   C.   benzoyl peroxide

   D.   prednisone

42. The nurse would instruct a patient with psoriasis to take which precautions to avoid exacerbation?

   A.   avoid overexposure to sun

   B.   avoid over-the-counter medications

   C.   wash hands frequently

   D.   avoid exposure to cold

43. Which nursing action would be a priority in treating a patient who has a known allergy to Hymenoptera? Monitor

   A.   skin integrity

   B.   for infection

   C.   breathing patterns

   D.   fluid status

44. Which of the following patients would have the greatest risk of developing a pressure ulcer?

    A.   female, 85, in assisted living facility

    B.   male, 66, with diabetes

    C.   female, 72, history of stroke, paralysis, anemia

    D.   male, 90, history of arthritis, pneumonia

45. The most appropriate treatment for the patient with a Stage II pressure ulcer would be to

    A.   apply transparent dressing

    B.   clean with Betadine, apply dry dressing

    C.   clean with saline, apply wet-to-dry dressing

    D.   debride wound, then pack tightly

Nursing Care Plans

46. Write a nursing care plan for the patient with a bacterial skin infection. Use the following nursing diagnosis.

    Nursing diagnosis: Impaired skin integrity

    Patient outcome:

    Interventions:

47. Write a nursing care plan for the patient with a benign skin lesion. Use the following nursing diagnosis.

    Nursing diagnosis: Anxiety related to procedures to be done and possibility of skin cancer

    Patient outcome:

    Interventions:

48. Write a nursing care plan for the patient with a malignant melanoma. Use the following nursing diagnosis.

    Nursing diagnosis: Impaired skin integrity

    Patient outcome:

    Interventions:

Case Studies

Case Study No. 1

Mrs. P. is being treated for Crohn's disease. She is receiving systemic antibiotics and steroids. Because of this, the nurse realizes that the patient is at risk for developing Candidiasis.

49. Factors that decrease host resistance and are present in this patient include

    A. immunosuppressive therapy

    B. nutritional problems

    C. diabetes

    D. cancer

50. If candidiasis is present, the nurse would notice what type of skin lesions?

    A. brownish-white with vesicles

    B. pink and surrounded by white scale and pustules

    C. red with purple patches and pustules

    D. whitish with pustules and cysts

51. Treatment would involve

    A. parenteral antibiotic agents

    B. oral antibiotic agents

    C. topical antifungal agents

    D. parenteral antiviral agents

52. The nurse recognizes that the patient has an understanding of the cause and treatment of this disorder when she states

    A. "I understand that this is contagious."

    B. "I will leave the shampoo on 10 minutes before I rinse."

    C. "I will take my antibiotics for 10 days."

    D. "I will avoid sunlight in the future."

Case Study No. 2

Mr. G., age 18, is seen by a dermatologist for treatment of severe acne vulgaris.

53. As the nurse assesses Mr. G., she would expect to see which type of characteristic lesions?

    A. papules, pustules, cysts, and erythema

    B. macules, suppurative cysts, scaling

    C. vesicles, erythema

    D. cysts, abscess formation

54. Mr. G. has been treated with topical keratolytic agents and systemic antibiotics. The physician now recommends using low-dose glucocorticoids. The reason is to

    A. suppress estrogen formation

    B. decrease the inflammatory reaction

    C. suppress androgen secretion

    D. speed turnover of epithelial cells

55. Which of the following nursing diagnoses would have priority?

    A. Potential for infection

    B. Altered skin integrity

    C. Body image disturbance

    D. Altered health maintenance

56. The nurse would instruct Mr. G. on principles of skin care. These would include

    A. clean the skin with abrasive soap four times daily

    B. wash face with mild soap twice a day

    C. eat a healthy diet with no restrictions

    D. shampoo hair only twice a week

57. The physician is also using isotretinoin (vitamin A derivative) to treat Mr. G. The nurse is aware that side effects of this medication often include

    A. nausea, vomiting, diarrhea

    B. visual changes, dizziness

    C. cheilitis, dry skin, nosebleeds

    D. postural hypotension

Case Study No. 3

Ms. M., age 35, has had psoriasis for many years. She has another flare-up, and is being evaluated in a clinic to determine other possible therapies.

58. The nurse asks Ms. M. if she knows what factors aggravate this problem. Ms. M. answers correctly

   A.   using alcohol, trauma to the skin

   B.   exposure to people with the disease

   C.   reaction to insect bites

   D.   allergic reaction to chemical irritants

59. The nurse reviews the current treatment protocol which involves

   A.   use of occlusive dressing over infected areas

   B.   therapeutic baths once a week

   C.   using coal tar or corticosteroid three times a day

   D.   all of the above

60. A nursing diagnosis which is a priority for Ms. M. at this time would be

   A.   High risk for individual ineffective coping

   B.   Risk for infection

   C.   Potential for alteration in skin integrity

   D.   Alteration in skin integrity

61. Using the priority diagnosis, an appropriate nursing intervention would be

   A.   provide Ms. M. with information about support groups

   B.   refer Ms. M. to another dermatologist

   C.   give Ms. M. some written material on this disorder

   D.   suggest Ms. M. see a psychiatrist

62. The goal of medical management in the treatment of Ms. M.'s condition would be to

   A.   put the disease into remission

   B.   control the pain and itching

   C.   reduce the amount of scarring

   D.   decrease epidermal proliferation and dermal inflammation

Case Study No. 4

Mr. O., age 88, is admitted to the surgical unit for treatment of squamous cell carcinoma. He has a history of diabetes, anemia, and hypertension, and is anorexic and depressed.

63. The nurse is aware that the most common and effective method of treatment for this disorder is

   A.   cryotherapy

   B.   laser therapy

   C.   curettage and desiccation

   D.   radiation therapy

64. Which information in Mr. O.'s history would give the nurse information about the etiology of this disorder? The patient

   A.   had actinic keratosis for several years

   B.   has a history of sebaceous cysts

   C.   has a history of psoriasis

   D.   has peripheral vascular disease

65. Because of his age and other medical problems, surgical resection is too risky. Another treatment option would include

   A.   radiation therapy

   B.   chemotherapeutic agents

   C.   steroidal agents

   D.   immunosuppressive agents

66. On the second hospital day, the nurse notices that the area over his coccyx is reddened and does not blanch. She suspects that the patient

    A.   is developing a Stage I pressure ulcer

    B.   is developing contact dermatitis

    C.   has signs of malnutrition

    D.   has a Stage III decubitus ulcer

67. Appropriate nursing intervention(s) would be

    A.   turn every hour

    B.   provide nutritional management

    C.   prevent shearing or friction

    D.   all the above

Learner Self-Evaluation

Do I fully understand the content? If no, then the areas I need to review are:

I need more information from my instructor on:

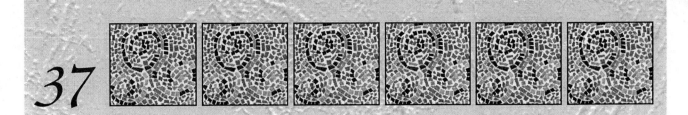

37

Nursing Care of Patients with Burns

Objectives

1.0 Demonstrate the ability to assess the patient with a burn injury.
   1.1 Identify factors that determine the severity of a burn.
   1.2 Match types of burns with identifying characteristics.
   1.3 Identify the physical examination data essential to the assessment of patients with burn injuries.

2.0 Demonstrate application of the nursing process when caring for the patient with a burn injury.
   2.1 Demonstrate an understanding of immediate care that is required following a burn injury.
   2.2 Demonstrate an understanding of patient needs during the emergent phase of the burn injury.
   2.3 Identify problems that can occur as a result of a burn injury.
   2.4 Demonstrate an understanding of patient needs during the acute phase of the burn injury.
   2.5 Demonstrate an understanding of patient needs during the rehabilitation phase.

3.0 Demonstrate an understanding of the interventions used to treat burn injuries.
   3.1 Identify ways to manage pain in the burn patient.
   3.2 Demonstrate an understanding of the metabolic needs of the patient with a burn.
   3.3 Write a nursing care plan for the burn patient.
   3.4 Identify types of wound care used in treating the patient with a burn.
   3.5 Identify the special considerations for special populations with burn injuries.

4.0 Demonstrate an understanding of the special needs of the patient with a severe burn.
   4.1 Demonstrate an understanding of the increased metabolic needs of the burn patient.
   4.2 Demonstrate an understanding of the fluid and electrolyte changes in the burn patient.
   4.3 Demonstrate an understanding of the psychosocial needs of the burn patient.

Learning Activities

Short Answers

1. List five important questions that the nurse should ask to obtain a history of the cause and circumstances of a burn injury.

    1.

    2.

    3.

    4.

    5.

2. List the factors that must be considered to classify the severity of a burn injury.

3. What is the purpose of using the rule of nines in relation to a burn injury?

4. During the first 48–72 hours after a burn,

    fluid shifts from _____ into _____.

5. Children under the age of _____ and adults

    over the age of _____ are considered to be

    high risk when burned.

6. Because the dermis of elderly patients is

    _____, they may suffer a _____ deeper

    burn after exposure to the heat source.

7. _____ failure is a major cause of death from a burn injury in the emergent phase.

8. Diuresis begins _____ days after a burn injury.

9. On the admission to a burn unit, all loose

    and nonviable tissue will be _____.

10. _____ is the use of water to clean burn wounds.

11. The focus of the nursing care for a patient

    with a burn injury is to maximize _____,

    minimize _____, and promote _____

    _____.

Identification

The ability of the nurse to correctly assess and interpret findings is an important skill. Use your skills to match the characteristics with the type of burn.

A. Superficial partial thickness burn

B. Deep partial thickness burn

C. Full thickness burn

12. _____ Caused by prolonged contact with flame or hot object

13. _____ Pink to red in color with dry surface and minimal edema

14. _____ Involves total destruction of epidermis and dermis

15. _____ Can result from contact with a hot object

16. _____ May appear black, waxy white, cherry red, or tan. Appears leathery, dry, and hard

17. _____ Appears red, mottled, or waxy white in color, fluid-filled surface vesicles form

18. _____ Burn is painless due to destruction of the nerves

19. _____ May blister and peel after 24 hours

20. _____ Heals spontaneously without scarring

21. _____ Spontaneous healing will not occur

True/False

22. _____ A minor burn has a partial thickness injury of less than 25% in adults.

23. _____ A patient with a major burn should be transported to the nearest hospital.

24. _____ A major burn is a partial thickness injury of > 25% total body surface area (TBSA) in adults.

25. _____ A major burn is one that involves the face and eyes.

26. _____ Burns > 20% will require parenteral fluid resuscitation.

27. _____ Diuretics are usually given during the early burn period.

28. _____ Debridement is painless.

29. _____ Chemical burns have the same appearance as any burn.

Knowledge Application

30. If a patient suffered a burn in a small enclosed area, the nurse would assess for signs of
    A. cardiac complications
    B. acute airway obstruction
    C. severe fluid imbalances
    D. stress reaction

31. The nurse is aware that it is important to determine the size of the body area burned in order to
    A. medicate for pain appropriately
    B. prevent serious complications
    C. determine amount of parenteral fluid replacement
    D. determine chance of survival

32. The reason that the Lund and Browder chart is a more accurate method of determining burn injury than other methods is that it
    A. can be used with children
    B. takes into account changes in body proportion that occur with age
    C. can predict serious complications
    D. all of the above

33. If a patient has a severe burn that damages the stratum germinativum, this would be very significant because
    A. this is the site where new cells are produced
    B. this tissue cannot regenerate
    C. respiratory complications are inevitable
    D. fluid shifts cannot be controlled

34. The acute phase of the burn injury is defined as the
    A. first 48–72 hours after injury
    B. period of time that begins with reabsorption of interstitial fluid
    C. period of time when the fluid shifts from the vascular to interstitial space
    D. period of time when the patient is unstable

35. The priority in treatment during the immediate care period of a burn is to
    A. stop the burning process
    B. assess for other injuries
    C. assess circulation
    D. maintain skeletal alignment

36. After the treatment priority has been accomplished, the next essential step is to
    A. cover the burned area
    B. establish a patent airway
    C. assess for other life-threatening injuries
    D. transport to a burn center

37. The emergent phase of burn care is also known as the

    A.   acute phase of the injury

    B.   critical phase of therapy

    C.   fluid resuscitation stage

    D.   life-threatening stage

38. On assessment, the nurse finds that a burn patient has a pink, flushed appearance and is restless, irritable, and confused. This suggests

    A.   impaired airway

    B.   smoke inhalation

    C.   carbon monoxide poisoning

    D.   massive fluid shifts

39. A patient has a burn of over 40% TBSA. If this patient exhibits anxiety, restlessness, labored breathing, and cyanosis, the nurse would suspect

    A.   inhalation injury

    B.   carbon monoxide poisoning

    C.   restrictive disease

    D.   decreased cardiac output

40. If carbon monoxide poisoning is suspected, the nurse would anticipate which of the following treatments to be ordered?

    A.   low flow oxygen and IPPB treatments

    B.   100% oxygen

    C.   mechanical ventilation

    D.   50% oxygen and frequent suctioning

41. Following a burn injury, the nurse would expect to see which serum lab changes during the emergent phase?

    A.   high sodium, low potassium

    B.   high sodium, high potassium

    C.   low sodium, high potassium

    D.   low sodium, low potassium

42. If a nurse suspects burn shock in a patient, the patient would exhibit which symptoms?

    A.   dehydration, increased urine output, hypotension

    B.   hypotension, tachycardia, decreased cardiac output

    C.   hypertension, increased urine output, tachycardia

    D.   decreasing consciousness, bradycardia, hypotension

43. Which of the following factors DO NOT contribute to the fluid shift from intravascular to interstitial space, leading to burn shock?

    A.   Capillaries at the site of the burn injury become more permeable.

    B.   Histamine is released from damaged cells.

    C.   Lymphatic system becomes overwhelmed by the interstitial edema.

    D.   Large protein molecules leak into the intravascular space.

44. After a severe burn, acid products including lactic acid accumulate in the blood, resulting in

    A.   respiratory acidosis

    B.   respiratory alkalosis

    C.   metabolic acidosis

    D.   metabolic alkalosis

45. When burn shock develops, the nurse would monitor the laboratory studies carefully. Which of the following are consistent with burn shock?

    A.   increased hematocrit, hyponatremia, hyperkalemia, high BUN

    B.   low serum osmolality, high urine specific gravity, hypernatremia, and hyperkalemia

    C.   hyperkalemia, hyperproteinemia, metabolic acidosis

    D.   hypokalemia, hypernatremia, high BUN, and creatinine

46. To determine the amount of fluid to be replaced following a burn injury, most authorities advocate administration of _____ of the volume in the first eight hours and _____ during each of the next eight hours.

    A. 33%, 33%

    B. 25%, 37%

    C. 50%, 25%

    D. 75%, 12%

47. The nurse is aware that the fluid shifts stop after the first 24 hours because

    A. capillary permeability increases

    B. hydrostatic pressure in interstitial space increases

    C. intravascular volume decreases

    D. leakage of protein has reached a maximum

48. In caring for the patient with a burn injury, the nurse would be aware that fluid mobilization is occurring when urine output is greater than

    A. 30 mL/hour

    B. 50 mL/hour

    C. 75 mL/hour

    D. 100 mL/hour

49. Because burn patients often have severe pain, the nurse would assist in pain management. This would include administration of _____ to control pain.

    A. aspirin

    B. Tylenol

    C. codeine

    D. morphine

50. Nursing care of the burn patient is aimed at preventing _____, which is the leading cause of death in the acute burn period.

    A. sepsis

    B. dehydration

    C. electrolyte imbalance

    D. respiratory failure

51. During the acute phase of the burn injury, the nurse is responsible for assessing metabolic needs of the patient, which can increase by

    A. 50%

    B. 100%

    C. 200%

    D. 300%

52. The main reason that the metabolic rate increases after a burn injury is thought to be

    A. the inability of the skin to conserve heat

    B. the loss of protein in wound exudate

    C. excessive nitrogen loss

    D. all of the above

53. Which lab finding, if low, would indicate that a burn patient has an alteration in nutrition?

    A. sodium

    B. potassium

    C. albumin

    D. creatinine

54. If the nurse detects an absence of bowel sounds in a burn patient, she or he would suspect

    A. Curling's ulcer

    B. paralytic ileus

    C. hypovolemic ileus

    D. bowel obstruction

55. Hypertrophic scar formation is often a problem with burn patients. To help prevent this problem, the nurse would assist in

    A. applying pressure garments

    B. debriding wounds daily

    C. providing adequate nutrition

    D. splinting all extremities

56. Chemical burns cause destruction of tissue by

   A.   burning

   B.   coagulation

   C.   heating

   D.   irritation

57. Initial medical management of a chemical injury would involve

   A.   stopping the burn by covering with sterile dressings

   B.   flushing the wound with copious amounts of water

   C.   covering with analgesic ointment as soon as possible

   D.   transporting to burn unit immediately

58. When a pregnant woman suffers a burn injury of TBSA of 60% or more, loss of pregnancy is a risk due to

   A.   infection

   B.   stress

   C.   fluid overload

   D.   hypoxia

59. The elderly often have a higher burn mortality from less extensive burns, due in part to

   A.   thinner skin with less elasticity

   B.   muscle tissues and bone are closer to surface

   C.   many have preexisting disorders

   D.   all of the above

Nursing Care Plans

60. Write a nursing care plan for the patient with altered respiratory function following a burn injury. Use the following nursing diagnoses.

   Nursing diagnoses:
   Impaired gas exchange
   High risk for ineffective airway clearance

   Patient outcome:

   Interventions:

61. Write a nursing care plan that addresses the needs of the patient with hypovolemia and electrolyte imbalance following a major burn injury. Use the following diagnosis.

   Nursing diagnosis: High risk for fluid volume deficit

   Patient outcome:

   Interventions:

62. Write a nursing care plan for the patient with pain following a burn injury. Use the following diagnosis.

    Nursing diagnosis: Pain related to open burn wounds

    Patient outcome:

    Interventions:

Case Studies

Case Study No. 1

Mr. J., age 28, was burned in a garage fire. He has burns on 43% of his body, including his face and upper body. He is admitted to the burn unit.

63. The initial exam classified this as a

    A. minor burn injury

    B. moderate burn injury

    C. major burn injury

64. The nurse working in the burn unit realizes that Mr. J. is at risk for hypovolemia and electrolyte imbalance during the emergent phase which occurs during the first

    A. 12 hours

    B. 24–48 hours

    C. 48–72 hours

    D. week

65. When assessing the severity of Mr. J.'s burns, the nurse notices soot around his mouth. The nurse should take special precautions because of the risk for

    A. respiratory complications

    B. cardiovascular complications

    C. gastrointestinal complications

    D. electrolyte imbalances

66. The nurse realizes that fluid shifts from the intravascular to the interstitial spaces because of

    A. decrease in the amount of histamine

    B. loss of red blood cells and hemoglobin

    C. increase in capillary permeability

    D. loss of healthy tissue

67. The nurse realizes the patient is in the _____ phase of the burn injury when _____ fluid is reabsorbed.

    A. critical, vascular

    B. emergent, extracellular

    C. acute, interstitial

    D. rehabilitation, vascular

68. Signs that indicate that Mr. J. is in the emergent phase of the burn injury would be

    A. edema, hypotension

    B. bradycardia, hypertension

    C. increased urine output

    D. increased cardiac output, tachycardia

69. The nurse reviews the lab results and notes that Mr. J.'s serum potassium is 6.0. The nurse would observe carefully for

    A. renal failure

    B. cardiac arrhythmias

    C. hypovolemic shock

    D. loss of consciousness

Case Study No. 2

Ms. S. has a severe burn over 50% of her body from a car accident. She is in the burn unit. It has been eight hours since her injury.

70. The nurse is aware of the importance of fluid resuscitation during the emergent phase of the injury. If Ms. S. has lost 2000 cc of fluid, how much parenteral fluid would the nurse be replacing?

    A.   500 cc

    B.   1000 cc

    C.   2000 cc

    D.   3000 cc

71. The type of fluid that will most likely be ordered is

    A.   5% dextrose

    B.   .9% sodium chloride

    C.   lactated Ringer's

    D.   albumin

72. Ms. S. has a full thickness burn on her upper thighs with eschar formation. Nursing care would include assessing for signs of

    A.   hypovolemia

    B.   impaired peripheral circulation

    C.   respiratory insufficiency

    D.   infection

73. It is the third postburn day and Ms. S. is in the acute phase of the burn injury. Nursing responsibilities during this period include observing for

    A.   increase in urine output, vital signs return to normal

    B.   decrease in urine output, hypertension

    C.   increase in cardiac output, hypotension

    D.   changing level of consciousness, hypertension

74. Ms. S. has the eschar debrided from her legs. The nurse is to apply closed wound dressings. This might include

    A.   silver sulfadiazine and sterile gauze

    B.   Bacitracin ointment and leaving wound open

    C.   Betadine wet-to-dry dressings

    D.   saline wet-to-dry dressings

75. Because of the full thickness burn injury on her thighs, the nurse anticipates that a _____ will be used.

    A.   homograft

    B.   heterograft

    C.   autograft

Case Study No. 3

Mr. F., age 70, was burned when he fell asleep while smoking. His wife died of smoke inhalation in the fire. He has burns of 38% TBSA on his chest and lower body.

76. Because of the cause of the burn injury, the nurse will monitor carefully for

    A.   cardiac standstill

    B.   respiratory failure

    C.   burn shock

    D.   infection

77. The nurse would assess which of the following during the emergent period? (Check all that apply.)

    A.   _____ assess skin for flushing, pallor, or cyanosis

    B.   _____ check arterial blood gases

    C.   _____ check urine output

    D.   _____ assess voice quality

    E.   _____ assess breathing pattern and breath sounds

Fortunately, Mr. F. improves rapidly and enters the next stage.

78. During the acute phase of his recovery, Mr. F. has a serum albumin of 2.0 and has lost 4 lbs. in 2 days. The priority nursing diagnosis would be

    A.   Alteration in fluid and electrolytes

    B.   Alteration in urinary elimination

    C.   Alteration in nutrition

    D.   Alteration in comfort

79. Mr. F. is unable to tolerate his diet, he is pale, has absent bowel sounds, and severe pain. An appropriate diet would be

    A.   high protein, high fat

    B.   tube feeding with Osmolite at 100 cc/hr

    C.   intravenous hyperalimentation

    D.   high protein, high carbohydrate diet with supplements

80. Mr. F. is depressed and withdrawn, and he refuses to talk about what happened. An appropriate nursing diagnosis would be

    A.   Post-trauma response

    B.   Self-concept disturbance

    C.   Ineffective coping

    D.   Impaired home management

81. To meet Mr. F.'s psychosocial needs, the nurse would (Check all that apply.)

    A.   _____ determine the circumstances of the accident

    B.   _____ ask him how he has coped with stressful situations in the past

    C.   _____ observe verbal and nonverbal cues

    D.   _____ encourage him to verbalize his feelings

82. To prevent the formation of scars during the rehabilitation period, the nurse would

    A.   do range-of-motion exercises four times daily

    B.   take patient to hydrotherapy

    C.   do dressing changes as ordered

    D.   give pain medication as ordered

Learner Self-Evaluation

Do I fully understand the content? If no, then the areas I need to review are:

I need more information from my instructor on:

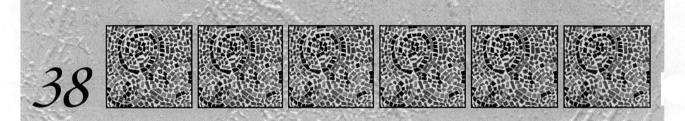

Knowledge Base for Men with Reproductive Dysfunction

Objectives

1.0 Review the anatomy and physiology of the male reproductive system.
- 1.1 Identify the parts of the male reproductive system.
- 1.2 List the functions of external and internal genitalia.
- 1.3 Identify signs of reproductive system dysfunction.

2.0 Demonstrate an understanding of the assessment data related to men with reproductive system dysfunction.
- 2.1 Identify clinical manifestations of male reproductive system dysfunction.
- 2.2 Identify diagnostic procedures used to identify problems in the male reproductive system.
- 2.3 Plan the nursing care for the patient having a biopsy.

3.0 Demonstrate an understanding of the interventions used to treat men with reproductive system dysfunction.
- 3.1 Identify medical and surgical treatment options available for men with reproductive dysfunction.
- 3.2 Plan nursing interventions for the patient having surgery.
- 3.3 Plan nursing interventions for the patient having a penile implant.
- 3.4 Identify needs of the elderly male with altered male reproductive system function.

*L*earning Activities

Identification

1. On the following diagram, identify the parts
    of the male reproductive system.

    A.   Penile urethra

    B.   Glans

    C.   Scrotum

    D.   Ejaculatory duct

    E.   Prostate gland

    F.   Testis

    G.   Epididymis

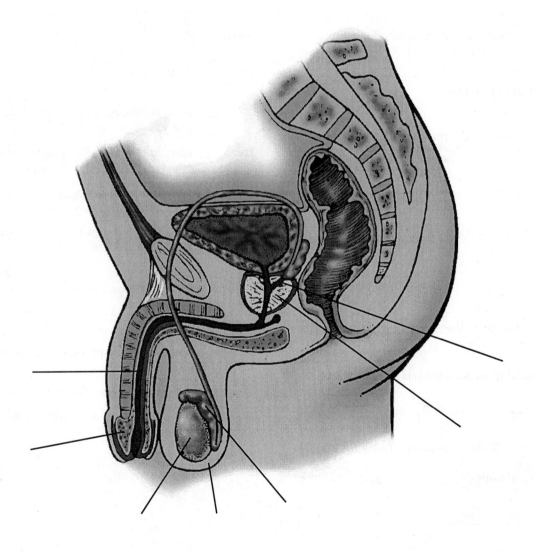

Match each of the following terms with the correct definition.

    A.   Spermatogenesis

    B.   Semen

    C.   Ejaculation

    D.   Impotence

    E.   Retrograde ejaculation

    F.   Infertility

2. _____ The process by which the germ cells become transformed into mature sperm

3. _____ Persistent inability to obtain or maintain erection

4. _____ Propulsion of seminal fluid from the posterior urethra into the bladder

5. _____ Milky viscid fluid that contains sperm

6. _____ Failure to conceive within a period of time

7. _____ Expulsion of the semen from the urethra

Short Answers

8. List two specific functions of the penis.
    1.

    2.

9. List two functions of the scrotum.
    1.

    2.

10. The testes are the _____ glands of the male.

11. Sperm from each testis is stored in the

    _____ and _____.

12. The urethra serves as a pathway for elimination of both _____ and

    _____.

13. Urinary _____ is the inability to empty the bladder with each voiding.

14. A digital rectal exam is done to examine the

    _____ _____.

15. A vasectomy is performed as a method of

    _____.

16. A testicular biopsy may be done on men with

    _____.

17. _____ is the most common manifestation for men with reproductive system dysfunction.

18. Prostatic enlargement is found in ____ % of males over the age of 65.

True/False

19. _____ Testosterone production begins during infancy.

20. _____ Testosterone production stops at about age 50.

21. _____ The vas deferens connects the epididymis with the ejaculatory duct.

22. _____ The seminal vesicles secrete an acidic fluid that helps sperm motility.

23. _____ The urethra passes through the prostate gland.

24. _____ Erection can occur by way of a spinal cord reflex mechanism.

25. _____ Impotence is a common problem with elderly males.

26. _____ Patients are hospitalized for 48 hours after vasectomy.

27. _____ A vasectomy can always be reversed.

28. _____ Bladder spasms are normal following prostatectomy.

Knowledge Application

29. The male sex hormone is

    A. progesterone

    B. testosterone

    C. spermatozoan

    D. estrogen

30. After ejaculation, the sperm live approximately _____ hours in the female reproductive tract.

    A. 6–8 hours

    B. 12–15 hours

    C. 24–28 hours

    D. 46–48 hours

31. The prostatic specific antigen (PSA) blood test is done to

    A. screen for prostate cancer

    B. screen for prostatic hypertrophy

    C. screen for bladder cancer

    D. rule out organic cause of impotence

32. The cause of premature ejaculation is believed to be

    A. organic

    B. psychologic

    C. neurogenic

33. Treatment for premature ejaculation would be

    A. surgery to correct defect

    B. medication such as testosterone

    C. sex therapy

34. Pain in the inguinal and lower abdominal area is most generally indicative of which condition?

    A. premature ejaculation

    B. prostatitis

    C. epididymitis

    D. urinary retention

35. Urinary retention is often associated with which of the following conditions?

    A. retrograde ejaculation

    B. benign prostatic hypertrophy

    C. epididymitis

    D. impotence

36. In obtaining a history from the patient with a sexual dysfunction, which of the following questions should the nurse ask? (Check all that apply.)

    A. _____ "Are you using any medications?"

    B. _____ "Are you circumcised?"

    C. _____ "Can you describe your symptom(s)?"

    D. _____ "Do you have any urinary problem(s)?"

    E. _____ "Do you have any gastric problem(s)?"

37. Prior to a male pelvic examination, which information would the nurse give to the patient?

    A. "You will need to move your bowels."

    B. "You will need to empty your bladder."

    C. "You will be examined in the prone position."

    D. "You will feel some pain during the exam."

38. When an infertility problem is suspected, the nurse would expect which diagnostic procedure to be done?

    A. rectal exam

    B. semen analysis

    C. radioimmunoassay

    D. prostatic specific antigen

39. Blood analysis is often done to diagnose male reproductive disorders. Measurement of the prostate acid phosphatase is used in the diagnosis of which condition?

    A. prostatic cancer

    B. penile cancer

    C. infertility

    D. epididymitis

40. The blood test for alpha-fetoprotein (AFP) will show an elevation in which of the following conditions?

   A.   prostatic cancer

   B.   benign prostatic hypertrophy

   C.   bowel cancer

   D.   testicular cancer

41. Laboratory results indicate that a 33-year-old patient has a testosterone level of 2.5 mg/dL. How would the nurse interpret this information?

   A.   normal for the patient

   B.   low and may be related to infertility

   C.   high and may be related to prostate cancer

   D.   high and may be related to testicular cancer

42. A patient has just returned from a transperineal biopsy of the prostate. Which manifestation indicates a possible side effect of this procedure? The patient

   A.   complains of discomfort in perineal area

   B.   voids 30 mL eight hours after procedure

   C.   states he is free from pain

   D.   complains of nausea

43. Which of the following nursing interventions would be appropriate following a testicular biopsy?

   A.   encourage the patient to drink fluids

   B.   schedule a physician appointment in six weeks

   C.   suggest the use of a scrotal support

44. A patient is to be discharged following cystourethroscopy and transurethral prostatic biopsy. Discharge instruction aimed at preventing infection would include (Check all that apply.)

   A.   _____   teach patient to take antibiotics if ordered

   B.   _____   teach patient to take analgesics if ordered

   C.   _____   teach patient to avoid contaminating biopsy site

   D.   _____   instruct patient on how to clean perianal area

   E.   _____   instruct patient to report chills, fever, or pain

45. Reasons that surgery may be done for dysfunctions of the male reproductive system include all of the following EXCEPT to

   A.   restore normal anatomy

   B.   repair structural abnormalities

   C.   treat epididymitis

   D.   restore normal sexual functioning

46. A patient is scheduled for prostate surgery because of an obstruction. Which of the following findings indicate a possible complication of the surgery? The patient

   A.   has a urinary output of 75 mL the first hour

   B.   complains of pain in his leg

   C.   has bloody urine during the first 12 hours

   D.   has respiratory rate of 24 and pulse of 92

47. For the patient who has had a TURP, which of the following complications should the nurse observe for?

   A.   bleeding

   B.   infection

   C.   wound dehiscence

   D.   cystitis

48. One of the disadvantages of the transurethral prostatectomy over other methods is that

    A. hemorrhage is more common

    B. infection is more common

    C. urethral stricture can occur

    D. pain is more severe

49. For the patient who has a very large prostate and abdominal surgery is contraindicated, which approach would be preferred for removal?

    A. perineal

    B. transurethral

    C. retropubic

    D. suprapubic

50. Following removal of the prostate, a patient becomes restless, disoriented, and nauseated. Which lab values should the nurse monitor?

    A. serum sodium, potassium, and osmolarity

    B. hemoglobin and hematocrit

    C. white blood count, sedimentation rate

    D. BUN and creatinine

51. Management for the patient with the above symptoms might include administration of

    A. IV of 5% dextrose and water, potassium bolus

    B. IV of 3% sodium chloride, Lasix

    C. transfusion of packed red blood cells

    D. antibiotics

52. A penile implant is generally used on patients with

    A. psychogenic impotency

    B. organic impotency

    C. anyone who wants one

53. To prevent a common postoperative complication following penile implant, which of the following interventions should the nurse implement?

    A. monitor for urinary bleeding

    B. assess for any respiratory distress

    C. monitor temperature every four hours

    D. assess for bowel sounds every eight hours

Nursing Care Plans

54. Plan the nursing care for the patient with a penile implant. Use the following nursing diagnosis.

    Nursing diagnosis: Anxiety related to effects of the surgery on his sexual functioning

    Patient outcome:

    Interventions:

55. Write a nursing care plan for the patient who has just returned from a prostatectomy.

    Nursing diagnosis:

    Patient outcome:

    Interventions:

Case Study

Mr. C. is 66 years old and is admitted with a diagnosis of benign prostatic hypertrophy. He is scheduled for surgery.

56. The nurse obtains the health history from Mr. C. Which of the following information is most likely related to his current condition? He

   A. is constipated

   B. gets up a night to urinate

   C. must sleep on two pillows

   D. complains of intermittent leg pain

57. Mr. C. is scheduled for a transurethral resection. The nurse should explain to him that this means

   A. under general anesthesia, the physician will make an abdominal incision and remove the tissue

   B. in the patient's room, the physician will use a cystoscopy to excise the tumor

   C. using local anesthesia, a resectoscope is inserted into the urethra to scrape out the enlarged gland

   D. using general anesthesia, the physician incises the perineal area to remove hypertrophied tissue

58. Mr. C. wonders why he needs to have an enema. He says, "I thought they didn't do that anymore." The nurse explains that the purpose of the enema is to

   A. clean the bowel

   B. prevent straining postoperatively

   C. prevent an infection in his incision

   D. reduce pain

59. In caring for this patient, which of the following nursing diagnoses would be the most important?

   A. Alteration in urination

   B. Alteration in comfort

   C. Potential for aspiration

   D. Alteration in mobility

60. As the primary nurse, you realize that it is important to explain to the patient that he should not try to urinate around the drainage catheter. What is the rationale for this? It may

   A. cause an infection

   B. precipitate bleeding

   C. precipitate bladder spasms

   D. cause TUR syndrome

61. Which information would it be important to relay to this patient on discharge?

   A. Normal urinary function will return immediately.

   B. Temporary urinary problems may occur such as dribbling or urgency.

   C. Bleeding during urination may occur for the next two weeks.

   D. Impotency is a common complication of this surgery.

Learner Self-Evaluation

Do I fully understand the content? If no, then the areas I need to review are:

I need more information from my instructor on:

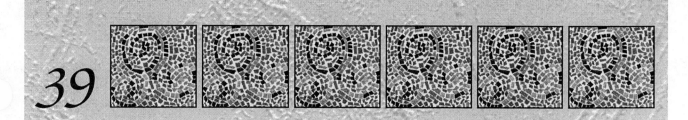

39

Nursing Care of Men with Reproductive Disorders

*O*bjectives

1.0 Demonstrate an understanding of the inflammatory processes of the male reproductive system.

    1.1 Identify several inflammations and infections of the male reproductive system.

    1.2 Identify the etiology and clinical manifestations associated with inflammatory processes.

    1.3 Plan nursing interventions for the patient with an infection.

    1.4 Identify the teaching needs of men with a reproductive system infection.

2.0 Demonstrate an understanding of the structural disorders of the male reproductive system.

    2.1 Identify several structural disorders.

    2.2 Identify the etiology and clinical manifestations of structural disorders.

    2.3 Plan nursing interventions for the patient with a structural disorder.

3.0 Demonstrate an understanding of the types of neoplasms that affect the male reproductive system.

    3.1 Identify the clinical manifestations of several neoplasms.

    3.2 Identify types of medical treatment used with neoplasms of the male reproductive system.

    3.3 Identify surgical interventions used to treat neoplasms of the male reproductive system.

    3.4 Apply the nursing process when planning care for the male patient with a neoplasm of the reproductive system.

$\mathcal{L}$earning Activities

Identification

Match each of these male reproductive disorders with the best definition.

A. Balanoposthitis

B. Hydrocele

C. Orchitis

D. Phimosis

E. Cryptorchidism

F. Priapism

G. Varicocele

1. _____ Foreskin is unable to retract over the penis

2. _____ Failure of one or both testicles to descend into the scrotum before birth

3. _____ Collection of clear fluid in the tunica vaginalis

4. _____ Inflammation of one or both of the testes

5. _____ Inflammation of the glans penis and the prepuce

6. _____ Cluster of dilated veins

7. _____ Prolonged, uncontrolled erection that is not associated with stimulation

Short Answers

8. Performing a _____ would be the appropriate treatment of phimosis in the adult.

9. To treat for paraphimosis, the physician would perform a _____ _____.

10. Two conditions that have been associated with infertility are _____ and _____.

11. Two complications that can occur following a varicocelectomy are _____ and _____.

12. Causes of problems with sexual function in older men include:

13. The most common solid tumor in men between the ages of 20 and 40 is _____ carcinoma.

14. Benign prostate hyperplasia (BPH) occurs only in _____ men with normal _____ function.

15. Prostatic cancer is the _____ leading cause of death among men.

True/False

16. _____ Orchitis usually results in sterility.

17. _____ Drainage of a hydrocele reduces the incidence of testicular atrophy.

18. _____ Chronic bacterial prostatitis is usually treated with Bactrim.

19. _____ Priapism is considered a urologic emergency.

20. _____ Painless swelling of the scrotum is the classical sign of a hydrocele.

21. _____ Conservative treatment of a varicocele involves using a scrotal support.

22. _____ Most of the men with BPH are asymptomatic.

23. _____ One of the symptoms associated with BPH is urinary retention.

24. _____ The most common form of prostatic cancer is adenocarcinoma.

25. _____ Prostate cancer can be palpated during a rectal exam.

Knowledge Application

26. The diagnosis of penile cancer is suggested by a small lesion on the glans, and is confirmed by _____.

    A. x-ray

    B. laboratory testing

    C. ultrasound

    D. biopsy

27. A contributing factor to the development of balanoposthitis would be

    A. poor nutrition

    B. poor hygiene

    C. sexual practices

    D. heredity

28. Epididymitis occurs as a result of an infection which often descends from the

    A. urinary tract

    B. gastrointestinal tract

    C. integumentary system

    D. vascular system

29. A possible complication of epididymitis is

    A. impotency

    B. hemorrhage

    C. sterility

    D. urinary retention

30. Mr. P. has been diagnosed with epididymitis. All of the following are possible treatments EXCEPT

    A. antibiotic therapy

    B. heat therapy

    C. analgesics

    D. cold therapy

31. All of the following are symptoms of prostatitis EXCEPT

    A. urinary frequency

    B. pain in the rectal area

    C. greenish ureteral discharge

    D. prostate swelling

32. What is the rationale for giving anticholinergic medications to the patient with prostatitis? To

    A. relieve discomfort associated with urination

    B. relieve gastrointestinal discomfort

    C. reduce the amount of ureteral discharge

    D. reduce swelling

33. A patient with epididymitis is having severe pain. An appropriate nursing intervention would be to

    A. elevate the scrotum

    B. apply a Bellevue bridge

    C. apply ice packs to the scrotum

    D. all of the above

34. A 23-year-old male has recently recovered from mumps. He is at risk for developing

    A. orchitis

    B. prostatitis

    C. epididymitis

    D. urinary infection

35. A patient has been admitted for incision and drainage of the scrotum. The most appropriate nursing diagnosis is

    A. Alteration in self-concept

    B. High risk for infection

    C. High risk for altered health maintenance

    D. Anxiety related to outcome of procedure

36. Medical management for acute bacterial prostatitis would include administration of

    A. penicillin G

    B. corticosteroid

    C. testosterone

    D. co-trimoxazole DS

37. A 28-year-old male is seen in the emergency room with pain, redness, and purulent discharge from his penis. The foreskin cannot be retracted and he states he is unable to urinate. The procedure that will most likely be performed is

A. phimosectomy

B. dorsal slit is made in penis

C. incision and drainage of abscess

D. transurethral resection

38. Unsuccessful treatment of paraphimosis might result in

A. urinary retention

B. impotency

C. necrosis of the penis

D. systemic infection

39. A complication of cryptorchidism would be

A. urinary tract infection

B. testicular cancer

C. impotency

D. phimosis

40. In the majority of cases, the cause of priapism is unknown. Which statement best describes the pathophysiology of this condition?

A. Penile enlargement results from an obstruction to the outflow of blood from the corpora cavernosa.

B. Penile enlargement results from a change in neurologic enervation.

C. Penile enlargement results from sexual overstimulation and delayed orgasm.

D. Penile enlargement results from an endocrine dysfunction.

41. Which serum tumor marker antigen becomes significantly elevated when penile cancer becomes metastatic?

A. CEA

B. TA-4

C. PSA

D. PC-1

42. A patient has had an orchiopexy performed. Because of the reason for, and possible outcome of, the surgery, the nurse should

A. monitor intake and output

B. administer antibiotics as ordered

C. medicate frequently for pain

D. assess emotional state

43. Which statement is most accurate about the male who has TIS primary cancer of the penis?

A. It is almost 100% curable.

B. The neoplasm spreads rapidly.

C. There is no known treatment.

D. Surgery involves a radical penectomy.

44. Following a total penectomy, what changes will be made in the patterns of urinary elimination? The patient will have

A. an abdominal urethrostomy

B. a perineal urethrostomy

C. an indwelling catheter

D. a suprapubic catheter

45. Because of the radical nature of a penectomy, which nursing diagnosis would be most appropriate?

A. Alteration in urination

B. Alteration in body image

C. Alteration in mobility

D. Alteration in breathing

46. Which statement is true about testicular cancer?

A. Pain is often the first symptom.

B. Most men detect the tumor.

C. Tumors can be palpated by bimanual exam of the scrotum.

D. The diagnosis is confirmed by biopsy.

47. A diagnosis of Stage B1 (IIA) testicular cancer would mean that the tumor

    A. is a hard localized mass

    B. has spread to the retroperitoneal lymph nodes

    C. has spread beyond the retroperitoneal lymph nodes

    D. has spread to the bone and abdominal organs

48. For the patient with Stage B1 (IIA) testicular cancer, treatment would most likely involve

    A. chemotherapy

    B. radiation therapy

    C. orchiectomy

    D. orchiectomy and radiation therapy

49. To reduce the risk of postoperative paralytic ileus for a patient having a retroperitoneal lymph node dissection to treat Stage II testicular cancer, the nurse would

    A. administer antibiotics

    B. hold all food for 24 hours

    C. administer mechanical bowel preparations

    D. teach use of incentive spirometer

50. Following a thoracoabdominal approach for retroperitoneal lymph node biopsy, nursing care would involve

    A. monitoring chest tube drainage system

    B. maintaining bed rest

    C. administering corticosteroids

    D. maintaining gastric tube.

51. A nurse is doing a community teaching session about the conservative treatment for benign prostatic hypertrophy (BPH). This would include information on

    A. increasing fluid intake, limiting alcohol

    B. prostate massage, mild tranquilizers

    C. sexual intercourse, limiting fluids

    D. application of heat, forcing fluids

52. Alpha blocker therapy is a treatment for benign prostatic hypertrophy. The rationale for the administration of this medication is that it

    A. will relieve painful bladder spasms

    B. increases testoterone, which slows the prostate overgrowth

    C. shrinks the prostate gland

    D. relaxes smooth muscle and facilitates urination

53. Surgical removal of the enlarged prostate is usually performed when symptoms of obstruction occur. An indication of this might be that the patient

    A. voids every two hours

    B. develops a hydrocele

    C. develops hydronephrosis

    D. develops a bladder infection

54. A prostatic specific antigen test will

    A. identify prostatic cancer

    B. monitor effectiveness of treatment regimens

    C. detect tumor progression

    D. all of the above

55. The accepted treatment for Stage B prostatic cancer would be

    A. orchidectomy

    B. radical prostatectomy

    C. chemotherapy

    D. radiation therapy

56. A possible side effect of radiation therapy used in the treatment of prostatic cancer would be that the patient

    A. develops alopecia

    B. develops a reddish discoloration on skin

    C. develops bruises on his buttocks

    D. complains of lethargy

57. Because of the high incidence of prostate cancer in elderly males, the nurse would stress the importance of

    A.   yearly physical exams

    B.   following a low-fat diet

    C.   quitting smoking

    D.   increasing exercise

58. A 68-year-old male with protastic cancer and bone metastasis who has cardiac problems would probably be treated by

    A.   radical prostatectomy

    B.   chemotherapy

    C.   radiation therapy

    D.   pain control

59. Following a radical prostatectomy, the nurse would monitor for complications such as

    A.   pulmonary embolus

    B.   rectal injury

    C.   thrombophlebitis

    D.   urinary infection

    E.   any of the above

Home Care

60. Mr. P. is being treated at home for epididymitis. The nurse is involved in teaching him self-care. What should be included in the plan?

Nursing Care Plans

61. Write a nursing care plan for a patient who is in the emergency room with paraphimosis. He is complaining of pain and his penis is bluish and swollen.

Nursing diagnosis:

Patient outcome:

Interventions:

62. Write a nursing care plan for a patient who has had a total penectomy for Stage III cancer.

Nursing diagnosis: Sexual dysfunction related to loss of penis

Patient outcome:

Interventions:

Food for Thought

What is the rationale for recommending PSA testing on all males over a certain age? What if treatment isn't even recommended; for example, elderly males who have early prostatic cancer but no evidence of spread? Is the emotional upset justified if the cancer won't be treated?

Case Studies

Case Study No. 1

Mr. H. is a 32-year-old male who is admitted with high fever and inguinal pain. The diagnosis is orchitis.

63. Which statement by Mr. H. would suggest the cause of his infection?

  A. "I had a swollen jaw last week."

  B. "I fell off my bike six weeks ago."

  C. "I have never been married."

  D. "I have severe allergies to pollen."

64. Which of the following interventions should the nurse implement?

  A. antibiotic therapy and warm, moist compresses

  B. bed rest, scrotal elevation, cold packs

  C. analgesics, antipyretics, steroids

65. Mr. H. wants to know why he is receiving diethylstilbestrol. The reason is

  A. to reduce swelling and inflammation

  B. as a prophylactic measure

  C. to control pain by inhibiting testicular function

  D. to prevent spread of infection

66. Mr. H. lives with a male roommate who has never had parotitis. Which precautions would his roommate take to avoid contracting this disease?

  A. have a dose of gamma globulin administered

  B. have a therapeutic dose of penicillin

  C. refrain from sexual relations for four weeks

  D. avoid contact with Mr. H. for two weeks

Case Study No. 2

Mr. S. is 33 years old and has a hard node in the left testicle. He is scheduled for an inguinal orchidectomy.

67. Before the surgery it would be important for the nurse to assess

  A. reproductive history

  B. understanding about surgery

  C. emotional status of patient

  D. all of the above

68. Mr. S. is very anxious about the surgery. A patient outcome related to this problem would be that the patient

  A. states that he does not have cancer

  B. asks questions about postoperative care

  C. states that he will be impotent

  D. can state diet restrictions

69. Mr. S. has recently married and has no children. Which information would it be important for him to know?

  A. If the remaining testis is normal, fertility is usually not affected.

  B. Sterility is usually an unfortunate side effect of this surgery.

  C. Many men have had the surgery without problems.

  D. The doctor can answer all of his questions.

70. Three days after his orchidectomy, Mr. S. is scheduled for a retroperitoneal lymph node dissection. Nursing care in preparation for the surgery would include

    A. mechanical bowel prep

    B. insertion of a nasogastric tube

    C. insertion of a central line

    D. all of the above

71. The surgeon uses a thoracoabdominal approach to perform the surgery. The nurse's responsibility in preventing complications following surgery include

    A. maintaining bed rest for 3–4 days

    B. maintaining patency of chest tubes

    C. giving Tylenol for pain as needed

    D. encouraging clear liquids as soon as possible

Case Study No. 3

Mr. B., age 50, has been recently diagnosed with T2B prostatic cancer. He is scheduled for treatment.

72. According to the TNM stage system, Mr. B.'s cancer is

    A. identified by needle biopsy

    B. no greater than 1.5 cm and in more than one lobe

    C. not fixed and has invaded prostatic apex

    D. fixed and has spread to lymph nodes

73. The recommended therapy would be

    A. transurethral resection

    B. radical prostatectomy

    C. radiation therapy

    D. hormonal therapy

74. Following the surgical intervention, Mr. B. asks the nurse if he will be impotent. The nurse replies

    A. "No, that is not a complication."

    B. "Impotence can occur occasionally."

    C. "Yes, impotency is a common side effect."

    D. "You need to talk to your doctor."

75. During the discharge teaching session, the nurse tells Mr. B. that the physician will monitor him and continue to watch his PSA level. The reason for this is to

    A. watch for a recurrence

    B. monitor for any spread

    C. check for effectiveness of treatment

    D. all the above

*L*earner Self-Evaluation

Do I fully understand the content? If no, then the areas I need to review are:

I need more information from my instructor on:

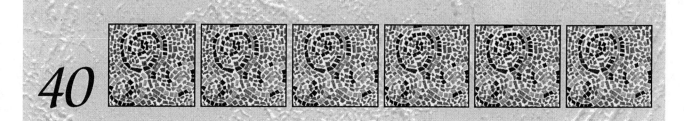

40

Knowledge Base for Women with Reproductive Dysfunction

*O*bjectives

1.0   Review the anatomy and physiology of the reproductive system.
     1.1   Identify the parts of the reproductive system.
     1.2   Identify the stages of menstruation.
     1.3   Demonstrate an understanding of the process of menopause.
     1.4   Identify symptoms associated with menopause.
     1.5   Write a care plan for the menopausal woman.

2.0   Demonstrate an understanding of the assessment data related to the female reproductive system.
     2.1   Identify symptoms of a reproductive dysfunction.
     2.2   Identify specific reproductive dysfunctions.
     2.3   Identify tests used to diagnose a reproductive dysfunction.

3.0   Demonstrate an understanding of interventions used to treat women with reproductive system dysfunction.
     3.1   Identify medical and surgical interventions used to treat reproductive system dysfunction.
     3.2   Plan the nursing care for the patient having medical or surgical intervention for a reproductive disorder.
     3.3   Identify complications following surgical treatment of reproductive disorders.
     3.4   Utilize the nursing process in planning the care for the patient who has had a hysterectomy.

*L*earning Activities

Identification

1. Identify the correct parts of the external genitalia.

   A. Mons pubis

   B. Clitoris

   C. Bartholin's glands

   D. Labia majora

   E. Vestibule

   F. Perineum

   G. Labia minora

   H. Hymen

   I. Urethral meatus

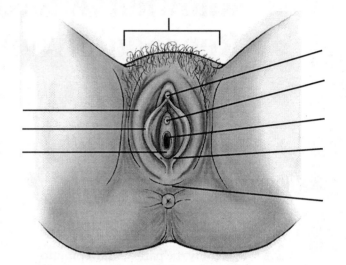

2. Identify the correct parts of the internal genitalia.

   A. Vagina

   B. Fallopian tubes

   C. Fundus

   D. Cervix

   E. Ovary

   F. Endometrium

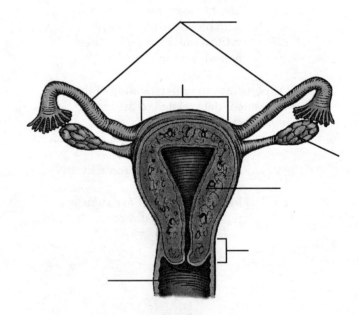

Short Answers

3. The _____ is a muscular tubelike organ lined with mucous membrane.

4. The _____ is a hollow, thick-walled, muscular organ shaped like an inverted pear.

5. The position of the uterus in the pelvic cavity is maintained by a series of _____.

6. The _____ transport ova from the ovaries to the uterus.

7. The _____ secrete the female sex hormones.

8. _____ is the period before, during, and after menopause.

9. List three things that can affect the frequency of the menstrual cycle.
   1.

   2.

   3.

10. List four symptoms associated with meno-pause.
   1.

   2.

   3.

   4.

Identification

Match each of the following stages of menstrua-tion with the best definition.

   A.   Ischemic phase

   B.   Menstrual phase

   C.   Proliferative phase

   D.   Secretory phase

11. _____ Occurs from the end of menstruation to ovulation.

12. _____ Occurs three days before next menses.

13. _____ The time of the menstrual flow.

14. _____ Occurs from ovulation until three days before next menses.

True/False

15. _____ Menopause most often occurs between ages 35 and 55.

16. _____ Pregnancy can occur during meno-pause.

17. _____ Hot flashes are experienced by many women during menopause.

18. _____ Ovulation usually ends before the last menses.

19. _____ Research has found a potential link between estrogen therapy and cancer.

20. _____ Most women do not seek care for menopausal symptoms from traditional health-care providers.

21. _____ Urinary symptoms are common manifestations of gynecologic disor-ders.

22. _____ Pelvic examination assesses structural conditions of the reproductive organs.

23. _____ A Pap smear examines cells obtained in the uterus.

24. _____ Significant changes occur in the repro-ductive system as a result of aging.

Identification

Match each of the following reproductive dysfunc-tions with the best definition.

   A.   Dysmenorrhea

   B.   Metrorrhagia

   C.   Amenorrhea

   D.   Leukorrhea

   E.   Polymenorrhagia

   F.   Oligomenorrhea

   G.   Menorrhagia

25. _____ Absence of menstruation for six months.

26. _____ Frequent but regular episodes of bleeding.

27. _____ Bleeding that is excessive in amount and duration.

28. _____ Infrequent, irregular episodes of bleeding.

29. _____ Cyclic pain associated with menstruation.

30. _____ Vaginal discharge other than blood.

31. _____ Normal bleeding that is irregular.

True/False

32. _____ Cryosurgery is a technique that uses exposure to cold to destroy tissue.

33. _____ Cryosurgery may be performed in an office without anesthesia.

34. _____ Electrocautery is done to burn away abnormal tissue.

35. _____ Tubal ligation may be done 24 hours after delivery.

36. _____ A vaginal approach for a tubal ligation is the preferred procedure.

37. _____ Sexual intercourse is restricted for two weeks following tubal ligation.

Knowledge Application

38. What is the current recommended treatment for the individual who is having severe menopausal symptoms?

    A. estrogen therapy 5 mg daily until symptoms subside

    B. progesterone 20 mg daily and estrogen 2 mg b.i.d. for six months, then daily

    C. estrogen therapy .625 mg daily, which can be combined with medroxyprogesterone therapy

39. Estrogen therapy is contraindicated with individuals who have had which of the following disorders?

    A. breast cancer

    B. endometrial cancer

    C. recurrent thrombophlebitis

    D. all of the above

40. The nurse is helping a patient cope with the psychologic effects of menopause. Evidence of success would be which of the following statements by the patient?

    A. "I realize that I can no longer get pregnant."

    B. "I realize that I can still work and be a wife."

    C. "I realize that the symptoms are all in my mind."

    D. "I realize that gaining weight is inevitable."

41. Abnormal uterine bleeding can be caused by

    A. ectopic pregnancy

    B. threatened abortion

    C. intrauterine devices

    D. anticholinergic agents

    E. all but D

    F. all of the above

42. Findings suggest that primary dysmenorrhea is due to

    A. excessive vaginal discharge

    B. excessive uterine contractility

    C. excessive exercise during menstruation

    D. dietary habits

43. Recent research indicates which of the following as being responsible for the symptoms of primary dysmenorrhea?

    A. high levels of prostaglandins

    B. high level of progesterone

    C. high levels of estrogen

    D. low levels of estrogen

44. Which nursing intervention is likely to be effective in relieving symptoms associated with dysmenorrhea?

    A. administration of analgesics

    B. application of heat

    C. increase in exercise at start of menses

    D. bed rest with hot fluids

    E. any of the above

45. One reason that a physician may perform a colposcopy would be

    A. the patient is having vaginal bleeding

    B. the cervix is normal but the Pap test is atypical

    C. the patient has symptoms and abdominal pain

    D. all of the above

46. Why is a conization (cone biopsy), NOT performed on women who plan on bearing children?

    A. There is a great risk of infection.

    B. It can cause prolapse of the uterus.

    C. It can lead to spontaneous abortion.

    D. It can cause incompetence of the cervix.

47. The nurse is discharging a patient who had a cone biopsy. All of the following would be emphasized EXCEPT

    A. resume normal activity as soon as possible

    B. avoid using tampons unless directed otherwise

    C. don't remove vaginal packing until instructed to do so

    D. do not douche until told to do so

48. Which of the following diagnostic tests allows for direct visualization into the intrauterine cavity?

    A. ultrasonography

    B. hysteroscopy

    C. endometrial smear

49. Which group of women have an increased risk of developing postoperative depression following a hysterectomy?

    A. women in their early thirties

    B. women with less than two children

    C. women who are unmarried

    D. all of the above

50. All of the following statements are true about laparoscopy EXCEPT that it

    A. allows for visualization of the internal pelvic organs

    B. is done through an incision in the vaginal wall

    C. is used as a diagnostic procedure to evaluate abdominal pain

    D. can be used to determine patency of the fallopian tubes

51. When assessing the patient two hours after having a laparoscopy, the nurse finds her complaining of shoulder pain and soreness in her chest. The nurse should

    A. immediately notify the physician

    B. monitor vital signs and if the heart rate is elevated, administer a narcotic

    C. record the findings and reassess in one hour

    D. reassure patient that these are common symptoms and offer analgesics

52. A patient had a dilation and curettage early in the morning. Later that day, she tells the nurse that she has changed her pad twice in the last hour. The nurse is aware that

    A. this amount of bleeding is normal during the first day

    B. this is excessive; pads should not require changing more than once every hour

53. What intervention would be appropriate based on the above information?

    A. reassure her that everything is fine

    B. call the physician immediately

    C. check the amount of saturation on the pads

54. The vaginal route is considered a preferred route for a hysterectomy when

    A. there is a diagnosis of cancer

    B. the patient is young and in good health

    C. vaginal repair is being done

    D. a salpingectomy is also performed

55. Which of the following is a frequent postoperative complication following abdominal hysterectomy?

    A. cystitis

    B. bladder fistula

    C. evisceration

    D. nerve damage

56. Which patient would have the highest risk for development of an incisional infection following an abdominal hysterectomy?

    A. 23 years old with cervical cancer

    B. 44 years old with uterine cancer, history of asthma

    C. 35 years old with benign tumors, history of cystitis

    D. 68 years old with ovarian cancer, history of diabetes

57. Following gynecologic surgery, patients have a high risk for development of _____.

    A. thromboembolism

    B. depression

    C. sepsis

    D. nutritional deficiency

Nursing Care Plans

58. Write a care plan for a woman entering menopause. Use the following nursing diagnosis.

    Nursing diagnosis: Knowledge deficit: menopause and related self care

    Patient outcome:

    Interventions:

59. Write a nursing care plan for the patient who has had a total hysterectomy. Use the following nursing diagnosis.

    Nursing diagnosis: Anxiety related to the physical and psychosocial effects of impending surgery

    Patient outcome:

    Interventions:

Case Studies

Case Study No. 1

A 19-year-old female is seen in the clinic with a complaint of severe menstrual pain. She has had menstrual pain since age 15, but never this severe.

60. During the history she says, "My mother thinks I must have contracted VD because I have such severe pain." An appropriate response by the nurse would be

    A. "Painful menstruation does not have to be associated with any other problem."

    B. "Painful menstruation is often related to secondary VD."

    C. "Painful menstruation is usually caused by endometriosis."

    D. "Painful menstruation is something women have to live with."

61. The nurse will discuss treatment options. Severe menstrual pain is often treated with

    A. analgesics, antibiotics, anticholinergics

    B. antibiotics, sedatives, antispasmodics

    C. analgesics, antispasmodics, heat, rest

    D. relaxation therapy, narcotics

62. One medication ordered for this patient is Motrin (ibuprofen). Side effects which you will discuss include

    A. rapid heart rate, hypertension

    B. gastric upset, headache

    C. constipation, urinary frequency

    D. any of the above

63. The patient asks if it is advisable for her to use oral contraceptives to help with the dysmenorrhea. An appropriate reply would be

    A. "No, that is not a recommended therapy."

    B. "Yes, that is probably a good idea."

    C. "Yes, if you also desire them as a contraceptive."

    D. "No, there are too many side effects."

Case Study No. 2

Ms. S., 28 years old, has chronic pelvic pain. She is scheduled for a laparoscopy in the morning in the same-day surgical care center.

64. The nurse would talk to Ms. S. the day before to include information about the preoperative care. This would include (Check all that apply.)

    A. _____ nothing by mouth after midnight

    B. _____ laxative as prescribed

    C. _____ shave abdomen from nipple line to knees

    D. _____ discuss general anesthesia

65. Ms. S. has a diagnosis of possible endometriosis and blocked fallopian tubes. How is the patency of the tubes evaluated? By

    A. intravenous injection of a dye

    B. injecting a dye via a cannula through the cervix

    C. abdominal ultrasound

    D. the use of the laparoscope

66. Following the procedure, the nurse is aware that the most serious complication of laparoscopy is

    A. hemorrhage

    B. sepsis

    C. intestinal burns

    D. embolism

67. Ms. S. has done well and is ready for discharge. It is apparent that she has a good understanding of her instructions when she states (Check all that apply.)

    A. _____ "I must avoid sexual intercourse for six weeks."

    B. _____ "I should not experience any discomfort."

    C. _____ "I should avoid heavy lifting for a week."

    D. _____ "I may experience pain in my chest or shoulder."

Case Study No. 3

Mrs. D. is scheduled for a total abdominal hysterectomy (TAH) and bilateral salpingo-oophorectomy (BSO) for a malignancy. She has a history of breast cancer and diabetes.

68. Mrs. D. asks if she will continue to menstruate after this procedure. The nurse would reply

    A. "No, you will no longer menstruate."

    B. "Yes, you may have slightly irregular periods."

69. Mrs. D. wonders why she is not having a vaginal approach like her friend had. How should the nurse respond?

    A. Tell her that she needs to talk to her physician.

    B. Tell her that everyone is different.

    C. Tell her that her approach is preferred when the adnexae and uterus are to be removed.

70. Mrs. D. is crying and says, "I know I no longer will feel like a woman. The doctor says he won't even prescribe estrogen for me. Why not?"

    A.   You explain that she needs to talk to the physician.

    B.   You ask her if she is upset about the surgery.

    C.   You explain that estrogen therapy may be contraindicated for individuals with her history.

    D.   You tell her that she is lucky to be alive.

71. On the second postoperative day, Mrs. D. tells the nurse that she had to get up to urinate six times last night. Her urine output is 300 mL. This suggests that Mrs. D.

    A.   is in pain and should be medicated

    B.   is probably bleeding which is putting pressure on the bladder

    C.   probably has urinary retention

    D.   is very anxious and needs to talk

72. During the assessment, you find that Mrs. D. has no bowel sounds. The physician orders an abdominal scan which reveals a paralytic ileus. The reason that this complication occurs is that the patient has

    A.   been immobilized

    B.   had nerve trauma from handling the viscera

    C.   had too much anesthesia

    D.   not had any food or drink for 48 hours

73. How can the nurse evaluate Mrs. D.'s psychologic response to the surgery?

    A.   check vital signs every four hours, monitor the wound

    B.   ask her if she has any questions

    C.   monitor any changes in behavior

Learner Self-Evaluation

Do I fully understand the content? If no, then the areas I need to review are:

I need more information from my instructor on:

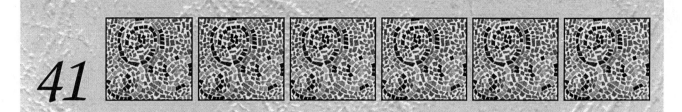

41

Nursing Care of Women with Reproductive Disorders

*O*bjectives

1.0 Demonstrate an understanding of the infections and inflammatory processes within the female reproductive system.

    1.1 Define several of the inflammatory disorders.

    1.2 Identify the causes and signs and symptoms of several infectious disorders of the female reproductive system.

    1.3 Identify the teaching needs of the patient with an inflammatory process.

    1.4 Identify appropriate nursing interventions for a patient with an infection.

2.0 Demonstrate an understanding of functional disorders of the reproductive system.

    2.1 Identify symptoms related to premenstrual syndrome.

    2.2 Describe current treatment options for the patient with a functional disorder.

    2.3 Describe the emotional problems of a female with a functional abnormality.

    2.4 Write a nursing care plan for the patient with premenstrual syndrome.

3.0 Demonstrate an understanding of the structural disorders of the female reproductive system.

    3.1 Define several structural disorders.

    3.2 Identify clinical manifestations of a structural abnormality of the reproductive system.

    3.3 Identify medical interventions used for a patient with a weakened pelvic structure.

    3.4 Plan the nursing care for a patient having surgical repair of a structural disorder.

4.0 Demonstrate an understanding of the types of neoplasms that affect the female reproductive system.

    4.1 Identify clinical manifestations of neoplasms.

    4.2 Review treatment options for the patient with a neoplasm.

    4.3 Identify the psychologic needs of a woman who has a disorder of the reproductive system.

    4.4 Plan the nursing care for the woman with a radioactive implant.

    4.5 Plan the nursing care for the woman with a neoplasm of the reproductive system.

*L*earning Activities

Identification

Match these common disorders of the female reproductive system with the appropriate definition.

- A. Vaginitis
- B. Vulvitis
- C. Endometriosis
- D. Colpocele
- E. Rectocele
- F. Toxic shock syndrome
- G. Cystocele

1. _____ Inflammation of the membrane that lines the inner surface of the uterus
2. _____ Inflammation of the vagina
3. _____ Vaginal mucosa protrudes outside vagina
4. _____ Rectum protrudes into vagina
5. _____ Inflammation of the external genitalia
6. _____ Bladder protrudes into the vagina
7. _____ Acute illness caused by *Staphylococcus aureus*

Short Answers

8. The most common symptom of vaginitis is

   _____.

9. List four clinical manifestations of toxic shock syndrome.
   1.
   2.
   3.
   4.

10. Symptoms of premenstrual syndrome (PMS)

   disappear during _____.

11. List some of the symptoms that have been associated with PMS.

12. The symptom most frequently associated with endometriosis is _____.

13. One of the primary causes of weakened pelvic support is damage due to

   _____.

14. A genital fistula can be between the

   _____ or the _____

   and the vagina.

15. Cancer of the _____ is the most common cancer of the female reproductive system.

True/False

16. _____ Symptoms of PMS are similar for most women.
17. _____ PMS is thought to be caused by an estrogen-progesterone imbalance.
18. _____ The cause of endometriosis is unknown.
19. _____ During pregnancy, there is often an increase in symptoms related to PMS.
20. _____ Damage during childbirth is the main cause of weakened pelvic support.
21. _____ Uterine prolapse is visible on inspection.
22. _____ Repairs of pelvis relaxation can be done anytime.
23. _____ Pessaries should be recommended for patients with pelvic relaxation.
24. _____ Genital fistulas often result from labor trauma.
25. _____ Cervical cancer is almost always curable in the early stages.

Identification

Match the following neoplasms with the best definition.

    A.   Polyp

    B.   Leiomyoma

    C.   Vulvar carcinoma

    D.   Dermoid cyst

26. _____ Benign smooth muscle tumor

27. _____ Benign ovarian neoplasm

28. _____ Tumor that has stalks

29. _____ Neoplasm in the vulvar epidermis

Knowledge Application

30. A classic clinical manifestation of vulvitis that the nurse would assess for is

    _____.

    A. pruritus

    B. vaginal discharge

    C. dribbling of urine

    D. perineal pain

31. When working with an individual who has vaginitis an important nursing measure would be to

    A. provide pain medication

    B. teach proper hygiene

    C. explain treatment options

    D. make sure antibiotics are taken

32. Organisms that have been found to cause vaginitis include

    A. *Escherichia coli*

    B. *Trichomonas vaginitis*

    C. *Treponema pallidum*

    D. herpes simplex

    E. any of the above

33. There are many factors that predispose a woman to developing vaginitis. These would include all of the following EXCEPT

    A. malnutrition

    B. stress

    C. pregnancy

    D. exercise

34. Culture results show that a patient has vaginitis caused by *E. coli*. The nurse knows that the patient understands how to prevent a recurrence of this problem when she

    A. describes the proper way to wipe after a bowel movement

    B. states that she should avoid tight clothing

    C. states that she cannot have sexual relations

    D. states that she is starting a new diet

35. The reason that atrophic vaginitis occurs in postmenopausal women is thought to be the

    A. drop in estrogen levels

    B. drop in progesterone levels

    C. loss of vaginal mucosa

    D. decrease in vaginal secretions

36. Which of the following clinical manifestations would indicate that a woman has atrophic vaginitis?

    A. itching and yellow discharge

    B. burning and brownish discharge

    C. thin, yellow discharge and burning

    D. itching and foul-smelling discharge

37. Treatment for the patient with vaginitis might involve baths containing

    A. antibiotics

    B. tannic acid

    C. baby oils

    D. hydrogen peroxide

38. An effective therapy for a 65-year-old postmenopausal woman who has severe vaginitis might be

    A. estrogen creme

    B. topical ointment

    C. antibiotics

    D. cessation of intercourse

39. Nursing care for the patient with toxic shock syndrome is designed to enable the woman to

    A. control the long-term side effects

    B. return to psychosocial stability

    C. return to physiologic stability

    D. effect a cure rapidly

40. Primary medical treatment for toxic shock syndrome would be

    A. life support

    B. antibiotic therapy

    C. intravenous therapy

    D. nutritional support

41. A patient recovering from toxic shock syndrome exhibits the following symptoms: petechiae, hematoma on legs, cool extremities, and cyanotic nailbeds. These findings suggest

    A. acute renal failure

    B. peripheral vascular collapse

    C. disseminated intravascular coagulation

    D. cardiogenic shock

42. The nurse is discharging a patient who has recovered from toxic shock syndrome. Which statement indicates she understands a contributory factor and ways to prevent a recurrence?

    A. "I will see my physician in six weeks."

    B. "I will change tampons every four hours."

    C. "I will stop using birth control pills."

    D. "I will only take tub baths."

43. A patient has a diagnosis of endometriosis. She asks for an explanation of this disorder. The nurse explains

    A. "It is an inflammation of the endometrium."

    B. "It is a condition where tissue similar to endometrium is found in other locations."

    C. "It is a condition that causes severe abdominal pain and cessation of menstruation."

    D. "It is a condition where the lining of the endometrium is shed and passed as large clots."

44. In the absence of significant clinical manifestations, the reason that women who have endometriosis often seek medical attention is

    A. lack of interest in sexual activity

    B. frequent mood changes

    C. infertility

    D. changes in activity

45. One of the newest therapies to treat endometriosis is synthetic androgen therapy with Danazol. A disadvantage of this treatment is that

    A. serious side effects occur

    B. it is not approved by the FDA

    C. symptoms recur when discontinued

46. When a woman with endometriosis no longer desires children, surgery may be recommended to

    A. relieve symptoms

    B. remove the scar tissue

    C. cure the disease

    D. prevent disease from becoming malignant

47. The nurse would teach the patient with endometriosis which of the following to help her cope with symptoms? (Check all that apply.)

    A. _____ correct use of analgesics

    B. _____ correct use of hormone therapy

    C. _____ correct application of heat

    D. _____ correct application of cold packs

    E. _____ pelvic exercises

    F. _____ increased periods of rest

48. Identify the clinical manifestations of a weakened pelvis support. (Check all the symptoms that may occur.)

    A. _____ lump protruding from vagina

    B. _____ foul-smelling vaginal discharge

    C. _____ constipation

    D. _____ pruritus

    E. _____ changes in urination

    F. _____ pain on intercourse

49. The primary reason that patients with a cystocele seek medical help is

    A. constipation

    B. stress incontinence

    C. abdominal pain

    D. diarrhea and vomiting

50. The medical treatment for a patient with a weakened pelvic structure will most often involve

    A. muscle relaxant medications

    B. antibiotic therapy

    C. surgical intervention

    D. aggressive exercise program

    E. insertion of a pessary

51. After posterior repair for a rectocele, a common problem is

    A. infection

    B. constipation

    C. vaginal stenosis

    D. respiratory disorders

52. Following an anterior colporrhaphy, which symptom should be reported to the physician at once?

    A. inability to void

    B. refusal to get up

    C. nausea and vomiting

    D. constipation

53. For a patient with retrodisplacement of the uterus, which intervention might help alleviate the discomfort?

    A. warm sitz baths

    B. daily douching

    C. Tylenol as ordered

    D. postural therapy

54. A patient is admitted with leakage of urine from the vagina. The nurse suspects

    A. vaginitis

    B. vesicovaginal fistula

    C. urinary infection

    D. prolapse of uterus

55. An appropriate nursing diagnosis for this patient would be

    A. High risk for impaired skin integrity

    B. Pain related to infectious process

    C. Alteration in fluid and electrolytes

    D. Alteration in mobility

56. An important part of the teaching for this patient would involve ways to

    A. control discomfort

    B. maintain adequate nutrition

    C. cope with constipation

    D. decrease discharge

57. The first symptom of cervical cancer is often

    A. abdominal pain

    B. excessive menstrual bleeding

    C. thin, watery discharge

    D. vaginal pain and foul discharge

58. One of the main reasons that many women do not have routine gynecologic examinations after menopause is that they

    A.   are no longer at risk

    B.   have limited resources

    C.   lack knowledge

    D.   lack transportation

59. One of the primary symptoms of vulvar carcinoma is

    A.   pruritus

    B.   thin, watery discharge

    C.   painless bleeding

    D.   protruding mass

60. All of the following would be ordered postoperatively for the patient who has had a radical vulvectomy EXCEPT

    A.   Hemovac

    B.   intravenous therapy

    C.   high-residue diet

    D.   Foley catheter

61. The most common complication after a radical vulvectomy is

    A.   pulmonary embolus

    B.   wound breakdown

    C.   loss of sexual functioning

    D.   stress incontinence

62. The nurse is aware that the patient who has had a radical vulvectomy is at risk for developing an infection. To prevent this, the nurse would

    A.   get the patient up as soon as possible

    B.   change dressing frequently and clean wound with sterile solution

    C.   provide a diet low in fiber and high in protein

    D.   medicate as ordered every four hours

63. The classic symptom of cervical cancer is

    A.   intermittent, painless bleeding

    B.   thick, foul-smelling discharge

    C.   heavy bleeding with clots

    D.   painful periods with heavy flow

64. Risk factors associated with cervical cancer include all of the following EXCEPT

    A.   age of first sexual activity

    B.   age of first pregnancy

    C.   number of pregnancies

    D.   ethnic background

    E.   nutritional status

    F.   socioeconomic status

65. The usual treatment for the woman who has a diagnosis of carcinoma in situ would be

    A.   radiation therapy

    B.   chemotherapy

    C.   conization or hysterectomy

    D.   hysterectomy with bilateral salpingo-oophorectomy

66. A patient is admitted for insertion of an internal radiation device. A possible effect of this therapy is?

    A.   nausea, vomiting

    B.   malaise

    C.   radiation enteritis

    D.   cystitis

    E.   any of the above

67. When caring for the patient with a radiation implant, which nursing action is of primary importance?

    A.   maintain patient on strict bed rest

    B.   keep patient on NPO status

    C.   administer narcotics for pain control

    D.   maintain patency of nasogastric tube and IV therapy

68. When reviewing a patient's chart, the nurse notices that the diagnosis is Stage III adeno-carcinoma of the uterus. This means that the cancer

    A. is confined to the uterus and the cervix

    B. extends outside the uterus but not outside the pelvis

    C. involves the uterus and either the bladder or rectum

    D. has spread beyond the uterus to the brain

69. The recommended treatment for the patient with Stage III uterine cancer would include

    A. total abdominal hysterectomy with bilateral salpingo-oophorectomy followed by hormonal therapy

    B. radiation therapy followed by hormonal therapy

    C. hysterectomy followed by chemotherapy

    D. palliative therapy only

Nursing Care Plans

70. Write a nursing care plan for the woman with PMS. Use the following nursing diagnosis.

    Nursing diagnosis: Potential for ineffective coping

    Patient outcome:

    Interventions:

71. The nurse is aware that women with PMS need specific information on lifestyle changes shown to have some impact on the control of symptoms. Write appropriate interventions under each area that would be appropriate to discuss at a community focus session on this disorder.

    Rest and activity:

    Diet:

    Fluids:

    Anxiety:

72. Plan the nursing care for the patient who has had a radical vulvectomy. Use the following diagnosis.

    Nursing diagnosis: Potential for impaired tissue integrity related to disruption of suture line

    Patient outcome:

    Interventions:

73. Plan the nursing care for a patient who has had a total hysterectomy. Use the following nursing diagnosis.

Nursing Diagnosis: Potential for ineffective coping

Patient Outcome:

Interventions

74. Plan the nursing care for the patient with a radioactive implant using the following nursing diagnosis.

Nursing diagnosis: Knowledge deficit related to restrictions and safety precautions to be followed

Patient outcome:

Interventions:

Case Studies

Case Study No. 1

Mrs. W. has severe symptoms of PMS. She has severe mood swings and can't control her emotions. She has tried many methods of medical treatment without any success.

75. Nursing care for Mrs. W. would include all of the following EXCEPT

A. teach her to accept a disease that has no known cure

B. teach ways to implement changes in lifestyle

C. provide information on surgical alternatives

D. provide information on support groups

76. Mrs. W. states that she feels fat and often gains five pounds prior to beginning menstruation. What advice would be appropriate?

A. reduce or eliminate alcoholic beverages

B. reduce intake of food high in sodium

C. eat food high in protein

D. reduce intake of water

77. The nurse is evaluating the teaching plan. Which statement by Mrs. W. shows she has some misunderstandings?

A. "I will try to stop eating potato chips."

B. "I am going to try to walk daily."

C. "I hope the new medication will cure me."

D. "I will try to sleep eight hours each night."

Case Study No. 2

Mrs. C. is admitted because of weakened pelvic support. She has four children, is overweight, and spends all her time caring for her family. She says, "it feels like my insides are falling out."

78. Mrs. C. is scheduled for anterior and posterior surgical repair. She wonders if this surgery will interfere with her ability to have any more children. An appropriate response would be

    A. "Yes, you will be sterile after the surgery."

    B. "Not always, but infertility may be a problem."

    C. "No, in fact it will help any future deliveries."

    D. "You need to discuss this with your doctor."

79. Which information from Mrs. C. would it be important to report to the physician?

    A. she has been using birth control pills

    B. she doesn't exercise regularly

    C. she received antibiotics preoperatively

    D. she has no known allergies

80. Postoperatively, nursing interventions should include all of the following EXCEPT

    A. clean perineal area with warm water every four hours

    B. encourage the patient to cough and deep breathe

    C. assess for adequate urinary output

    D. monitor for positive Homans' sign

Case Study No. 3

Mrs. P. has ovarian cancer and is admitted for a total abdominal hysterectomy, with bilateral salpingo-oophorectomy. She is anxious and needs emotional support and teaching prior to her surgery. The surgery will be followed by radiation therapy.

81. Mrs. P. wonders if all patients receive radiation therapy after surgery. The nurse replies

    A. "As far as I know, that is the best treatment."

    B. "That is the usual treatment, although some physicians may use chemotherapy or hormonal therapy."

    C. "For your kind of cancer, you must have radiation therapy in order to be cured."

    D. "Radiation therapy is not usually done, but your doctor must have a reason for suggesting it."

82. Mrs. P. is crying and says, "I am no longer going to be a woman. I may as well die." The nurse responds

    A. "What do you mean? Of course you are still a woman."

    B. "Don't be silly; you aren't going to die."

    C. "You seem concerned about having this procedure."

    D. "Let me call your husband; you know he loves you."

83. Counseling for which of the following should be an important part of the discharge planning?

    A. self breast examination

    B. side effects of chemotherapy

    C. cough and deep breathe

    D. refer her to Reach for Recovery

Case Study No. 4

Mrs. S., 55, has been diagnosed with advanced adenocarcinoma of the uterus with metastasis to the bowel and bladder. She is scheduled for a total pelvic exenteration.

84.   Prior to the surgery, extensive diagnostic testing is done to

   A.   rule out any metastasis beyond the pelvis

   B.   determine the usage of radiation therapy

   C.   determine if her bowels will function well after surgery

   D.   all of the above

85.   During the preoperative preparation the nurse will be administering which of the following?

   A.   laxatives and antibiotics

   B.   anticholinergics and analgesics

   C.   antiemetics and antibiotics

   D.   antacids and antibiotics

86.   The nurse explains to Mrs. S. that she will be kept in the ICU for several days after the surgery. The reason for this is the risk of

   A.   sepsis

   B.   shock or cardiac problems

   C.   respiratory failure

   D.   fluid overload

87.   Following this radical surgery, the patient will be discharged with

   A.   NG tube for feeding, Foley catheter

   B.   Hickman catheter and antibiotic therapy

   C.   colostomy, ileal conduit

   D.   jejunostomy tube

*L*earner Self-Evaluation

Do I fully understand the content? If no, then the areas I need to review are:

I need more information from my instructor on:

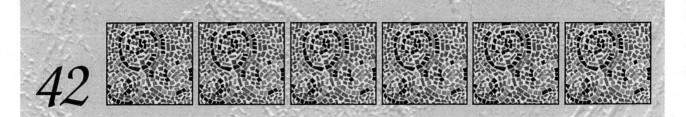

42

Nursing Care of Patients with Breast Disorders

*O*bjectives

1.0   Review the anatomy and physiology of the breast.
    1.1   Identify the structure of the breast.
    1.2   Identify changes in breast structure.

2.0   Demonstrate an understanding of assessment data related to breast disorders.
    2.1   Identify information and examination procedures essential to the assessment of the breast.
    2.2   Identify clinical manifestations of breast disorders.
    2.3   Match basic diagnostic tests with the appropriate definition.

3.0   Demonstrate an understanding of the infections and inflammations of the breast.
    3.1   Identify clinical manifestation of infectious disorders.
    3.2   Identify treatment modalities for infectious disorders.
    3.3   Identify nursing interventions for the patient with an infectious disorder of the breast.

4.0   Demonstrate an understanding of the structural disorders of the breast.
    4.1   Identify characteristics of structural disorders.
    4.2   Identify the collaborative management techniques for the structural disorders of the breast.
    4.3   Identify nursing interventions used for patients with structural disorders of the breast.

5.0   Demonstrate an understanding of the neoplasms that affect the breast.
    5.1   Identify the etiology and pathophysiology of several breast neoplasms.
    5.2   Identify the clinical manifestations of neoplasms of the breast.
    5.3   Identify the treatment protocols for the patient with a neoplasm of the breast.
    5.4   Write a nursing care plan for the patient with breast cancer.

𝓛earning Activities

Short Answers

1. The breast is composed of _____,

   _____, and _____ tissue.

2. The _____ tissue has the ability to elongate in response to pregnancy and lactation.

3. Normal breast development requires the

   production of _____ and

   _____ hormone by the anterior

   pituitary.

4. Structural change in the older female breast after menopause is known as

   _____.

5. When the breasts are examined, the patient

   should be in _____ position.

6. List four of the risk factors associated with the development of breast cancer.
   1.

   2.

   3.

   4.

7. Women should be taught breast self-exami-

   nation and should practice it _____.

8. The most common causative agent of masti-

   tis is _____ _____.

9. Painless, movable breast masses with well-defined borders are known as

   _____.

10. Hormones, especially _____, have been linked to the development of breast cancer.

11. _____ is a surgical procedure that creates a natural-looking breast shape.

Identification

Match each of these diagnostic tests with its definition.

   A. Mammography
   B. Xeroradiography
   C. Thermography
   D. Ultrasonography
   E. Breast biopsy

12. _____ Takes pictures of infrared emissions.

13. _____ Provides an x-ray picture of the internal breast structure.

14. _____ May be used to differentiate a breast cyst from a tumor.

15. _____ X-ray which can reveal circulation around a tumor.

16. _____ Done to provide a definitive diagnosis of a breast mass.

True/False

17. _____ About 90% of all breast masses are found by women themselves.

18. _____ Approximately 50% of breast masses are malignant.

19. _____ A baseline mammography should begin at age 50.

20. _____ If a breast biopsy is positive, surgery is performed immediately.

21. _____ If a lactating patient develops mastitis, she should stop nursing.

22. _____ Fibrocystic disease can affect half of premenopausal women.

23. _____ Breast cancer is the most common form of cancer among American women.

24. _____ Elderly women have a higher risk of developing breast cancer.

25. _____ Patients with breast disorders seek help in a variety of health-care delivery settings.

Knowledge Application

26. A woman who must discontinue nursing her infant abruptly to return to work is at risk for developing
    A. fibrocystic breast disease
    B. mastitis
    C. breast cancer
    D. gynecomastia

27. The etiology of gynecomastia is thought to be
    A. disturbance in the ratio of sex hormones
    B. disturbance in growth hormone
    C. normal process of growth
    D. normal process of aging

28. Patient education for the patient with fibrocystic disease would include information on all the following EXCEPT
    A. avoid sleeping in the prone position
    B. use heating pad for pain relief
    C. limit use of caffeine
    D. reduce intake of sodium

29. Clinical manifestations of fibrocystic breast disease include
    A. breast swelling that begins after menstruation
    B. fever, lethargy, and breast tenderness
    C. discharge from breast; a hard, firm mass
    D. aching pain in breast before menstruation

30. Medical treatment of fibrocystic breast disease may include medications that inhibit anterior pituitary production of FSH and LH such as
    A. progesterone
    B. Danazol
    C. estrogen
    D. thyroxin

31. The primary symptom of intraductal papilloma is
    A. pain in both breasts
    B. change in breast size
    C. bleeding from the nipple
    D. enlargement of lymph nodes

32. The most common site of breast cancer is the
    A. nipple area
    B. lower quadrant
    C. upper outer quadrant
    D. inner quadrants

33. If a patient with breast cancer is found to have noninvasive tumor cells confined to the duct in which they originated, this is called
    A. early malignancy
    B. epithelial carcinoma
    C. carcinoma in situ
    D. metastatic disease

34. If a woman has a breast tumor less than 2 cm with tumor cells in two lymph nodes, she would be in which stage?
    A. Stage I
    B. Stage II
    C. Stage III
    D. Stage IV

35. The primary treatment of breast cancer is
    A. palliative therapy
    B. chemotherapy
    C. radiation therapy
    D. surgical removal

36. When a patient has a left radical mastectomy, which procedure would be contraindicated?

    A.   doing arm exercises with both arms

    B.   taking blood pressure in left arm

    C.   drawing blood from right arm

    D.   elevating arm and hand on pillow

37. When might a lumpectomy be a suggested treatment option for the patient with breast cancer? When

    A.   he or she is in Stage I or II

    B.   the tumor is small and has not spread

    C.   the tumor is localized in the nipple

    D.   this procedure is preferred by the patient

38. A recommended treatment after lumpectomy is

    A.   chemotherapy

    B.   hormonal therapy

    C.   antibiotic therapy

    D.   radiation therapy

39. The type of chemotherapeutic agent that interferes with DNA replication is known as a(n)

    A.   mitotic inhibitor

    B.   antimetabolites

    C.   alkylating agent

    D.   hormonal inhibitor

40. If a woman with Stage III breast cancer is found to be estrogen-receptor positive, she would most likely receive

    A.   estrogen

    B.   actinomycin

    C.   prednisone

    D.   tamoxifen

41. When a patient has a radioactive implant to treat breast cancer, the nurse would

    A.   provide frequent time for discussion

    B.   explain that this will cure the cancer

    C.   limit time spent in the room

    D.   explain that pain medication is scheduled

42. The safest breast implants used for reconstruction are those filled with

    A.   saline

    B.   silicone

    C.   foam gel

    D.   plastic

43. Following breast reconstructive surgery, the nurse would monitor for

    A.   bleeding

    B.   infection

    C.   scar formation

    D.   all of the above

44. A patient is being discharged from an outpatient surgery center following left breast reconstruction. The nurse would instruct her to

    A.   lie on her back

    B.   lie on her left side

    C.   lie in a prone position

    D.   sit up as much as possible

Nursing Care Plan

45. Write a nursing care plan for the patient who has had a modified radical mastectomy. Use the following diagnosis.

    Nursing diagnosis: Knowledge deficit: procedure and perioperative routines

    Patient outcome:

    Interventions:

Case Studies

Case Study No. 1

Ms. S., age 32, was diagnosed with fibrocystic breast disease six years ago. Her condition is worsening and she is seeking more information.

46. Typical symptoms that Ms. S. reports include

    A. irregularity of breast with pain and tenderness

    B. greenish discharge and pain at nipple

    C. sharp pain in breast radiating to back

    D. dimpling of breast tissue, nontender masses

47. Which one of the following behaviors by Ms. S. would the nurse recommend she change?

    A. "I follow a low cholesterol diet."

    B. "I drink tea instead of coffee."

    C. "I watch my salt intake."

    D. "I exercise every day."

48. In order to be sure that Ms. S. does not have a malignant process, the physician

    A. orders a mammogram

    B. orders an ultrasound

    C. orders breast biopsy

    D. prepares for surgery

49. One of the more important things that the nurse will discuss when talking with Ms. S. is the

    A. need for yearly mammograms

    B. need to perform SBE

    C. need to take entire course of antibiotics

    D. relationship between fibrocystic breast disease and breast cancer

Case Study No. 2

Ms. T., age 48, has just found out that she has breast cancer. She is scheduled for surgery in the morning.

50. What is the primary nursing diagnosis for the patient at this time?

    A. Pain related to surgery

    B. Anxiety related to uncertain outcome

    C. Body image disturbance

    D. Potential for infection

51. Because her tumor is 4 cm in size and the physician has found tumor cells in the lymph nodes, a decision is made to do a modified radical mastectomy. This means that the

    A. tumor itself is excised along with the blood vessels

    B. breast, pectoralis minor muscle, and lymph nodes are removed

    C. breast, pectoralis minor and major muscles, and all adjacent lymph nodes are removed

    D. tumor and most of the breast and lymph nodes are removed

52. Following surgery, the nurse would explain the purpose of

    A. IV therapy

    B. arm exercises

    C. drainage catheters

    D. all of the above

53. In order to inhibit swelling, the nurse would instruct the patient to

    A. sit with bed raised

    B. elevate legs when out of bed

    C. keep arm elevated on pillow

    D. do coughing and deep breathing every two hours

54.   The nurse is aware that if Ms. T. does not follow the recommended nursing intervention, she may develop

    A.   lymphedema

    B.   mastitis

    C.   infection

    D.   pneumonia

Ms. T. talks to the nurse. She was confused when the physician told her that her tumor is estrogen-receptor positive. He also suggested that she needs radiation therapy.

55.   The nurse would explain that estrogen receptor positive means

    A.   that the tumor is localized

    B.   the tumor has spread

    C.   the tumor can be treated with hormonal manipulation

    D.   you can't ever take hormones

56.   The nurse further explains that the rationale for radiation therapy is to

    A.   be sure that the cancer can never recur

    B.   locally control tumor cells that may have spread

    C.   shrink the size of the tumor

    D.   reduce any postoperative pain

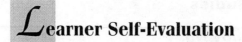

Learner Self-Evaluation

Do I fully understand the content? If no, then the areas I need to review are:

I need more information from my instructor on:

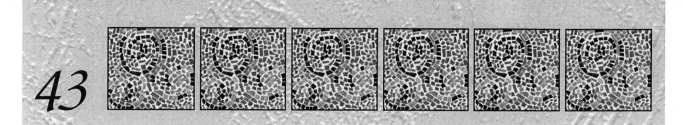

Nursing Care of Patients with Sexually Transmitted Diseases

Objectives

1.0 Demonstrate an understanding of several types of sexually transmitted diseases.
   1.1 Identify several sexually transmitted diseases.
   1.2 Identify the clinical manifestations of sexually transmitted diseases.
   1.3 Identify the current treatments for sexually transmitted diseases.

2.0 Plan the nursing care for the patient with a sexually transmitted disease.
   2.1 Write several nursing diagnoses and patient outcomes.
   2.2 Write nursing interventions for the patient with a sexually transmitted disease.
   2.3 Identify the teaching needs of the patient with a sexually transmitted disease.

Learning Activities

Identification

Match these common sexually transmitted diseases with the appropriate definition.

   A. Syphilis

   B. Genital herpes

   C. Gonorrhea

   D. Condylomata acuminata

1. _____ Sexually transmitted disease caused by gram-negative bacteria

2. _____ Warts in genital area caused by human papillomavirus

3. _____ Infectious, chronic, venereal disease caused by a spirochete that can affect any organ

4. _____ Infectious disease caused by the herpes simplex virus 2

Understanding cause and effect is part of nursing. Match each of the following organisms with the disease it produces.

   A. *Treponema pallidum*

   B. *Chlamydia trachomatis*

   C. Human papillomavirus

   D. *Pediculosis pubis*

   E. *Neisseria gonorrhoeae*

   F. *Ureaplasma urealyticum*

   G. *Sarcopted scabiei*

5. _____ Can cause nongonococcal urethritis

6. _____ Major cause of nongonococcal and postgonococcal urethritis in men

7. _____ Causes genital warts

8. _____ Can cause scabies

9. _____ Species of lice which is sexually transmitted

10. _____ Organism that causes syphilis

11. _____ Causes gonorrhea

Short Answers

12. The most common symptom of genital

    candidiasis is _____

    _____.

13. The normal vaginal environment is

    _____.

14. The drug of choice for the treatment of all

    stages of syphilis is _____.

15. Herpes simplex virus (HSV) is transmitted

    by _____ to _____ contact.

16. The recommended treatment for venereal

    warts is _____ or _____.

17. The primary symptom of lice infestation is

    _____.

18. The recommended treatment for pubic lice is

    _____.

19. Three factors that may precipitate a recur-

    rence of genital herpes are _____,

    _____, and _____.

20. In women, _____ has been
    implicated as one of the major causes of
    cervicitis and pelvic inflammatory disease
    (PID).

True/False

21. _____ Use of systemic antibiotics causes
    increased incidence of candidiasis.

22. _____ Candidiasis is rare during pregnancy.

23. _____ Flagyl is the only effective drug used to
    treat trichomoniasis.

24. _____ Herpes viruses have the ability to
    remain in the body and recur later.

25. _____ Most women with gonorrhea do not
    know they have it.

26. _____ Tetracycline is the best drug to treat
    gonorrhea.

27. _____ Using condoms will not prevent
    transmission of gonorrhea.

28. _____ Current treatment regimens can com-
    pletely eradicate genital herpes.

29. _____ Syphilis is inactive during the latent
    period.

30. _____ Tertiary syphilis is rare today.

31. _____ Sexual partners of the individual who
    has syphilis must be contacted.

32. _____ Infections by Chlamydia are more
    common than gonorrhea.

Knowledge Application

33. Which of the following questions elicits
    information concerning the *health history* of
    the individual suspected of having a vaginal
    infection? (Check all that apply.)

    A. _____ Ask the patient to describe the
    color, consistency, amount, and
    odor of discharge.

    B. _____ Ask the patient about history of
    other sexually transmitted dis-
    eases.

    C. _____ Ask the patient about her knowl-
    edge of normal vaginal function-
    ing.

    D. _____ Ask the patient about her per-
    sonal hygiene practices.

34. Choose the risk factors that often lead to the development of a fungal infection of the vagina. (Check all that apply.)

    A. _____ multiple sexual partners

    B. _____ change in the normal microbial environment

    C. _____ change in host resistance

    D. _____ poor nutrition

    E. _____ systemic antibiotic use

35. The most effective medication for the treatment of genital candidiasis would be

    A. miconazole

    B. ampicillin

    C. cefoxitin

    D. Micronase

36. One of the most common sexually transmitted urogenital infections is

    A. gonorrhea

    B. trichomoniasis

    C. *Candida*

    D. syphilis

37. Which of the following symptoms are generally associated with trichomoniasis?

    A. thin, watery discharge; itching

    B. hematuria, pruritus

    C. greenish-gray or purulent discharge, dysuria

    D. urinary frequency, brown drainage

38. In women that have been diagnosed with nonspecific vaginitis, the causative organism in 95% of them has been found to be

    A. Candidiasis

    B. trichomoniasis

    C. *Gardnerella vaginalis*

    D. *Neisseria gonorrhoeae*

39. During the assessment of a patient with vaginitis, the nurse reviews the personal hygienic habits because she or he realizes one of the practices that may predispose a woman to infection is

    A. frequent douching with solutions that alter vaginal pH

    B. wearing of cotton underwear

    C. taking a bath or shower immediately after intercourse

    D. urinating every four hours

40. Recurrence of herpes simplex can be precipitated by

    A. intercourse

    B. emotional stress

    C. menstruation

    D. any of the above

41. The nurse suspects primary genital herpes in a clinic patient. If herpes is present, the lesions would appear

    A. pustular, which crust and spread along linear tracts

    B. red, flattened lesions around genitals

    C. raised, scaly, and crusty

    D. multiple small papules that become vesicular or pustular

42. When a pregnant woman develops a primary infection with genital herpes, the nurse discusses the most serious problem encountered during pregnancy. This is

    A. possibility of spontaneous abortion

    B. transmission of herpes infection to neonate

    C. high risk of congenital anomalies

    D. risk of systemic problems

43. Herpes simplex virus has the ability to stay in the body in a latent state and cause recurrent disease. In caring for a patient with herpes the nurse is aware that

    A. herpes is infectious only during the first episode

    B. herpes is infectious during each episode of recurrence

    C. having herpes provides immunity against another attack

    D. having genital herpes prevents contacting herpes labialis

44. Major symptoms associated with genital herpes include

    A. pain, itching, dysuria, discharge, vesicles

    B. purulent drainage, vesicular formation, ulcers

    C. fever, nausea, lethargy

    D. localized lesions over perineum and trunk

45. In women the major site of infection by HSV is

    A. vulva

    B. vagina

    C. cervix

    D. uterus

46. In most individuals, there is a strong emotional reaction when they are told that they have contracted genital herpes. Which of the following reactions may occur?

    A. shock

    B. anger

    C. denial

    D. all of the above

47. Medical care for the patient with genital herpes would most likely include administration of

    A. ampicillin

    B. tetracycline

    C. acyclovir

    D. Leukeran

48. A patient with active genital herpes is admitted in labor. What would be an appropriate nursing action?

    A. monitor patient carefully because of the risk of birth defects

    B. set up for cesarean section

    C. prepare for normal labor routine

    D. contact the neonatal intensive care unit

49. When counseling patients with genital herpes, the nurse is aware that much of the anxiety that individuals experience is due to the

    A. potential for recurrent, unpredictable outbreaks of infection

    B. problems related to dealing with an ongoing continuous infectious process

    C. problems related to becoming sterile

    D. problems related to infertility

50. Which of the following medications is able to eradicate both gonorrhea and co-existent Chlamydia?

    A. procaine penicillin G

    B. ampicillin

    C. tetracycline

    D. acyclovir

51. The medical treatment of choice for trichomoniasis and *Gardnerella vaginitis* is

    A. gentamicin

    B. acyclovir

    C. ampicillin

    D. metronidazole

52. A patient complains of difficulty urinating. On further questioning he also states he has noticed he has a yellowish urethral discharge. This information suggests that he has

    A. a urinary tract infection

    B. genital herpes

    C. contacted gonorrhea

    D. contracted syphilis

53. What is the most common and serious complication of gonorrhea infection in women?

    A. pelvic inflammatory disease

    B. acute septicemia

    C. sterility

    D. kidney failure

54. What diagnostic test is done to verify the presence of gonorrhea in women?

    A. pelvic exam

    B. cervical culture

    C. cervical biopsy

    D. ultrasound of reproductive organs

55. What is the rationale for using probenecid along with penicillin to treat gonorrhea? Probenecid

    A. prevents allergic reactions to penicillin

    B. increases secretion of penicillin

    C. decreases renal secretion of penicillin

    D. has analgesic qualities to control discomfort

56. If the nurse suspects that disseminated gonococcal infection is present in an individual, which of the symptoms would probably be present?

    A. gastric upset, nausea, vomiting, diarrhea

    B. skin lesions on legs, arthritic symptoms, fever, anorexia

    C. diffuse rash on trunk, flushing on face, fever

    D. anorexia, vomiting, dehydration

57. The nurse has completed an education program to discuss risk factors associated with sexually transmitted diseases. Which statement by an 18-year-old female would indicate that the teaching was ineffective?

    A. "My boyfriend wouldn't give me any disease."

    B. "Abstinence will prevent STD."

    C. "Having sex can lead to a disease."

    D. "I didn't know how easy it was to get an STD."

58. Which statement provides valid information about primary syphilis?

    A. Multiple painful genital lesions are present.

    B. The infection heals spontaneously in 3–6 weeks.

    C. If the lesions disappear, no further treatment is needed.

    D. It includes lesions, discharge, fever, and lethargy.

59. When counseling a group of young men about STDs, the nurse would state

    A. "Latent syphilis is detected by physical exam."

    B. "Tertiary syphilis occurs in less than 5% of patients."

    C. "Repeated exposure is needed for syphilis to develop."

    D. "If left untreated, syphilis will ultimately produce systemic symptoms."

60. The nurse is aware that when a person has syphilis, there is a possibility for a false negative test to occur. What is the reason for this?

    A. The virus hasn't fully matured.

    B. It can take up to three weeks for the antibodies to form.

    C. The antigen-antibody reaction doesn't occur with this disease.

    D. The lab tests take two weeks to run.

61. Which statement is NOT true about *Chlamydia*? It

   A. has a high incidence of infecting the neonate at the time of delivery

   B. is a major cause of pelvic inflammatory disease

   C. is a potent virus that affects both men and women

   D. causes symptoms such as abdominal pain and vaginal bleeding and can lead to infertility

62. The patient with a suspected case of *Chlamydia* should have a thorough history taken. Which of the following is the most significant predictor for this infection?

   A. use of contraceptives

   B. socioeconomic status

   C. history of STDs

   D. sexual history, number of partners

63. Which of the following antibiotics have been found to be highly effective in the treatment of *C. trachomatis* infections?

   A. tetracycline and sulfisoxazole

   B. penicillin G and tetracycline

   C. doxycycline and ampicillin

   D. doxycycline and azithromycin

Nursing Care Plans

64. Write a nursing care plan for the individual with genital herpes.

   Nursing diagnosis: Ineffective coping related to the potential effects of having a chronic sexually transmitted disease

   Patient outcome:

   Interventions:

65. An important concern of the nurse is to prevent further transmission of sexually transmitted diseases. Write a plan that addresses how you would present this information in a teaching session. Use the following nursing diagnosis.

   Nursing diagnosis: Knowledge deficit related to disease process and prevention of transmission

   Class outcome:

   Interventions:

66. Noncompliance with the treatment of syphilis is a problem in society. Write a nursing care plan that relates to this. Use the following diagnosis.

   Nursing diagnosis: Potential noncompliance with the treatment regimen related to lack of knowledge, lifestyle, and distrust of health professionals

   Patient outcome:

   Interventions:

67. Write a nursing care plan for the patient who has her third vaginal infection with Candida this year.

    Nursing diagnosis:

    Patient outcome:

    Interventions:

68. The nurse is planning the home care for a woman with sexually transmitted vaginitis. Using the following diagnosis, write an outcome and several interventions.

    Nursing diagnosis: Pain related to inflammatory process

    Patient outcome:

    Interventions:

Case Studies

Case Study No. 1

Ms. S. is 23 and 3 months pregnant. She is seen in the clinic with lesions on her vulva, vagina, cervix, and perineum. She is diagnosed as having genital herpes.

69. How would the physician know if this is a primary or recurrent infection? Based on

    A. patient history alone

    B. history and absence of antibodies to HSV

    C. history of exposure from sexual partner

    D. the presence of high WBC and ANA

70. Ms. S. wonders how she could have developed this problem. What information does the nurse give her? Genital herpes is

    A. transmitted via sexual contact

    B. transmitted by contact with the virus

    C. transmitted because of poor hygienic practices

    D. always present; being pregnant caused her to have an outbreak

71. Ms. S. is crying when the nurse enters the room. She says, "The doctor told me there is no cure for this disease." An appropriate response is

    A. "You sound upset; I'm sure that's not true."

    B. "Don't worry, most people never have a recurrence."

    C. "While it is true there is no permanent cure, there are medications to treat the symptoms."

    D. "Don't cry, you will only cause more stress on your pregnancy."

72. Based on Ms. S.'s current health status, what would the nurse explain to her?

   A. She will have to be monitored closely and deliver her baby by cesarean section.

   B. She may have a spontaneous abortion because of the severity of her symptoms.

   C. She will need to have weekly cultures and if they are negative, she may be able to deliver vaginally.

   D. She will very likely have a child with birth defects.

Case Study No. 2

Ms. P. is seen in the clinic with cervical discharge and abdominal pain. Testing reveals she has an infection caused by Chlamydia. Assessment reveals she also has a fever, vomiting, and intermittent bleeding.

73. The presence of these symptoms suggests what other problem?

   A. ascending urinary tract infection

   B. pelvic inflammatory disease

   C. septicemia

   D. gonorrhea as well as Chlamydia

74. The nurse would assess the patient's knowledge of the disease and its mode of transmission. Which question would the nurse use to elicit this information?

   A. "What factors in your sexual lifestyle would have put you at risk for this infection?"

   B. "Explain to me how you contracted this disease."

   C. "Give me a list of all your sexual partners."

   D. "How many children do you have?"

75. Ms. P. is very upset and wants to know if this disease can be treated. Which information should be provided? The disease

   A. has no cure but symptoms can be treated

   B. can be treated and cured, but you could be reinfected

   C. will go into remission without treatment

   D. will have some recurring episodes, lessening in severity

76. Ms. P. is ready for discharge. Which statement indicates that she has a good understanding of the way this disease is spread?

   A. "I will tell my boyfriend I don't want to see him again."

   B. "I am going to find another boyfriend."

   C. "I am going to be more selective in my sexual partners."

   D. "I don't see why this happened to me."

Learner Self-Evaluation

Do I fully understand the content? If no, then the areas I need to review are:

I need more information from my instructor on:

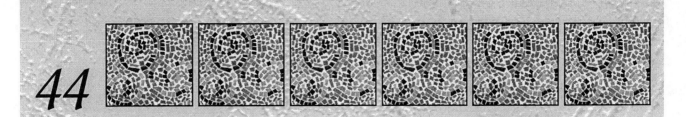

44

Knowledge Base for Patients with Eye Dysfunction

Objectives

1.0 Review the anatomy and physiology of the eye.
 1.1 Identify the structures of the eye.
 1.2 Explain the process of vision.
 1.3 Match the parts of the eye with their functions.

2.0 Demonstrate an understanding of the assessment data related to dysfunction of the eye.
 2.1 Review the assessment data specific to the eye.
 2.2 Identify clinical manifestations of eye dysfunction.
 2.3 Match diagnostic procedures used to identify visual dysfunctions with the correct definition.

3.0 Demonstrate an understanding of the interventions used to treat eye dysfunctions.
 3.1 Identify several medications used to treat eye dysfunctions.
 3.2 Identify surgical interventions used to treat eye dysfunctions.
 3.3 Demonstrate application of the nursing process when caring for a patient with a dysfunction of the eye.
 3.4 Demonstrate an understanding of the postoperative care for the patient who has undergone eye surgery.

*L*earning Activities

Identification

1. On the diagram below, label the structures of the eye.

   A. Cornea

   B. Ciliary body

   C. Vitreous humor

   D. Sclera

   E. Retina

   F. Lens

   G. Iris

   H. Optic disk

   I. Choroid

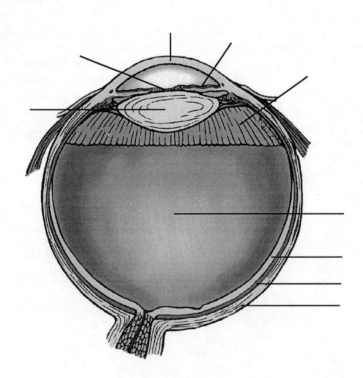

Short Answers

2. Tears are produced by the

    _____ gland.

3. The _____ is responsible for regulating the amount of light entering the eye.

4. The _____ is a vascular membrane that nourishes the retina.

5. The inner coat of the eye that forms the

    visual image is known as the _____.

6. The fluid responsible for maintaining the intraocular pressure is known as

    _____ _____.

7. The _____ refracts or bends light rays so that they converge on the retina.

8. Explain how the visual image is produced in the retina.

9. When you see the pupillary finding recorded as PERRLA in the patient record this means

    _____.

10. The muscles that control movement of the eye are under the control of cranial nerves

    _____, _____, and

    _____.

11. In the eye, drugs that cause sympathetic

    stimulation are called _____. They

    cause the pupil to _____.

12. Drugs that cause parasympathetic stimulation are called _____. They cause the

    pupil to _____.

13. Carbonic anhydrase inhibitors

    _____ intraocular pressure by

    causing a decrease in the amount of

    _____ _____.

14. Mannitol is an example of a drug which

    moves fluid rapidly by _____.

15. Another name for a corneal transplant or

    grafting is _____.

16. The complete removal of the globe is called

    _____.

Identification

Match each of the structures of the eye with the appropriate definition.

    A. Iris
    B. Choroid
    C. Retina
    D. Cones
    E. Rods

17. _____ Posterior portion of the middle coat, absorbs light rays to prevent reflection

18. _____ Responsible for color vision and visual acuity

19. _____ Regulates the amount of light entering the eye

20. _____ Covers the choroid, forms visual images

21. _____ Gives support to the posterior cavity

22. _____ Allow for vision in dim light

Identify these symptoms of eye dysfunction with the best definition.

- A. Floaters
- B. Photophobia
- C. Scotoma
- D. Diplopia
- E. Photopsia
- F. Nystagmus

23. _____ Involuntary twitching eye movements

24. _____ Appearance of flashing light in the visual field

25. _____ Seeing one object as two

26. _____ Unusual intolerance to light

27. _____ Fixed defects or "spots" in the visual field

28. _____ Moving spots in the visual field

Match each of the diagnostic tests with the best explanation of its purpose.

- A. Tonometry
- B. Fluorescein staining
- C. Gonioscopy
- D. Ultrasonography

29. _____ Measurement of intraocular pressure

30. _____ Used in the diagnosis of glaucoma

31. _____ Used to detect corneal abrasions

32. _____ Uses sound waves to detect tumors

True/False

33. _____ Eye surgery is generally done using local anesthesia.

34. _____ Miotic agents are given before surgery to dilate the pupil.

35. _____ Postoperatively, the operated eye is usually covered with an eye patch.

36. _____ Drainage following surgery is a cause for concern.

37. _____ Severe eye pain can indicate a complication such as hemorrhage.

38. _____ Laser therapy is a noninvasive procedure done on an outpatient basis.

39. _____ Peripheral vision generally narrows with aging.

Knowledge Application

40. During the admission process, a patient tells the nurse that he has blurred vision. Which information in his history may be related?
    - A. hypertension
    - B. ulcer
    - C. angina
    - D. leg cramps

41. Which of the following is a primary symptom of nonocular conditions such as meningitis or migraine headaches?
    - A. floaters
    - B. photophobia
    - C. scotoma
    - D. blurred vision

42. The most common cause of blurred vision is
    - A. drug overdose
    - B. congenital defect
    - C. refractory error
    - D. ocular muscle weakness

43. The sudden appearance of flashing lights in the visual field can be a symptom of _____.
    - A. retinal detachment
    - B. diabetes mellitus
    - C. hypertension
    - D. glaucoma

44. Sudden loss of vision is associated with which of the following?
    - A. retinal detachment
    - B. cataracts
    - C. glaucoma
    - D. diabetic retinopathy

45. Visual acuity is usually tested by use of a
    - A. ophthalmoscope
    - B. penlight
    - C. Snellen chart
    - D. otoscope

46. Legal blindness is defined as

    A. corrected vision of < 20/100

    B. corrected vision of < 20/200

    C. uncorrected vision of < 20/100

    D. uncorrected vision of < 20/300

47. Consensual response when testing the pupillary reaction to light is

    A. constriction of the pupil in response to light

    B. constriction of the pupil of opposite eye

    C. dilation of pupil when light is removed

    D. inward movement of eye in response to light

48. If a patient is unable to see any letters during a visual exam, the nurse should

    A. notify the physician

    B. check the ability to count fingers

    C. have him or her put on glasses

    D. use the ophthalmoscope

49. To test for _____, the nurse would hold a finger 6" from the patient's nose and have him or her look behind then back at the finger.

    A. direct response

    B. consensual response

    C. extraocular movement

    D. accommodation

50. Which of the following pharmacologic agents would be used for treatment of a foreign body in the eye?

    A. anesthetic

    B. anti-infective

    C. anti-inflammatory

    D. autonomic drug

51. After eye surgery, which of the following activities would be permitted during the postoperative period?

    A. smoking

    B. lying on the unaffected side

    C. lying on the stomach

    D. frequent coughing to expand lungs

52. The drug of choice to suppress hyperemia, photophobia, and pain is _____.

    A. analgesic

    B. antipyretic

    C. corticosteroid

    D. antibiotic

53. When a sympatholytic drug is to be used in treating an eye condition, it should be used cautiously for a patient with _____.

    A. diabetes

    B. cardiac disease

    C. hepatic disease

    D. skin disease

54. If a patient has angle-closure glaucoma, the preferred medical treatment would be

    A. carbonic anhydrase inhibitors

    B. sympathomimetic drugs

    C. parasympatholytic drugs

    D. sympatholytic drugs

Nursing Care Plan

55. Write a nursing care plan for the patient having eye surgery. Use the following nursing diagnosis.

    Nursing diagnosis: Knowledge deficit related to preoperative experience and the expected effect on vision

    Patient outcome:

Interventions:

Case Studies

Case Study No. 1

Ms. M. has had eye surgery to correct a visual deficit. The following questions relate to the postoperative period.

56. Why would the nurse encourage her to refrain from smoking following the surgery? It will

    A.   lower her blood pressure

    B.   irritate her vision

    C.   cause increased ocular pressure

    D.   increase her heart rate

57. Which of the following symptoms in the immediate postoperative period warrants immediate attention?

    A.   nausea

    B.   constipation

    C.   headache

    D.   thirst

58. The nurse tells Ms. M. that she should lie on her back and have the bed elevated slightly. What is the reason for this instruction? To

    A.   prevent hemorrhage

    B.   prevent an infection

    C.   avoid pressure on the eye

    D.   provide for effective coughing

Case Study No. 2

A patient is to have a corneal transplant because of degeneration.

59. Preoperatively, the nurse would administer

    A.   antibiotic eyedrops, pilocarpine HCl

    B.   antibiotics and analgesics

    C.   mydriatic and analgesics

    D.   osmotic diuretic

60. Which of the following information is true about the procedure?

    A.   It is done under general anesthetic.

    B.   Patients stay in the hospital for 3–5 days.

    C.   Local anesthetic is used, stay is overnight.

    D.   A living donor is used.

61. Postoperative teaching by the nurse would include (Check all that apply.)

    A.   _____   instruction on fluid restrictions

    B.   _____   information on use of eye patch and shield

    C.   _____   information on antibiotics

    D.   _____   information on activity limits

    E.   _____   information on how to instill eye drops

*L*earner Self-Evaluation

Do I fully understand the content? If no, then the areas I need to review are:

I need more information from my instructor on:

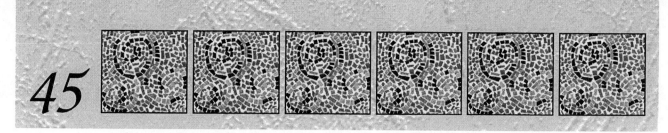

Nursing Care of Patients with Eye Disorders

$\mathcal{L}$earning Activities

Identification

Match these common eye disorders with the best definition.

- A.   Blepharitis
- B.   Chalazion
- C.   Conjunctivitis
- D.   Dacryocystitis
- E.   Keratitis
- F.   Endophthalmitis

1. _____ Chronic inflammation of the eyelid

2. _____ Infection or inflammation of the internal eye

3. _____ Infection of the nasolacrimal sac or duct

4. _____ Inflammation or infection of the conjunctiva

5. _____ Inflammation or infection of the cornea

6. _____ Chronic inflammation of the Meibomian gland

Short Answers

7.   Allergic conjunctivitis occurs after repeated exposure to _____ or from _____.

8.   Increased prominence of the conjunctival blood vessels is called _____.

9.   Refractory errors are treated by changing the _____ ability.

10.   Refractive errors can be treated surgically by altering the shape of the _____.

11.   Following cataract extraction, the individual will need a _____ replacement.

12.   An increased intraocular pressure can result in _____.

Identification

Match each of these clinical symptoms with the description.

- A.   Epiphora
- B.   Photophobia
- C.   Hypopyon
- D.   Hyperopia
- E.   Myopia
- F.   Entropion

13. _____ Excessive tearing

14. _____ Purulent material in anterior chamber

15. _____ Farsightedness

16. _____ Sensitivity to light

17. _____ Nearsightedness

18. _____ Inward turning of eyelid

True/False

19. _____ Evidence exists that cataracts can be seen in most patients over age 70.

20. _____ Surgery is needed to cure vision loss from cataracts.

21. _____ Pain is a symptom of glaucoma.

22. _____ Spontaneous healing is common after retinal detachment.

23. _____ Age-related macular degeneration is the leading cause of irreversible vision loss in persons over 65.

Knowledge Application

24. Patients in a hospital at risk for exposure to keratitis would include those

    A. on ventilators

    B. who are comatose

    C. with exophthalmos

    D. any of the above

25. Symptoms such as itching, burning, photophobia, and the sensation of a foreign body in the eye suggest

    A. blepharitis

    B. hordeola

    C. chalazia

    D. conjunctivitis

26. When assessing a patient with an allergic conjunctivitis, the primary symptom is usually

    A. drainage

    B. itching

    C. conjunctival edema

    D. redness

27. Which information would the nurse obtain from a patient who has recurrent conjunctivitis?

    A. history of hypertension

    B. use of antibiotics

    C. exposure to irritants

    D. recent loss of vision

28. The primary cause of corneal ulceration is

    A. herpes simplex virus

    B. *Streptococcus aureus*

    C. *Escherichia coli*

    D. *Staphylococcus*

29. All of the following symptoms may be present with bacterial keratitis EXCEPT

    A. reduced visual acuity

    B. photophobia

    C. mucopurulent discharge

    D. ocular pain

    E. scratchy feeling in eye

30. One of the main treatment objectives with keratitis is

    A. controlling pain

    B. protecting the cornea

    C. administering corticosteroids

    D. all of the above

31. A person who is experiencing visual fatigue, eye discomfort, or headache may have a

    A. corneal abrasion

    B. refractory error

    C. traumatic injury

    D. sensitivity to light

32. One of the problems with using rigid contact lenses is that they

    A. are easily damaged

    B. can harbor microorganisms

    C. are easily broken

    D. dry eyes or cause corneal warping

33. Following radial keratotomy, the nurse would discuss potential complications that might occur such as (Check all that apply.)

    A. _____ infection

    B. _____ corneal haze

    C. _____ bleeding

    D. _____ astigmatism

    E. _____ perceptions of halos

34. When providing discharge instruction following radial keratotomy, the nurse would instruct the patient to

    A. avoid driving for 72 hours

    B. use eyedrops as directed

    C. return to work in 24 hours

    D. wear an eye patch for 5 days

35. Which of the following eye medications should be used with caution in the elderly person with cardiac disease?

    A. Diamox

    B. Pilocar

    C. Tearisol

    D. Timoptic

36. The chief clinical manifestation of a cataract is

    A. gradual, painless blurring of central distance vision

    B. sudden loss of peripheral vision

    C. pain and mucoid discharge from the eye

    D. excessive tearing of eyes

37. The preferred method of treating patients with significant visual loss is

    A. surgical excision and intraocular lens implant

    B. laser surgery and contact lens

    C. cataract spectacles

    D. radiation therapy and lens implant

38. Which statement best describes the pathophysiology of glaucoma?

    A. Intraocular pressure decreases gradually.

    B. Vitreous humor is overproduced.

    C. Aqueous humor is produced faster than it can be drained.

    D. Obstructive processes in the eye canal occur.

39. A patient is complaining of sudden onset of severe unilateral ocular pain, nausea, vomiting, and seeing haloes. These symptoms suggest

    A. primary open-angle glaucoma

    B. angle-closure glaucoma

    C. secondary glaucoma

    D. unilateral cataract

40. Oral hyperosmotics may be used to reduce intraocular pressure (IOP) in a patient. Side effects that the nurse would observe for include

    A. cardiac arrhythmias

    B. ataxia, paresthesia

    C. bradycardia, hypotension

    D. headaches, confusion, disorientation

41. When pharmacologic treatment for primary open-angle glaucoma is ineffective, the physician may suggest

    A. adding a second medication

    B. argon laser trabeculoplasty

    C. intraocular surgery

    D. intraocular shunting

42. When a patient suddenly complains of seeing flashes of bright light or spots before their eyes, this suggests

    A. diabetic retinopathy

    B. macular degeneration

    C. retinal detachment

    D. conjunctivitis

43. Following a scleral buckling procedure, the nurse would administer antibiotic and steroid eyedrops such as

    A. Timoptic

    B. atropine

    C. Pred-G

    D. dextran

44. When educating the patient about macular degeneration, the nurse would explain

    A. "Treatment with miotic drugs can control symptoms."

    B. "Laser surgery may be used if medication is ineffective."

    C. "Total blindness is inevitable."

    D. "Vision loss is permanent but total loss is rare."

45. To help the patient with macular degeneration cope with sensory-perceptual alteration, the nurse would

    A. assist the patient to maximize existing vision

    B. explain how to instill eyedrops

    C. explain the use of an eye patch

    D. explain proposed surgical procedures

46. When a traumatic injury has been sustained, the first diagnostic procedure should be

    A. ophthalmoscopy

    B. fluorescein stain

    C. visual acuity

    D. ultrasonography

47. Emergency treatment of chemical burns of the eye would involve

    A. flushing eye with a large amount of water

    B. patching the eye immediately

    C. transport to emergency room

    D. instilling antibiotic eyedrops

Nursing Care Plans

48. Write a nursing care plan for the patient with a corneal ulcer. Use the following nursing diagnosis.

    Nursing diagnosis: Sensory perceptual alteration, vision; related to corneal transparency

    Patient outcome:

    Interventions:

49. Write a nursing care plan for the patient undergoing cataract surgery. Use the following nursing diagnosis.

    Nursing diagnosis: High risk for injury

    Patient outcome:

    Interventions:

Case Studies

Case Study No. 1

Ms. N. had cataract surgery this morning. The following questions relate to the surgery and follow-up care.

50. When providing Ms. N. with preoperative information, the nurse would ask about use of

    A.   antibiotics

    B.   aspirin

    C.   antihypertensives

    D.   laxatives

51. The nurse would also be sure that Ms. N.

    A.   has someone to drive her home

    B.   realizes she needs her glasses

    C.   brings an overnight bag

    D.   has no allergies to iodine

52. Which statement best describes the type of pain control that Ms. N. will need? (Check all that apply.)

    A.   _____ Narcotics will be used for the first 24 hours.

    B.   _____ Pain is unusual and Tylenol is usually effective.

    C.   _____ Pain may persist for 3–5 days.

    D.   _____ Pain unrelieved by Tylenol should be reported.

53. Which intervention would be included under the nursing diagnosis High risk for impaired home maintenance?

    A.   Use eyedrops every two hours.

    B.   Don't bend at the waist or lift more than 20 pounds.

    C.   Remove eye shield at night.

    D.   Resume normal activity.

54. Signs and symptoms of complications that Ms. N. would report immediately include

    A.   spots in vision

    B.   flashes of light

    C.   change in vision

    D.   all of the above

Case Study No. 2

A patient was diagnosed with primary open-angle glaucoma two years ago and is being treated medically. She is in for a routine checkup.

55. Which statement best describe the initial symptoms experienced by most patients with this condition?

    A.   onset is acute; severe eye pain is primary symptom

    B.   onset is slow with vision suddenly changing

    C.   patients often symptomatic with complaints of foggy vision

    D.   symptoms include headache, nausea, photophobia

56. Which of the following manifestations of this condition are evident during the eye exam?

    A.   Retinal vessels are tortuous.

    B.   Sclera is red, cornea looks steamy.

    C.   Lens is gray and bulging.

    D.   Optic disc is pale or gray.

57. Because of the many side effects of the medications which reduce IOP, presence of which of the following would contraindicate using Timoptic?

    A.   ulcerative colitis

    B.   diabetes

    C.   migraine headache

    D.   renal disease

58. Because medications have not been effective in controlling IOP, the patient is scheduled for laser surgery. Which statement best describes what the patient can expect?

   A. Following the procedure, medication is no longer necessary.

   B. IOP is lowered in 80% of patients, but effectiveness may be lost over time.

   C. If laser surgery is ineffective, the patient is immediately taken for intraocular surgery.

   D. Effects are immediate and often full vision is restored.

59. Following the laser surgery, the nurse would

   A. monitor vital signs every four hours

   B. keep patient flat in bed for eight hours

   C. monitor IOP on arrival and after giving Iopidine

   D. keep both eyes patched and room dim

$\mathcal{L}$earner Self-Evaluation

Do I fully understand the content? If no, then the areas I need to review are:

I need more information from my instructor on:

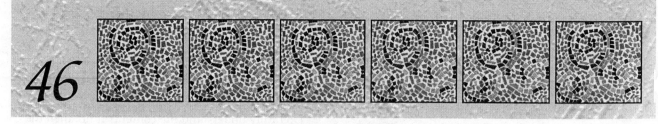

46

Knowledge Base for Patients with Ear Dysfunction

Objectives

1.0 Review the anatomy and physiology of the ear.
    1.1 Locate the parts of the external ear.
    1.2 Locate the parts of the internal ear.
    1.3 Explain the process of hearing.

2.0 Demonstrate an understanding of the assessment data related to ear dysfunction.
    2.1 Identify clinical manifestations of adults with dysfunction of the ear.
    2.2 Identify specific types of hearing loss.
    2.3 Define specific symptoms of hearing disorders.
    2.4 Match diagnostic procedures used to evaluate ear disorders with the definition.

3.0 Demonstrate an understanding of the interventions used to treat adults with ear dysfunction.
    3.1 Identify surgical procedures used to treat ear dysfunction.
    3.2 Identify medical treatments used for the patient with ear dysfunction.
    3.3 Write a nursing care plan for the patient having ear surgery.

*L*earning Activities

Identification

1. On the diagram below identify the structures
    of the ear.

    A. Malleus

    B. External ear

    C. Stapes

    D. Incus

    E. Tympanic membrane

    F. Eustachian tube

    G. Semicircular canals

    H. Cochlea

    I. Cochlear nerve

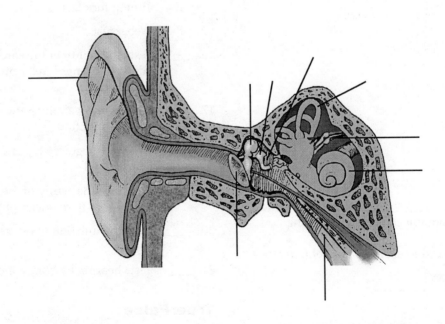

Match each of the following with the best definition.

 A. Otalgia

 B. Tinnitus

 C. Otorrhea

 D. Vertigo

 E. Presbycusis

2. _____ Pain in ear

3. _____ Drainage from the ear

4. _____ Sensation of imbalance, unsteadiness, or faintness

5. _____ Progressive sensorineural hearing loss associated with age

6. _____ Sensation of buzzing, ringing in one or both ears

Short Answers

7. The external ear includes the

 _____ and the _____.

8. Explain the process of hearing.

9. The _____ is a tubelike structure that contains the organ of hearing.

10. The term used to express a unit of frequency

 is _____.

11. Intensity of sound is measured in

 _____.

12. In assessing the auditory canal, an

 _____ is used to detect obstructions.

Identification

Match these common types of hearing loss with the best definition.

 A. Sensorineural hearing loss

 B. Conductive hearing loss

 C. Functional hearing loss

13. _____ Condition that interferes with transmission of sound waves from the external or middle ear to the sensorineural apparatus of the inner ear

14. _____ Psychogenic problem with no organic cause

15. _____ Results from a problem within the internal ear

Match the following diagnostic tests with the best description.

 A. Rinne test

 B. Caloric test

 C. Audiometry

 D. Pneumatoscopy

 E. Tuning fork test

 F. Weber test

16. _____ Tests the ability of the eardrum to adjust to changes in air pressure in the middle ear

17. _____ Tests hearing ability between air and bone conduction

18. _____ Used to categorize types and severity of hearing loss

19. _____ Measures the acuity of the sense of hearing for frequencies of sound waves

20. _____ Tests the function of the vestibular system

21. _____ Tests hearing by bone conduction

True/False

22. _____ Many ear disorders can be treated with medications.

23. _____ Tuning fork tests differentiate between conductive and sensorineural hearing loss.

24. _____ Hemorrhage is the major complication of ear surgery.

25. _____ A tympanoplasty may be done to improve hearing.

26. _____ Cochlear implants are a solution for the profoundly deaf.

27. _____ Hearing is restored after a cochlear implant.

28. _____ The elderly find it harder to distinguish high-pitched sounds.

Knowledge Application

29. The major clinical manifestation of ear disorders is
    A. pain in the ear
    B. dizziness
    C. drainage from ear
    D. loss of hearing

30. Which information in the medical history can be a cause of an ear disorder in adulthood? (Check all that apply.)
    A. _____ measles
    B. _____ allergies
    C. _____ chronic use of aspirin
    D. _____ listening to loud music

31. Repeated upper respiratory infections can predispose an individual to a _____ hearing loss.
    A. conductive
    B. sensorineural
    C. mixed
    D. functional

32. Repeated exposure to loud noise may result in a _____ hearing loss.
    A. conductive
    B. sensorineural
    C. mixed
    D. functional

33. When a patient with an ear disorder suffers from vertigo, the nurse would instruct him or her to
    A. avoid sudden changes in position
    B. use warm compresses on ear
    C. take analgesics as ordered
    D. take prescribed course of antibiotics

34. One of the medications that may be prescribed for the individual with mild vertigo is
    A. prednisone
    B. Dramamine
    C. Valium
    D. Tylenol

35. The nurse would closely monitor the patient taking _____ for signs of ear toxicity.
    A. gentamicin
    B. streptomycin
    C. furosemide
    D. all of the above

36. When a patient has a sensation of dizziness or vertigo, it may be due to
    A. pressure behind the tympanic membrane
    B. movement of fluid in the semicircular canals
    C. decreased fluid in the cochlea
    D. interference in conduction of sound waves

37. The function of the _____ is to amplify the force of sound.
    A. stapes
    B. auditory meatus
    C. ossicle
    D. cochlea

38. To visualize the auditory canal in an adult, the auricle should be pulled

    A. down and back

    B. up and forward

    C. up and back

    D. down and forward

39. When the Rinne test is positive, it indicates

    A. air conduction is longer than bone conduction

    B. bone conduction is longer than air conduction

    C. air conduction and bone conduction are equal

40. A patient who has been complaining of ataxia and dizziness would probably be given which test?

    A. Weber test

    B. past-pointing test

    C. caloric test

    D. Rinne test

41. A patient with a sensorineural hearing loss when given the Weber test will hear better in _____ ear.

    A. the affected

    B. the unaffected

    C. neither

42. A patient with a sensorineural hearing loss would score _____ during the speech discrimination test.

    A. low

    B. normal

    C. high

43. When the patient with a hearing disorder also has tinnitus, which test would be appropriate?

    A. impedance audiometry

    B. vestibular tests

    C. audiometric testing

    D. Rinne test

44. The normal response of the patient to a caloric test should be

    A. jerking movement of the eye toward or away from water instillation

    B. ringing in the ear when water is instilled

    C. sensation of dizziness and headache with water instillation

    D. no abnormal response should be noted if test is normal

45. For which of the following conditions would a myringotomy be an appropriate intervention?

    A. rupture of eardrum

    B. otorrhea

    C. presbycusis

    D. eustachian tube blockage

46. Following a mastoidectomy, the nurse would position the patient

    A. supine

    B. low-Fowler's

    C. Trendelenburg

    D. position of comfort

Nursing Care Plan

47. Write a nursing care plan for the patient who has had a tympanoplasty.

    Nursing diagnosis: Sensory/perceptual alteration related to vertigo secondary to surgical manipulation

    Patient outcome:

    Interventions:

Case Studies

Case Study No. 1

Ms. P. has been admitted with an infected mastoid bone and is scheduled for a radical mastoidectomy.

48. Ms. P. asks if she will have her hair shaved. The surgeon plans to use an endaural approach. The appropriate response would be

    A. "No, that isn't necessary."

    B. "Yes, we will shave a small area behind the ear."

    C. "Yes, we shave 6" around the ear for asepsis."

49. A correct explanation of the surgical procedure is

    A. the air cells in the mastoid process will be removed

    B. a bone graft will be sutured in place and then packing inserted

    C. the wall of the external canal, the tympanic membrane, and most of the middle ear structure is removed

50. Following the surgery the nurse would monitor for damage to cranial nerve

    A. II

    B. III

    C. V

    D. VIII

51. It is apparent that Ms. P. has a good understanding of her discharge instructions when she states

    A. "I will follow my special diet."

    B. "I am glad that I don't have any physical restriction."

    C. "I know I should avoid blowing my nose."

    D. "I will lie flat in bed after the procedure."

Case Study No. 2

Mr. J. is 20 years old. He has had severe otitis media for several years. Current medical treatment has been ineffective.

52. On assessment, findings consistent with otitis media would be

    A. retracted membrane, gray in color

    B. bulging of the membrane, whitish in color

    C. absence of the membrane, pus in the canal

53. The nurse notes that Mr. J. has a perforated eardrum. The procedure to repair this is called a(n)

    A. myringoplasty

    B. ear reduction

    C. labrintectomy

    D. spadectomy

54. Mr. J. will have the above surgery on an outpatient basis. The nurse calls him to explain the procedure. A correct explanation of this surgery would be

    A. "A local anesthetic is used and an incision is made into the eardrum."

    B. "A short-acting general anesthetic is used and an incision is made into the eardrum, followed by a graft."

    C. "A general anesthetic is used and several incisions will be made into the eardrum."

55. To repair the perforation, a graft will be harvested and held in place by

    A. stapling

    B. sutures

    C. Gelfoam

    D. sterile dressing

56. Discharge instructions should include information about complications such as

   A.   primary infection

   B.   secondary infection

   C.   hearing loss

   D.   hemorrhage

57. Discharge instruction would involve giving Mr. J. information on which of the following? (Check all that apply.)

   A. _____ wipe away any excess drainage

   B. _____ change the dressing frequently

   C. _____ shower as desired

   D. _____ avoid lifting or straining

   E. _____ take antihistamine as prescribed

   F. _____ report fever or increased pain

58. The nurse would be sure that Mr. J. understands that hearing improvement may not be apparent for

   A.   one week

   B.   two weeks

   C.   four weeks

   D.   six weeks

Learner Self-Evaluation

Do I fully understand the content? If no, then the areas I need to review are:

I need more information from my instructor on:

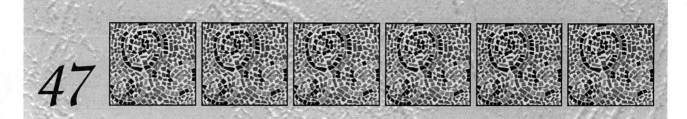

47

Nursing Care of Patients with Ear Disorders

Objectives

1.0 Demonstrate an understanding of the infections and inflammations of the ear.

   1.1 Define several inflammatory processes of the ear.

   1.2 Identify the clinical manifestations of several inflammatory processes of the ear.

   1.3 Identify the medical treatment of infections and inflammations of the ear.

   1.4 Identify nursing interventions for a patient with an ear disorder.

   1.5 Write a nursing care plan for the patient with an infection of the ear.

2.0 Demonstrate an understanding of structural disorders of the ear.

   2.1 Identify clinical manifestations of structural disorders.

   2.2 Identify medical treatment of structural disorders.

   2.3 Review the surgical treatment of structural disorders.

   2.4 Plan the nursing care for a patient with a structural disorder.

Learning Activities

Identification

Match each of the following ear disorders with the appropriate definition.

   A.   External otitis

   B.   Otomycosis

   C.   Furuncle

   D.   Otitis media

   E.   Mastoiditis

   F.   Labyrinthitis

   G.   Meniérè's disease

   H.   Presbycusis

1. _____ Fungal infection of the outer ear

2. _____ Inflammation of the skin of the auricle and/or the outer ear

3. _____ Infection of the inner ear

4. _____ Progressive sensorineural hearing loss seen with aging

5. _____ Recurrent attacks of severe vertigo, sensorineural hearing loss, and tinnitus

6. _____ Inflammation of the labyrinth of the inner ear

7. _____ Inflammation of the spongy cells of the mastoid bone

8. _____ Localized suppurative inflammation of the skin and underlying tissue

Based on your understanding of the clinical manifestations of the various disorders, match the assessment findings with the disorder.

    A.   External otitis

    B.   Serous otitis media

    C.   Acute otitis media

    D.   Mastoiditis

9. _____ Eardrum is red and bulging with fluid

10. _____ Eardrum is dull, thickened, swollen

11. _____ Eardrum is retracted

12. _____ Red, swollen external ear canal

Short Answers

13. _____ is a common symptom of generalized external otitis.

14. A tympanic perforation is a

_____ in the eardrum.

15. Otosclerosis is an overgrowth of spongy bone that prevents movement of the

_____.

16. The cause of Meniérè's disease is

_____.

17. More than _____ % of older people residing in nursing homes have hearing loss.

True/False

18. _____ Otitis media is usually caused by a bacteria.

19. _____ Acute otitis media is frequently associated with an upper respiratory infection.

20. _____ Prednisone is the treatment of choice for acute otitis media.

21. _____ Sudden changes in atmospheric pressure can result in occlusion of the ear canal.

22. _____ Chronic otitis media often results in perforation of the eardrum.

23. _____ Tympanic membrane perforations often heal spontaneously.

24. _____ Brain infection is a major complication of mastoidectomy.

25. _____ Stapes replacement surgery is done under local anesthetic.

Knowledge Application

26. Which ear condition often results from swimming in contaminated water?

    A.   external otitis

    B.   otomycosis

    C.   otitis media

    D.   mastoiditis

27. Medical management of external otitis involves

    A.   intravenous antibiotics

    B.   oral antibiotics and warm compresses

    C.   topical antibiotics and steroids

    D.   analgesics and Betadine soaks

28. Symptoms of acute otitis media include

    A.   severe earache and total hearing loss

    B.   earache and mild hearing loss, fever, nausea

    C.   purulent drainage, vertigo, hypertension

    D.   ear pain, severe headache, sore throat

29. Symptoms of serous otitis media include

    A.   earache, fever, nausea

    B.   earache, fever, tinnitus

    C.   purulent drainage, pain, tinnitus

    D.   tinnitus, conductive hearing loss

30. In viral labyrinthitis, the hearing loss is usually

    A.   sudden, profound, and permanent

    B.   sudden and profound but temporary

    C.   gradual and permanent

    D.   gradual but temporary

31. _____ may be administered intravenously to control dizziness for the patient with labyrinthitis.

    A.   Valium

    B.   Vistaril

    C.   Demerol

    D.   Haldol

32. Which information in the health history might explain why a patient has a perforation of the tympanic membrane?

    A.   ear infection

    B.   ear trauma

    C.   recent diving competition

33. The most common cause of progressive conductive hearing loss when there is no history of ear infection is

    A.   otitis media

    B.   labyrinthitis

    C.   mastoiditis

    D.   otosclerosis

34. Medical treatment for Meniérè's disease would include

    A.   antibiotics and steroids

    B.   analgesics and sedatives

    C.   sedatives and vestibular suppressants

    D.   all of the above

35. During an acute attack of Meniérè's disease the patient would be advised to

    A.   stay in bed

    B.   follow a low-sodium diet

    C.   restrict fluids

    D.   all of the above

36. The reason that the patient with Meniérè's disease should avoid use of nicotine or caffeine is

    A.   vasodilation can result in fluid in the inner ear

    B.   they cause the person to be overstimulated

    C.   vasoconstriction decreases circulation to the inner ear

    D.   they will lower the pain threshold

37. Patient education for the individual with serous otitis media would include which information?

    A.   blow nose vigorously several times a day

    B.   take decongestants as indicated

    C.   avoid exposure to allergens

    D.   all of the above

38. Discharge instructions for the patient following stapedectomy would include all of the following EXCEPT

    A.   no showers for six weeks

    B.   avoid forceful coughing

    C.   avoid tub baths for two weeks

    D.   avoid airplane travel as ordered

39. The reason that the patient must avoid bending or lifting after a stapedectomy is to

    A.   prevent infection

    B.   prevent displacement of prosthesis

    C.   prevent rupture of eardrum

    D.   help drain the ear

40. Presbycusis, a progressive hearing loss that is part of aging, is a result of

    A.   decreased movement of stapes

    B.   chronic ear infections

    C.   loss of hair cells in the cochlea

    D.   destruction of tympanic membrane

Nursing Care Plans

41. Write a nursing care plan for a patient with serous otitis media. Use the following nursing diagnosis.

    Nursing diagnosis: Knowledge deficit related to prevention of recurrence of problem

    Patient outcome:

    Interventions:

42. Write a nursing care plan for the patient who has a traumatic perforation of the eardrum.

    Nursing diagnosis:

    Patient outcome:

    Interventions:

43. Write a nursing care plan for the patient with Meniérè's disease. Use the following nursing diagnosis.

    Nursing diagnosis: Potential ineffective coping related to the chronic nature of the disease

    Patient outcome:

    Interventions:

44. Write a nursing care plan for an elderly individual with presbycusis. Use the following nursing diagnosis.

    Nursing diagnosis: Impaired communication related to hearing loss

    Patient outcome:

    Interventions:

Case Studies

Case Study No. 1

Ms. W. has had four episodes of otitis media during the past two years. She is now scheduled for a tympanoplasty.

45. Prior to surgery, you would expect that her treatment involves

    A. antibiotic therapy for two weeks

    B. cleansing of the ear canal and topical antibiotics

    C. systemic sympathomimetic agents

46. As the primary nurse, how do you explain this surgery?

    A. "It is a surgical repair of structure of the inner ear."

    B. "There is an insertion of a tube in the inner ear canal."

    C. "It is the removal of cholesteatoma."

47. Following the surgery, the patient complains of vertigo. What nursing diagnosis is appropriate at this time?

    A. Alteration in comfort

    B. Sensory-perceptual alteration

    C. Alteration in self-concept

    D. Potential for infection

48. Part of your nursing interventions include discharge instructions. These would include

    A. clean the ear with Q-tip daily

    B. blow nose vigorously every four hours

    C. avoid touching the ear, keep dressing dry

    D. avoid driving for eight weeks

Case Study No. 2

Mr. P. is scheduled for a stapedectomy in the outpatient surgical center. He has progressive otosclerosis and reports he has had periods of dizziness and a hearing loss.

49. Based on the diagnosis, when a Rinne test is done, results that confirm the diagnosis would be

    A. air conduction is greater than bone conduction

    B. bone conduction is greater than air conduction

50. Mr. P. is apprehensive about the proposed surgery. How would the nurse explain the procedure?

    A. "The diseased bone is removed and tubes are inserted."

    B. "The stapes is removed and replaced with a prosthesis."

    C. "The stapes is scraped and a bone graft inserted."

51. How does the nurse explain the anesthetic?

    A. "It is done under local anesthesia."

    B. "It is done using conscious sedation."

    C. "It is done using regional anesthesia."

52. When Mr. P. asks why he can't be put to sleep, the nurse would explain

    A. there are too many side effects

    B. the doctor wants to see if hearing improves

    C. it is such a minor procedure, you don't need very much anesthetic

    D. the anesthetic might depress breathing

53. The nurse is aware that the most common complication of stapedectomy is

    A. vomiting

    B. hemorrhage

    C. infection

    D. vertigo

54. Providing discharge instruction for Mr. P. is part of the nursing care. What information should be emphasized?

   A. no swimming or showers for six weeks

   B. no heavy lifting or strenuous exercise

   C. avoid coughing or nose blowing

   D. all of the above

Learner Self-Evaluation

Do I fully understand the content? If no, then the areas I need to review are:

I need more information from my instructor on:

Answer Key

CHAPTER I

Introduction to the Practice of Medical-Surgical Nursing

1. reduce

2. shorter

3. clinical pathway

4. diverse, multicultural

5. risk factors

6. acute care medical centers, ambulatory care, clinics, outpatient department, urgent care setting, home care

7. nurse practitioner, clinical specialist, nurse anesthetist

8. a profession built on art and science, nursing involves caring for individuals with acute and chronic health-care needs, and both illness and wellness where the individual is viewed holistically

9. a measure used to evaluate competency of care and quality of service, used to hold members of the health-care profession accountable

10. American Nurses' Association

11. aging society, care of the chronically ill, changes in reimbursement patterns, rising health-care costs, technological advances, expansion of nursing roles

12. reimbursement for nursing services, define levels of nursing practice, promote advances in nursing education through career paths, support health-care reform, use technology, such as computer in practice

13. listen carefully, be empathetic, recognize the patient's self interest, be flexible, have a sense of timing, use appropriate resources, provide relevant information

14. Increase the span of healthy life for Americans. Reduce health disparities among Americans. Achieve access to preventive services for all Americans.

15. North American Nursing Diagnoses Association (NANDA)

16. patient assessment, establishment of nursing diagnosis, developing care plan, implementation of plan, evaluation of plan

17. a clinical judgment about actual or potential health problems that can be alleviated or prevented by a nursing intervention

18. The first part is the diagnostic label or category. The second part is the etiology that deals with the reason for the alteration. The third part includes the defining characteristics.

19. 1. Setting priorities

    2. Establishing expected patient outcomes

    3. Selecting nursing interventions

    4. Documenting the plan of care

20. by comparing the patient status against the stated outcome

21. the problem that poses the greatest threat to the patient's well-being

22. Was the assessment complete? Was the nursing diagnosis correct? Was the expected outcome realistic? Were the nursing interventions appropriate? Have the priorities or situation changed?

23.   true
24.   true
25.   false
26.   true
27.   false

CHAPTER 2

Medical-Surgical Nursing in Multiple Settings

1.   health-care costs, technology, change in demographics, more poor and uninsured people, most people with chronic illness
2.   out-of-pocket, private insurance, Medicare, Medicaid
3.   36.4
4.   15%
5.   domestic
6.   80–90%
7.   education, research
8.   hospice
9.   providing comfort; promotion, maintenance, and restoration of health; and assisting with a peaceful death
10.   schools, homes, same-day surgery centers, ambulatory care centers, clinics, industry
11.   true
12.   true
13.   false
14.   true
15.   false
16.   true
17.   true
18.   B
19.   D
20.   A
21.   B
22.   D
23.   D
24.   B
25.   B
26.   D
27.   C
28.   all

CHAPTER 3

Death, Dying, and Bereavement

1.   death
2.   growth
3.   depression
4.   hope
5.   immortality
6.   acceptance
7.   guilt
8.   developmental
9.   denial, anger, bargaining, depression, acceptance
10.   Developing awareness of impending death; balancing hope and fear; relinquishing the will to live; letting go of autonomous control; detaching from former relationships; achieving spiritual preparation.
11.   It should be autonomous and offer a comprehensive program of care by a health team educated in thanatology. The goal should be to control symptoms and enable the patient to complete his or her life work and die in peace and dignity.
12.   Sense of peace, freedom from pain, awareness of leaving the physical body, sense of floating, movement through a tunnel into a light, finally viewing of one's life in a non-critical way.
13.   1.   Unresponsiveness even to pain
      2.   No spontaneous breathing for one hour, no breathing if off ventilator for three minutes
      3.   No reflexes
      4.   Flat EEG
      5.   Tests are the same 24 hours later
      6.   Cannot have hypothermia or central nervous system depression from drug overdose
14.   C
15.   D
16.   A
17.   B
18.   A
19.   C
20.   B
21.   B
22.   C

23. A

24. D

25. false

26. false

27. true

28. false

29. false

30. false

31. Outcome: Ms. H. can openly express unre-solved feelings of guilt, anger, and despair and actively seek ways to complete mourn-ing.

     Interventions: Listen actively. Provide opportunities for Ms. H. to express her feelings. Offer referrals for counseling as appropriate. Refer to support groups.

32. Outcome: Mrs. N. can openly express religious concerns and seek answers from clergy, nurses, or other members of her faith.

     Interventions: Act as an advocate in regard to religious practices. Explore ways to share religious rituals as appropriate. Engage in open, nonjudgmental, empathetic communi-cation. Encourage family visits by loved ones and other members of the religious commu-nity.

33. Outcome: Ms. D. openly ventilates, projects, and displaces anger and guilt feelings. Ms. D. gradually demonstrates acceptance of the death.

     Interventions: Provide opportunity for the family to say farewell with visual and tactile contact. Demonstrate empathy, patience, and tolerance during the anger phase. Encourage contact with self-help organizations. Provide opportunities to discuss the deceased. Actively listen and offer emotional support.

34. A

35. B

36. C

37. D

38. D

39. C

CHAPTER 4

Special Considerations for Nursing Care of Elderly Patients

1. 23%

2. gerontology

3. normal, abnormal

4. coping

5. 20–25%

6. decreased sweat production; loss of subcuta-neous fat; diminished peripheral circulation

7. 50%

8. 1. reduced gastric and intestinal motility increase the opportunity for drug interactions

    2. increased adipose tissue and impaired capillary function can affect absorption

    3. reduction in hepatic and renal function changes excretion

9. 1. instruction on how and when to take each medication

    2. information on expected effects and adverse effects

    3. importance of monitoring effects of medication

    4. importance of reporting adverse reactions or lack of expected response

    5. any food or drugs to avoid

    6. avoiding OTC medication without consulting physician

10. E

11. B

12. A

13. C

14. B

15. C

16. C

17. A

18. D

19. A

20. B

21. C

22. B

23. D

24. A

25. C

26. A

27. C

28. true

29. true

30. true

31. false
32. true
33. B, C, G, and H are part of normal aging
34. Nursing diagnosis: Altered health maintenance related to lack of knowledge of
medication regimen.

Patient outcome: Patient verbalizes understanding of need to follow prescribed
medication regimen prior to discharge.

Interventions: Determine patient's readiness
and ability to learn. Teach patient the name,
dose, frequency, expected action, and unto-
ward side effects of medication. Instruct
patient to notify physician if side effects
occur.
35. B
36. B
37. A
38. D
39. A
40. A
41. Instruct the patient that visual changes occur
with aging. Suggest glasses be kept at
bedside and put on before arising. Explain
circulatory changes that may cause episodes
of orthostatic hypotension. Teach patient to
rise slowly to sitting position and sit at
bedside for several minutes before rising.
42. D
43. Teach that constipation is a long-term effect
of laxative use due to decreased intestinal
muscle tone. Teach that regular exercise,
adequate fluids, and a high-fiber diet will
prevent constipation. Encourage adequate
fluid intake. Encourage that a regular time be
established for defecation.
44. A
45. Explain that immobility increases pressure
over bony prominences and impairs circulation. Instruct patient to sit in chair with
padded seat. Use egg crate or air mattress on
bed. Instruct patient to change position every
two hours.
46. E

CHAPTER 5

Knowledge Base for Patients with Fluid, Electrolyte, and Acid-Base Imbalances

1. high, low
2. hypovolemia
3. 60%
4. water, sodium
5. thirst
6. diuretics, digitalis, diet
7. arterial blood gases
8. FVD
9. FVE
10. FVD
11. FVE
12. FVD
13. FVE
14. hypernatremia
15. hypokalemia/hypernatremia
16. hypocalcemia
17. hyperkalemia
18. hypomagnesemia
19. hyponatremia
20. A
21. B
22. C
23. B
24. C
25. A
26. B
27. B
28. C
29. C
30. A
31. B
32. B
33. C
34. C
35. A
36. D
37. C
38. A
39. A
40. C
41. A

42. B
43. B
44. C
45. A
46. B
47. A
48. C
49. A
50. A
51. D
52. C
53. B
54. B
55. B
56. B
57. true
58. true
59. false
60. true
61. true
62. false
63. false
64. false
65. Potassium: 3.5–5.3 mEq/L
66. Sodium: 135–145 mEq/L
67. Serum calcium: 4.5–5.5 mEq/L
68. Ionized calcium: 2.2–2.5 mEq/L
69. Magnesium: 1.5–2.5 mEq/L
70. A
71. C
72. B
73. Nursing care plan

Nursing diagnosis: FVE related to excessive fluid retention

Patient outcome: Vital signs are within patient baseline. Breath sounds are clear. Extremities are free from edema.

Interventions: Monitor vital signs and breath sounds. Check for presence of edema. Monitor weight daily. Restrict fluid and sodium intake. Administer medications as ordered.

74. A
75. A
76. A
77. C

78. Oranges *
    Spinach *
    Potatoes *
    Yellow squash
    Turkey
    Fish
    Broccoli *
    Tomatoes *
79. C
80. A
81. B
82. A
83. A
84. B
85. C
86. C
87. A
88. C
89. A
90. C
91. C
92. B

CHAPTER 6

Knowledge Base for Patients Undergoing Surgery

1. ambulatory or short stay
2. advocate and educator
3. physician
4. microorganisms
5. void and defecate
6. malignant hyperthermia
7. hypoxia
8. impaired, impaired, diminished
9. before surgery
10. patient-controlled analgesia
11. evisceration
12. Implies that the patient or legal guardian has been informed by the physician of the nature, risks, desired results, and possible complications associated with the procedure.
13. Refers to emergency treatment that is performed without written permission when it is believed that the individual would have given permission if competent.

14. As a witness, the nurse is verifying that the patient has signed the form voluntarily and understands the procedure for which he or she is signing consent.

15. Extent of the surgery; urgency of the surgery; surgical approach

16. CBC; electrolytes; coagulation studies; chest x-ray; electrocardiogram

17. narcotics: to minimize pain and supplement the action of general anesthesia; barbiturates: to provide sedation; tranquilizers: to provide sedation and reduce anxiety; antihistamines: to provide sedation; anticholinergic: to reduce oral, respiratory, and gastric secretions

18. surgeon, surgical assistant, anesthesiologist, scrub assistant, circulating nurse

19. topical: sprays, gargles to surface area to be anesthetized; local infiltrate: injection of agent into subcutaneous tissue; nerve block: injection of agent into and around nerve; epidural block: injection of agent into epidural space for rectal or vaginal procedures; spinal: injection of agent into subarachnoid space

20. hypothermia, hypotension, hypoxia

21. C
22. A
23. D
24. B
25. D
26. A
27. C
28. D
29. A
30. B
31. B
32. C
33. C
34. D
35. C
36. B
37. A
38. C
39. D
40. A
41. B
42. C

43. false
44. true
45. false
46. true
47. true

48. Patient outcomes

1. Patient asks questions and verbalizes concerns.

2. Patient states feelings of apprehension have decreased.

49. Interventions

1. Provide opportunity for the patient to express thoughts and concerns.

2. Encourage questions to demonstrate interest and concern.

3. Reinforce the physician's explanation of planned surgery.

4. Provide appropriate referrals if indicated.

50. A,B,D
51. A
52. B
53. A
54. B
55. C
56. C
57. D
58. A

59. Nursing diagnoses

1. High risk for ineffective breathing patterns

2. High risk for fluid volume deficit

3. Pain related to surgical incision

4. High risk for injury

5. High risk for altered nutrition

60. C
61. C
62. B
63. C
64. A
65. E

CHAPTER 7

Knowledge Base for Patients with Cardiac Dysfunction

1.–11.

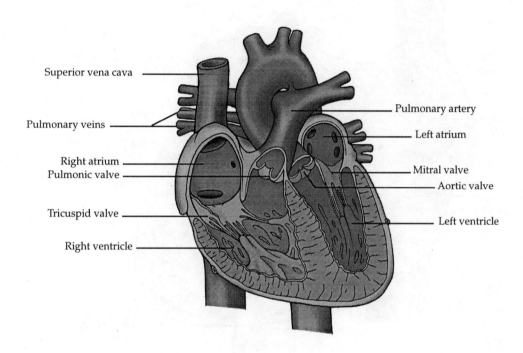

Superior vena cava

Pulmonary veins

Right atrium
Pulmonic valve

Tricuspid valve

Right ventricle

Pulmonary artery

Left atrium

Mitral valve
Aortic valve

Left ventricle

12. The heart's function is to pump blood through the vessels to all body tissues.

13. Venous (unoxygenated) blood returns to the right atrium, passes through the tricuspid valve to the right ventricle through the pulmonary valve, pulmonary artery, and into lungs where carbon dioxide is exchanged for oxygen. Oxygenated blood returns by the pulmonary veins to the left atrium, through the mitral valve, to the left ventricle. It is then pumped through the aortic valve through the aorta to the body.

14. coronary arteries

15. 1. intrinsic method of control: the more blood in the ventricles, the more blood will be pumped during systole

    2. neutral control: results from a combination of sympathetic, parasympathetic, and baroceptor reflex nerve function

    3. humoral control: accomplished by release of epinephrine and norepinephrine

16. Nonmodifiable: positive family history, increasing age, male sex

    Modifiable: hyperlipidemia, high blood pressure, diabetes mellitus, obesity, smoking, use of oral contraceptives, sedentary lifestyle, stress

17.

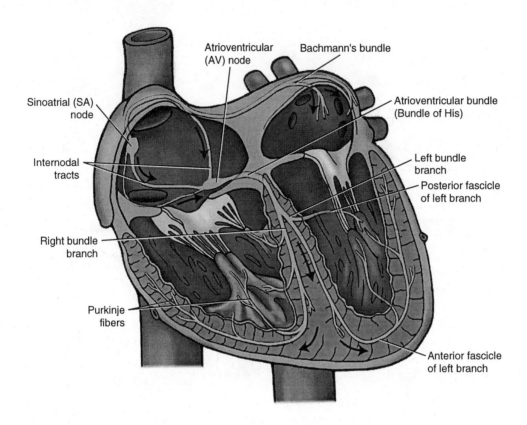

Atrioventricular (AV) node

Bachmann's bundle

Sinoatrial (SA) node

Atrioventricular bundle (Bundle of His)

Internodal tracts

Left bundle branch

Posterior fascicle of left branch

Right bundle branch

Purkinje fibers

Anterior fascicle of left branch

18. P wave: atrial depolarization

PR interval: time it takes impulse to pass from SA node to AV node to ventricular myocardium

QRS complex: ventricular depolarization, as well as the period of atrial repolarization

T wave: repolarization (recovery) of ventricular muscle

19. pericardium

20. contractile, electrical

21. contractility, preload, afterload

22. dyspnea, chest pain, syncope, palpitations, edema

23. right sided heart failure

24. C

25. A

26. D

27. B

28. C

29. CVP: right atrial pressure

30. PAP: gives information about pressure in left side of heart

31. PWP: indication of left ventricular end diastolic pressure

32. CO: amount of blood propelled forward by the heart

33. the volume of blood within each ventricle at the end of diastole

34. the tension that develops in the ventricular wall during systole

35. true

36. true

37. false
38. false
39. false
40. true
41. true
42. true
43. true
44. C
45. B
46. D
47. A
48. B
49. A
50. D
51. A
52. B
53. D
54. A
55. B
56. C
57. B
58. B
59. C
60. A
61. E
62. D
63. C
64. C
65. A,C,E
66. A
67. B
68. A
69. A
70. B
71. Patient outcome: Patient maintains adequate cardiac output as evidenced by hemodynamic monitoring.

    Interventions: Monitor vital signs and hemodynamic indicators q2–4h. Encourage frequent rest periods. Instruct patient to stop activity if pain occurs. Monitor cardiac rhythm. Monitor intake and output. Monitor peripheral pulses.
72. Patient outcome: Patient verbalizes decreased feelings of fatigue and demonstrates an increased activity level.

    Interventions: Instruct patient on energy-saving techniques. Allow for planned periods of rest. Encourage good nutrition. Administer medications that improve oxygen supply.
73. Patient outcome: Patient relates accurate information about signs and symptoms and when to seek medical attention.

    Interventions: Describe potential complications of surgery such as bleeding, cardiac arrhythmias, respiratory distress, or infection. Explain home care restrictions. Explain the need to avoid lifting heavy objects. Explain the need for good nutrition.
74. C
75. B
76. C
77. B
78. A
79. D
80. D
81. A
82. C
83. D
84. C
85. D
86. A
87. D
88. A, B, D
89. all
90. A

CHAPTER 8

Nursing Care of Patients with Cardiac Disorders

1. A
2. D
3. F
4. B
5. E
6. C
7. cardiopulmonary resuscitation
8. planning, teaching
9. dysrhythmias
10. SA node
11. synchronized cardioversion
12. low cardiac output

13. defibrillation

14. Frank-Starling mechanism, increase in heart rate, ventricular hypertrophy, ventricular dilation

15. the renin-angiotensin system is activated

16. sinus tachycardia, rate about 110, PR .16, QRS .08

17. sinus rhythm with PACs, rate about 90, PR .16, QRS .06

18. ventricular tachycardia, rate about 150, no P wave

19. ventricular fibrillation

20. true

21. true

22. false

23. true

24. true

25. true

26. true

27. C

28. A

29. E

30. B

31. D

32. B

33. A

34. D

35. B

36. D

37. D

38. C

39. A

40. B

41. A

42. A

43. C

44. B

45. C

46. A

47. B

48. D

49. C

50. B

51. D

52. D

53. A

54. C

55. B

56. A

57. C

58. B

59. D

60. A

61. C

62. A

63. D

64. B

65. C

66. C

67. D

68. Patient outcome: Patient's vital signs are within acceptable range for patient. Patient is free from dysrhythmias.

   Interventions: Monitor vital signs at rest and upon activity. Encourage rest periods. Keep environment quiet. Monitor cardiac status. Monitor intake and output. Monitor urine output.

69. Patient outcome: Patient verbalizes understanding of heart disease and current condition. Patient verbalizes understanding of need to make lifestyle changes.

   Interventions: Explain cause and effects of MI. Instruct patient on medication, diet, and any lifestyle changes. Alert patient to signs and symptoms of complications.

70. D

71. B

72. A

73. A

74. A

75. C

76. D

77. A

78. B

79. D

80. A

81. B

CHAPTER 9

Knowledge Base for Patients with Vascular Dysfunction

1. tunica adventitia, tunica media, tunica intima
2. diameter of the vessel, elastic recoil, viscosity of blood
3. pain
4. ischemic neuropathy
5. cyanosis
6. sympathectomy
7. embolectomy
8. endarterectomy
9. amputation
10. elderly
11. E
12. B
13. A
14. F
15. D
16. C
17. A
18. A
19. C
20. C
21. A
22. C
23. D
24. A
25. C
26. B
27. B
28. B
29. B
30. A
31. C
32. D
33. C
34. D
35. Patient outcome: Person verbalizes a decrease in the level of pain.

    Interventions: Assess causes of pain. Discuss appropriate positions for pain relief (extremities dependent for arterial insufficiency; extremities elevated for venous disorders). Discuss reason for and evaluate effectiveness of analgesics. Teach relaxation exercises. Teach gradual exercise program.

36. Patient outcome: Patient exhibits palpable pulse, adequate temperature sensation and color in extremities.

    Interventions: Monitor neurocirculatory status for signs of reocclusion, assess pulses, assess extremities for color, sensation, temperature. Keep extremity straight for 24 hours and position patient off the graft site. Notify physician of any abnormalities.
37. C
38. B
39. B
40. D
41. D
42. D
43. A
44. D
45. C
46. C
47. A
48. D

CHAPTER 10

Nursing Care of Patients with Vascular Disorders

1. diet high in sodium, fats, smoking, sedentary lifestyle, obesity, heredity
2. nicotine causes vasoconstriction
3. constricting
4. arteriosclerotic heart disease
5. to develop collateral circulation and improve blood flow
6. 1. Avoid exposure to cold or damp temperatures.
   2. Wear protective clothing when out in the cold.
   3. Use relaxation exercises to reduce stress.
   4. Cease smoking.
   5. Stop activity during an episode of vasospasm.
7. aging
8. rubor
9. home
10. lifestyle changes
11. G

12. D

13. H

14. A

15. B

16. E

17. F

18. C

19. A

20. B

21. C

22. C

23. C

24. B

25. D

26. D

27. B

28. B

29. A

30. C

31. B

32. C

33. A

34. A

35. C

36. A

37. C

38. B

39. C

40. D

41. B

42. A

43. A

44. A

45. C

46. A

47. C

48. B

49. true

50. true

51. true

52. false

53. false

54. true

55. true

56. Patient outcome: Patient has increased perfusion as evidenced by warm, dry skin, strong pulses, absence of edema and cyanosis in the extremities.

Interventions: Encourage balanced period of rest and activity. Discourage smoking. Remove constricting clothing. Administer vasodilators as ordered. Teach lifestyle changes that will promote good circulation.

57. Patient outcome: Patient describes cause, effects, and risk factors associated with thrombophlebitis. Patient can describe self-care methods to treat disorder and prevent complications.

Interventions: Explain cause, effects and course of disease. Teach signs and symptoms of disease and possible complications. Teach type, dose, and side effects of medications. Teach comfort and therapeutic measures. Discuss when to call physician.

58. C

59. B

60. C

61. A

62. B

63. C

64. B

65. D

66. B

67. B

68. D

69. A

70. C

CHAPTER 11

Knowledge Base for Patients in Shock

1. hypovolemic; cardiogenic; distributive

2. adequate blood volume; effective pumping ability of the heart; blood vessels that constrict and dilate normally

3. heart rate and stroke volume

4. harder

5. decreased renal perfusion, decreased urine

6. vascular

7. extracellular

8. gram-negative bacteria

9.   antigen

10. 4–8 L/min.

11. 4–10 cm H_2O

12. C

13. E

14. A

15. D

16. B

17. A

18. C

19. D

20. A

21. D

22. C

23. A

24. C

25. A

26. C

27. B

28. D

29. B

30. D

31. A

32. Patient outcome: The patient will demonstrate hemodynamic stability as evidenced by heart rate < 100; BP > 110 systolic; cardiac output 4–8 L/min.

Interventions: Assess for signs of progressive ventricular failure. Assess hemodynamics. Monitor arterial blood gases. Monitor respiratory status. Administer oxygen as ordered. Administer medications as ordered. Notify physician if condition worsens.

33. A

34. C

35. A

36. D

37. B

38. A

CHAPTER 12

Knowledge Base for Patients with Hematologic Dysfunction

1.   blood, lymph nodes, bone marrow, spleen, and liver

2.   oxygen, carbon dioxide

3.   hematopoiesis

4.   hemoglobin

5.   coagulation

6.   protects the body from stressors through purification process; stores large quantities of blood; produces lymphocytes, plasma cells, and antibodies; removes injured cells, filters microorganisms from the blood

7.   fatigue, weakness, dyspnea, pallor

8.   granulocytes

9.   platelet count

10. direct Coombs' test

11. D

12. B

13. E

14. A

15. F

16. C

17. B

18. WBC 5000-10000 mm^3

19. RBC 4.2–5.4 million/mm^3 (male) 3.6–5.0 million/mm^3 (female)

20. Hematocrit 40–54% (male) 37–47% (female)

21. Hemoglobin 15–16.5 (male) 12–15 (female)

22. Platelet count 150,000–350,000 mm^3

23. Prothrombin time 8–12 seconds

24. PTT 30–45 seconds

25. Serum iron 80–160 mcg/dL (males) 50–150 mcg/dL (females)

26. D

27. C

28. E

29. A

30. C

31. B,D,E

32. B

33. B,C,D

34. D

35. A

36. C

37. B

38. A

39. D

40. C

41. A

42. A

43. D
44. C
45. D
46. B
47. B
48. D
49. B
50. A
51. A
52. E
53. C
54. B
55. B
56. Hemolytic reaction: caused by an infusion of ABO incompatible blood
57. Nonhemolytic reaction: caused by sensitivity to the donor's platelets, proteins, or white blood cells \
58. Allergic reaction: caused by sensitivity to plasma protein
59. Anaphylactic reaction: caused by the infusion of a specific protein to a patient deficient in the protein but who has antibodies to it
60. Septic reaction: occurs when a patient receives contaminated blood
61. true
62. false
63. false
64. true
65. true
66. true
67. Patient outcome: Patient follows regimen of planned activities and rest periods. Patient can complete daily activities without signs of fatigue.

    Interventions: Instruct the patient to develop a regimen of activity with frequent rest periods. Teach patient energy-saving techniques and ways to conserve energy. Encourage good nutrition.
68. Patient outcome: Patient's extremities are warm with good color and palpable pulses. Patient's laboratory studies are within normal limits.

    Interventions: Encourage rest periods to conserve oxygen. Administer oxygen if needed. Elevate the bed. Use range of motion exercises to stimulate circulation. Discourage smoking. Avoid constrictive clothing.

69. B
70. A
71. C
72. D
73. A
74. B
75. A
76. B
77. C
78. B
79. A
80. B
81. A

CHAPTER 13

Nursing Care of Patients with Hematologic Disorders

1. acute; chronic
2. red blood cell
3. shortened
4. polycythemias
5. Epstein-Barr virus
6. F
7. C
8. A
9. D
10. G
11. B
12. E
13. H
14. D
15. C
16. B
17. A
18. A
19. D
20. B
21. B
22. C
23. C
24. B
25. D
26. B
27. B

28. C
29. A
30. A
31. D
32. D
33. C
34. C
35. B
36. C
37. B
38. A
39. B
40. A
41. D
42. C
43. A
44. A
45. B
46. C
47. B
48. Patient outcomes: Patient's vital signs and laboratory studies are within normal limits for the patient. Patient exhibits no signs of infection.

    Interventions: Restrict visitors. Use protective isolation. Monitor vital signs frequently. Promote good nutrition. Provide good oral care. Teach patient signs of infection.
49. Patient outcomes: Patient's vital signs are within normal ranges for patient with no signs of cyanosis, dyspnea, tachypnea, or tachycardia. Patient can perform activities of daily living without respiratory distress.

    Interventions: Instruct patient to turn, cough, and deep breathe q1h to prevent respiratory infection and increase oxygen intake. Teach patient to use full chest expansion. Keep head of bed elevated. Promote good nutrition. Administer oxygen as needed.
50. C
51. B
52. A
53. B
54. D
55. B
56. A
57. C
58. B

59. C
60. A
61. D
62. B

CHAPTER 14

Knowledge Base for Patients with Respiratory Dysfunction

1.

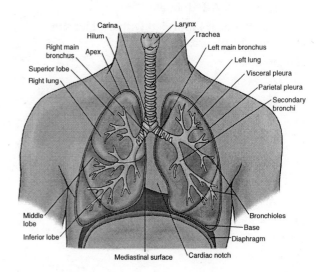

2. trachea, bronchi, bronchioles
3. nasal cavity, sinuses, nasopharynx, pharynx, larynx
4. active
5. passive
6. expands downward
7. elastic
8. stretched
9. alveolar membrane/cellular level
10. hemoglobin
11. coughing
12. cyanosis
13. vibration
14. postural drainage
15. C
16. A
17. B
18. B
19. A
20. C
21. C
22. B

23. A
24. D
25. increase in the depth of respirations
26. increase in both the depth and rate of respiration
27. rapid, deep breathing
28. cycle of apnea and hyperpnea
29. respirations which vary in depth with irregular apnea periods
30. abnormal prominence of the sternum with increased A-P diameter
31. chest appears rounded with the sternum pulled forward
32. B
33. A
34. C
35. D
36. E
37. F
38. A
39. A
40. E
41. C
42. A
43. D
44. D
45. B
46. B
47. B
48. A
49. A
50. A
51. E
52. C
53. B
54. C
55. D
56. B
57. A
58. A
59. A
60. D
61. A
62. B
63. A

64. C
65. B
66. C
67. B
68. E
69. C
70. D
71. B
72. E
73. C
74. C
75. A
76. A
77. A
78. D
79. C
80. A
81. B
82. D
83. B
84. B
85. C
86. A
87.

Drainage tube

Suction control device

UWS chamber

Tube to suction

Collection chamber

88. Nursing diagnosis: Ineffective breathing patterns

Patient outcome: Arterial blood gases are within patient's normal range.

Interventions: Maintain oxygen, keep head of bed elevated, explain all procedures, maintain ventilator function, assess breathing patterns frequently.

89. Nursing diagnosis: Ineffective breathing patterns

Patient outcome: Normal breath sounds, full lung reexpansion.

Interventions: Maintain airtight, patent, functioning chest drainage system. Maintain sterile, dry, occlusive dressing. Encourage patient to cough and deep breathe.

90. Nursing diagnosis: Knowledge deficit: breathing exercises, effective coughing, wound splinting, arm and shoulder exercises.

Patient outcome: Patient describes the role of breathing, coughing, and exercises as they relate to recovery.

Interventions: Explain rationale for coughing and breathing to remove secretions and facilitate ventilation. Demonstrate effective diaphragmatic and pursed-lip breathing. Demonstrate splinting of the chest. Demonstrate arm exercises and rationales for them.

91. B
92. B
93. A
94. C
95. C
96. B
97. B
98. C
99. D
100. A
101. B
102. D
103. C
104. D
105. D

CHAPTER 15

Nursing Care of Patients with Upper Respiratory Disorders

1. hospitalization
2. chronic disease
3. obstruction
4. tonsillitis
5. nosebleed
6. nasal polyp
7. submucous resection
8. rhinoplasty
9. heavy smoking and ingestion of alcohol
10. aspiration
11. D
12. B
13. E
14. F
15. C
16. A
17. false
18. true
19. false
20. true
21. true
22. true
23. A
24. C
25. A
26. C
27. B
28. D
29. B
30. C
31. D
32. D
33. A
34. C
35. B
36. A
37. A
38. D
39. B
40. B
41. C

42. A
43. B
44. D
45. B
46. Patient outcome: Patient can cough up secretions. Patient has normal respiratory rate and patterns.

Interventions: Have patient cough and deep breathe every two hours. Use lint-free wipes to remove secretions. Suction as needed to keep airway clear. Administer humidified air or oxygen. Provide tracheostomy care as needed.

47. D
48. B
49. A
50. D
51. A
52. C
53. B
54. D
55. C
56. B
57. A
58. B
59. C
60. B
61. C

CHAPTER 16

Nursing Care of Patients with Lower Respiratory Disorders

1. G
2. F
3. B
4. E
5. C
6. J
7. D
8. I
9. A
10. H
11. viral
12. pus
13. Mycobacterium
14. chemotherapy

15. prolonged
16. elderly
17. status asthmaticus
18. antibiotics
19. hypoxemia
20. dyspnea
21. hypoxemia, decreased
22. chest tube, intrapleural
23. radiation
24. 90%
25. all but C
26. B
27. D
28. A
29. D
30. A
31. C
32. C
33. C
34. C
35. B
36. C
37. A
38. B
39. D
40. A
41. C
42. B
43. A & D
44. B & C
45. B
46. A
47. C
48. D
49. B
50. D
51. E
52. A
53. A
54. A
55. B
56. A
57. C
58. E
59. B

60. D
61. D
62. A
63. B
64. B
65. A
66. A
67. D
68. A,C,D
69. C
70. C
71. B
72. C
73. C
74. D
75. A
76. D
77. A,B,D
78. A,B,D
79. A
80. B
81. D
82. C
83. Patient with pneumonia

Patient outcome: Patient will have normal blood gases. Patient will have normal breathing patterns, as evidenced by normal respiratory rate and rhythm and clear breath sounds.

Interventions: Turn the patient q2h; encourage coughing and deep breathing q2h; suction if needed; promote adequate fluid intake; administer supplemental oxygen as ordered

84. Patient with active tuberculosis

Patient outcome: Patient can state when disease is infectious. Patient can explain the method of transmission. Patient can describe precautions to prevent transmission.

Interventions: Teach patient how tuberculosis is spread and how to protect others from it. Explain principles of hand washing, avoiding face-to-face contact, and ways to prevent droplet transmission.

85. Patient with COPD

Nursing diagnosis: Ineffective airway clearance

Patient outcomes: Patient uses nebulizer and medication as ordered. Patient uses effective breathing techniques.

Interventions: Administer bronchodilator drugs as needed. Administer aerosol as needed. Instruct patient on proper use of medication. Explain the need to monitor therapeutic effect of medication. Force fluids to 2–3 liters per day to replace fluid loss.

Nursing diagnosis: Ineffective breathing patterns

Patient outcomes: Patient practices consciously controlling I:E ratio when short of breath. Patient uses diaphragmatic breathing to control dyspnea.

Interventions: Teach breathing techniques that promote good ventilation, ease the work of breathing, and control dyspnea.

86. Patient with spontaneous pneumothorax

Patient outcomes: Patient will exhibit arterial blood gases within normal range.

Interventions: Position patient in semi-Fowler's; encourage coughing and deep breathing; administer oxygen therapy; maintain proper setup of intrapleural drainage system

87. Patient with lung cancer

Patient outcome: Patient discusses concerns and feelings with support person.

Interventions: Provide opportunities for patient to express anxieties. Instruct the patient in relaxation techniques. Provide diversional therapy. Assist patient to identify available support systems.

88. C
89. A
90. B
91. A
92. B
93. A
94. D
95. A
96. B
97. C
98. B
99. A
100. B,C,D
101. D
102. C
103. B

CHAPTER 17

Knowledge Base for Patients with Neurologic Dysfunction

1.

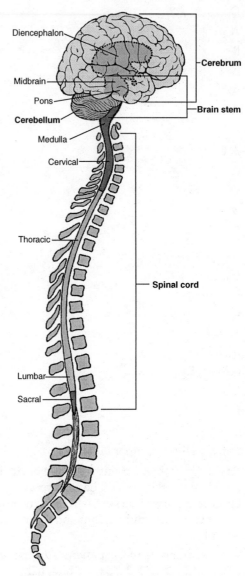

2.   brain and spinal cord

3.   cranial nerves, spinal nerves, autonomic nervous system

4.   dendrites, axons

5.   meninges

6.   choroid plexus

7.   to provide a cushion for the central nervous system, prevent injury

8.   venous system

9.   ascending, descending

10.   dermatones

11.   A

12.   F

13.   B

14.   C

15.   G

16.   H

17.   I

18.   D

19.   E

20.   J

21.   B

22.   A

23.   C

24.   C

25.   B

26.   C

27.   C

28. A
29. C
30. A
31. C
32. C
33. A
34. B
35. C
36. B
37. D
38. B
39. B
40. B
41. A
42. A
43. C
44. A
45. B
46. D
47. D
48. A
49. C
50. B
51. A
52. D
53. A
54. A
55. D
56. B
57. C
58. B
59. A
60. A
61. C
62. A
63. D
64. B
65. C
66. Patient outcome: Patient demonstrates adequate cerebral perfusion.

Interventions: Assess patient every 1–2 hours. Elevate head of bed 30–45 degrees as ordered. Instruct patient to refrain from any activity that can increase ICP. Minimize the number of invasive procedures.

67. Patient outcome: Patient maintains joint mobility.

Interventions: Perform range of motion for all joints q4h. Position properly in side-lying position. Turn and reposition every two hours. Teach family to participate in care.

68. Nursing diagnosis: Impaired verbal communication related to expressive aphasia

Patient Outcome: Patient demonstrates alternative methods of communication.

Interventions: Use alternative communication devices such as pantomime, communications board, flash cards, computers. Provide patient with choices that can be answered with yes or no. Allow patient time to answer. Allow patient to ventilate frustrations and provide accepting atmosphere to learn and test communication skills.

69. Patient outcome: Patient uses assistive devices and compensatory techniques to compensate for sensory dysfunction.

Interventions: Maintain a consistent environment. Keep personal belongings within reach. Explore use of assistive devices that will increase awareness of the environment. Teach patient that his or her awareness and visualization of activities are essential.

70. Patient outcome: Patient verbalizes satisfactory level of comfort.

Interventions: Medicate as needed and at least one-half hour prior to position changes. Log-roll from side to side to avoid tension on operative area. Monitor for side effects of analgesics.

71. C
72. B
73. B
74. C
75. D
76. C
77. C
78. A
79. D
80. B
81. C
82. A

CHAPTER 18

Nursing Care of Patients with Neurologic Disorders

1. antibiotics
2. establish a baseline of the neurologic status
3. dopamine
4. dementing
5. vascular
6. infection
7. aneurysm
8. trauma
9. dementia
10. delirium
11. F
12. A
13. E
14. G
15. C
16. H
17. D
18. B
19. true
20. false
21. false
22. false
23. true
24. true
25. true
26. true
27. false
28. true
29. A
30. C
31. D
32. B
33. C
34. A
35. C
36. B
37. A
38. C
39. C
40. B
41. B

42. A
43. C
44. A
45. E
46. C
47. A
48. C
49. C
50. A
51. B
52. A, D
53. C
54. D
55. A
56. C
57. C
58. B
59. A
60. D
61. C
62. C
63. B
64. D
65. A
66. B
67. B
68. A
69. D
70. B
71. A
72. A
73. C
74. C
75. A
76. C
77. B
78. C
79. B
80. A
81. A
82. C
83. B
84. A
85. B

86. Nursing diagnosis: Potential for alteration in nutrition related to anorexia, nausea, and vomiting.

    Patient outcome: Nausea and vomiting are minimized and adequate nutritional status is maintained.

    Interventions: Administer IV fluids as necessary to prevent dehydration. Provide supplemental feedings by nasogastric tube or total parenteral nutrition. Monitor intake and output, weight. Monitor laboratory values. Administer antiemetics.

87. Nursing diagnosis: Impaired physical mobility

    Patient outcome: Patient maintains current level of mobility with assistance as needed.

    Interventions: Encourage patient to be as physically independent as possible. Provide active and passive range of motion q6h. Allow for sufficient time to perform ADLs. Administer medication to control symptoms. Provide assistive devices as needed.

88. Patient outcome: Patient participates in ADLs.

    Interventions: Perform range of motion every six hours. Assist patient to be as independent as possible. Obtain supportive and assistive devices. Provide good skin care.

    Patient outcome: Patient can successfully communicate needs.

    Interventions: Identify alternate strategies to facilitate communication. Decrease environmental distraction when communicating. Allow patient time to interpret message and express needs.

89. Patient outcome: Deviations in baseline neurologic functioning will be identified.

    Interventions: Establish baseline neurologic status and reevaluate every two hours. Monitor patient according to the Glasgow coma scale. Monitor for signs of increased ICP. Administer medication to decrease cerebral edema.

90. Patient outcome: Baseline neurologic function is maintained.

    Interventions: Maintain cervical traction as ordered. Log-roll patient when positioning. Monitor neurologic status frequently and report changes immediately.

91. B

92. B

93. D

94. B
95. A
96. C
97. A
98. A
99. B
100. B
101. A
102. D
103. B
104. B
105. A
106. C
107. C
108. A
109. D
110. C
111. D
112. C

CHAPTER 19

Knowledge Base for Patients with Musculoskeletal Dysfunction

1. bones, joints, ligaments, muscles, tendons

2. produce locomotion, support and protect body structures

3. 1. Formation of clot or hematoma forms. Fibroblasts and capillaries invade the clot to form granulation tissue.

   2. Proliferation of cell formation where the periosteum is torn. Fibroblasts develop and osteogenic cells proliferate at the site to form a callus across damaged bone.

   3. Cells differentiate into bone or cartilage.

   4. Ossification stage. Inorganic salts are deposited in the new bone matrix to calcify the bone.

   5. Consolidation and remodeling of the new bone occurs.

4. age, physical condition of individual, type of injury, degree of displacement of bone fragments, presence of infection, adequate immobilization after injury, vascular sufficiency, functional periosteum

5. ossification

6. puberty

7. osteoblasts, osteoclasts

8. periosteum

9. compact, cancellous

10. central nervous system

11. movement

12. ATP

13. energy

14. joint

15. goniometer

16. B

17. C

18. A

19. C

20. G

21. D

22. A

23. E

24. C

25. F

26. B

27. true

28. true

29. false

30. true

31. false

32. true

33. false

34. B

35. A

36. D

37. B

38. C

39. C

40. A

41. D

42. C

43. B

44. D

45. B

46. B

47. C

48. A

49. D

50. B

51. D

52. B

53. B

54. E

55. A

56. Patient outcome: Patient can state accurate information about the potential problems related to immobility. Patient can state the signs of complications of immobility. Patient can relate the measures necessary to lessen the risk of complications.

Interventions: Instruct patient about effects of immobility such as elimination difficulty, discoloration of the skin, diminished pulses, and symptoms of infection. Teach patient when to seek medical assistance. Explain safety measures. Teach patient to drink adequate fluids. Teach patient to follow high-fiber diet.

57. Patient outcome: Patient states appropriate information about care and management of device. Patient can demonstrate correct pin site care. Patient moves safely with fixation device intact.

Interventions: Teach patient how to care for device. Demonstrate pin care. Reinforce information about activity. Teach proper use of assistive devices. Provide information on ways to modify clothing.

58. B

59. D

60. C

61. A

62. B

63. A

64. C

65. A

66. A

67. D

CHAPTER 20

Nursing Care of Patients with Musculoskeletal Disorders

1. unknown

2. autoimmune

3. 80–90%

4. osteoarthritis

5. Lyme disease

6. crepitus

7.	G
8.	A
9.	H
10.	D
11.	B
12.	F
13.	C
14.	I
15.	E
16.	false
17.	true
18.	true
19.	false
20.	true
21.	true
22.	B
23.	D
24.	A
25.	C
26.	B
27.	A
28.	A
29.	C
30.	D
31.	A
32.	D
33.	C
34.	C
35.	A
36.	B
37.	B
38.	A
39.	A
40.	B
41.	D
42.	A
43.	B
44.	C
45.	C
45.	D
46.	B
47.	B
48.	D
49.	B
50.	D

51.	C
52.	B
53.	A
54.	C
55.	D
56.	A
57.	A
58.	C
59.	D
60.	B
61.	A
62.	D
63.	A
64.	D
65.	B
66.	A
67.	B
68.	C
69.	A

70. Patient outcome: Patient can perform passive range of motion exercises to maintain strength. Patient maintains mobility with the assistance of an ambulatory aid.

   Interventions: Teach the patient passive and active range of motion (ROM) exercises. Instruct patient to change position frequently. Use ambulatory aids to assist with mobility. Involve patient in a physical therapy program. Give analgesics to decrease pain levels.

71. Patient Outcome: Patient's extremity has good color, sensation, and pulses with no signs of compromised circulation.

   Interventions: Help conserve oxygen by encouraging rest. Monitor for signs of compromised circulation. Prevent edema by elevating extremity. Use ROM exercise.

72.	B
73.	A
74.	C
75.	A
76.	D
77.	B
78.	B
79.	A
80.	C
81.	B

82. all
83. C
84. B
85. D
86. C

CHAPTER 21

Knowledge Base for Patients with Gastrointestinal Dysfunction

1. saliva
2. peritoneum
3. peristalsis
4. pyloric sphincter
5. vitamin B_{12}
6. negative/pH
7. chyme
8. duodenum, jejunum, ileum
9. small intestine
10. bile
11. large intestine
12. storage and metabolism of nutrients, detoxication of noxious substances, production of bile
13. store and concentrate
14. pancreas
15. E
16. B
17. A
18. D
19. C
20. D
21. F
22. B
23. E
24. B
25. C
26. G
27. D
28. A
29. C
30. E
31. B
32. A
33. C
34. C

35. A
36. B
37. D
38. C
39. C
40. B
41. C
42. A
43. B
44. C
45. B
46. B
47. B
48. A
49. C
50. C
51. B
52. D
53. B
54. D
55. C
56. B
57. D
58. A
59. B
60. C
61. A
62. A
63. A
64. C
65. D
66. B
67. A
68. D
69. A
70. C
71. E
72. C
73. B
74. B
75. Nursing diagnosis: Knowledge deficit related to appearance and function of colostomy, and need for learning self-care measures.

    Patient outcome: Patient will be able to demonstrate how to care for colostomy.

Interventions: Provide the patient with basic information about the function of the colostomy, including a drawing. Define terms such as stoma, appliance, pouch. Explain the daily routine for self care. Demonstrate the procedure. Allow the patient time to ask questions. Have patient practice the procedure.

76. Patient outcome: Patient practices relaxation as instructed. Patient expresses an optimistic view about the surgical outcome.

Interventions (Anxiety): Reassure patient that anxiety is normal. Reassure patient about surgical outcome, if appropriate. Discuss surgery in general terms, the frequency that the surgeon performs the operation, and positive outcomes. Review relaxation techniques. Maintain a quiet, calm environment.

Patient outcome: Patient describes pre- and postoperative procedures. Patient describes importance of coughing and deep breathing.

Interventions (Knowledge deficit): Review the preoperative preparation. Explain all tests and procedures as appropriate. Explain the specifics of the postoperative course, including the equipment (IV, NG, Dsg, etc.). Explain the usual diet and activity orders.

77. Nursing diagnosis: Pain

Patient outcome: Patient moves without signs of severe pain. Patient rests quietly without sign of discomfort. Patient states pain is relieved.

Interventions: Administer pain medications as ordered. Keep bed elevated to decrease pull on the incision. Splint incision when turning, coughing. Encourage relaxation.

Nursing diagnosis: Breathing

Patient outcome: Patient can cough and deep breathe as instructed. Patient has no cyanosis. Patient has normal respiratory rate and normal ABGs.

Interventions: Turn, cough, and deep breathe every two hours. Splint incision. Medicate as needed. Encourage ambulation.

78. Patient outcome: Patient consumes a 1200 calorie diet per day.

Interventions: Offer foods that are well-liked and meet the patient's nutritional needs. Encourage family to provide favorite food. Serve food in small portions in attractive setting. Keep environment calm, neat, and free from odors or offensive sights.

79. Patient outcome: Oral mucous membrane is pink and moist. Lips are supple, moist, and free from cracks.

Interventions: Provide good mouth care. Use a soft toothbrush to avoid trauma. Avoid lemon and glycerin swabs and mouthwash that contains alcohol. Apply a water-soluble lubricant to lips. Use saline gargle and anesthetic throat lozenges as ordered.

80. A
81. B
82. C
83. B
84. C
85. A
86. B
87. A
88. B
89. A
90. D
91. A
92. C
93. A
94. A
95. B

CHAPTER 22

Nursing Care of Patients with Disorders of the Upper Gastrointestinal System

1. esophagus
2. smoking, intake of alcohol, spicy food, ingestion of caustic agents, reflux of acidic gastric contents
3. gastritis
4. *Helicobacter pylori*
5. pain
6. increased intra-abdominal pressure
7. heartburn
8. dysphagia
9. D
10. F
11. C
12. A
13. E
14. B

15. D

16. B

17. C

18. A

19. all

20. A,C,D

21. B

22. D

23. C

24. A

25. B

26. C

27. A

28. C

29. B

30. C

31. A

32. A

33. C

34. C

35. A

36. D

37. A

38. B

39. A,B,C

40. C

41. D

42. B, C

43. D

44. B

45. A

46. B

47. C

48. A

49. D

50. A

51. B

52. C

53. D

54. A

55. all are factors

56. C

57. B

58. C

59. D

60. B

61. B

62. Patient outcome: Patient can state proper self-administration of medications. Patient states the discomfort is decreased.

Interventions: Administer antacids or other prescribed medications. Encourage use of relaxation techniques. Teach patient not to smoke or drink. Have patient follow a diet that includes nonirritating foods.

63. Nursing diagnosis: Pain related to the irritating effects of gastric juices on injured tissue

Patient outcome: Patient states pain is relieved (acute phase of illness).

Interventions: Administer medications as ordered (antacids, histamine antagonists, analgesics). Encourage patient to avoid smoking. Teach patient to avoid those foods which cause exacerbation of pain. Teach patient to drink 6–8 glasses of water daily.

64. Nursing diagnosis: Potential alteration in nutrition: less than body requirements

Patient outcome: Patient will take in enough calories to meet basic body requirements. Patient will maintain normal body weight. Patient will maintain normal nitrogen balance.

Interventions: Provide high-protein, high-calorie diet. Provide supplemental tube feeding or TPN if needed. Teach patient to eat slowly and eat small amounts. Provide privacy and environment conducive to eating.

65. A

66. C

67. B

68. A

69. A

70. B

71. C

72. D

73. A,B,C

74. B

75. A

76. B

77. A

78. A

79. A

80. B
81. C

CHAPTER 23

Nursing Care of Patients with Disorders of the Lower Gastrointestinal System

1. peritoneum
2. intraluminal; bacterial
3. surgically
4. palliative
5. cobblestone
6. hemorrhoids
7. peristalsis; obstruction
8. hydrogen breathe test
9. bowel habits
10. constipation
11. G
12. B
13. A
14. F
15. D
16. E
17. C
18. true
19. false
20. true
21. false
22. false
23. true
24. false
25. true
26. false
27. true
28. D
29. A
30. D
31. B
32. B
33. D
34. B
35. A
36. D
37. A
38. C

39. C
40. A
41. B
42. D
43. D
44. C
45. C
46. E
47. D
48. B
49. C
50. A
51. C
52. A
53. B
54. B
55. C
56. A
57. C
58. B
59. B
60. B & C
61. D
62. B
63. A
64. B
65. C
66. C
67. B
68. C
69. B
70. D
71. C
72. A
73. Patient outcome: Patient can tolerate a sitting position 24 hours postoperatively.

   Interventions: administer prescribed analgesics, keep patient in side-lying position for 24 hours, give sitz baths or warm compresses, administer high-fiber diet, stool softeners
74. Patient outcomes: Vital signs within normal range for patient, urine output is > 30 mL/ hour, serum electrolytes are normal

   Interventions: Administer replacement fluids and electrolytes, monitor CVP, vital signs, I/O, urine output, hydration status.

75. Nursing diagnosis: Alteration in bowel elimination (constipation) related to scant stool with prolonged transit time in colon.

Patient outcome: Patient passes soft-formed stool of normal size.

Interventions: Explain the importance of high-fiber diet. Teach importance of food and fluid intake, need for scheduled time for food intake and defecation to promote good bowel function. Instruct patient to use bulk-forming laxatives and stool softeners

76. Nursing diagnosis: Knowledge deficit related to surgery, postoperative course, and routines

Patient outcome: Patient can describe the surgery and its expected effects.

Interventions: Review the surgical procedure and the expected effect on the cancer. Include information on preoperative preparation and postoperative routines. Provide information about pain control. Provide information about colostomy care.

77. Nursing diagnosis: Pain related to surgical trauma to anal area.

Interventions: Tell patient to administer analgesics as ordered. Obtain floatation pad. Take sitz baths. Apply ice packs, warm compresses, or analgesic ointments as needed. Call physician with any questions.

78. D
79. A
80. C
81. A
82. A
83. C
84. B
85. C
86. A
87. A
88. D
89. D
90. B
91. A
92. B
93. A
94. C
95. C
96. C
97. C

98. D
99. D
100. A

CHAPTER 24

Nursing Care of Patients with Disorders of the Accessory Organs of Digestion

1. gall bladder
2. stones
3. intolerance to fatty foods
4. bile, cholesterol, infection
5. trypsin
6. 80%
7. true
8. true
9. true
10. true
11. false
12. true
13. true
14. false
15. false
16. true
17. true
18. C
19. A,C,D
20. C
21. C
22. A
23. C
24. D
25. A
26. D
27. B
28. A
29. B
30. A
31. D
32. B
33. B
34. B
35. D
36. C
37. D

38. D

39. C

40. A

41. D

42. B

43. C

44. D

45. D

46. Patient outcome: Vital signs, hemodynamic measures within normal limits for patient.

    Interventions: Monitor vital signs q1h or as ordered. Monitor serum electrolytes. Monitor fluid status, I & O. Measure NG drainage, urine output. Maintain IV and administer as ordered.

47. Nursing diagnosis: Potential for noncompliance related to medication regimen and diet

    Patient outcome: Patient correctly explains administration of medication and rationale. Patient correctly describes dietary regimen.

    Interventions: Review the prescribed medications. Review the diet. Explain rationale for taking pancreatic enzymes and antacids. Explain that pain will subside and stools will return to normal when regimen is followed. Involve family in teaching sessions.

48. Nursing diagnosis: Alteration in nutrition: less than body requirements

    Patient outcome: Patient will take in calories needed to maintain weight.

    Interventions: Administer parenteral fluid, electrolytes, and nutrients as ordered. Administer TPN or diet as ordered. Offer small meals in a clean environment. Assess factors that affect metabolic rate.

49. B

50. B

51. A

52. B

53. A

54. A

55. B

56. B

57. A

58. B

59. C

60. D

61. C

62. D

63. A

CHAPTER 25

Knowledge Base for Patients with Hepatic Dysfunction

1.

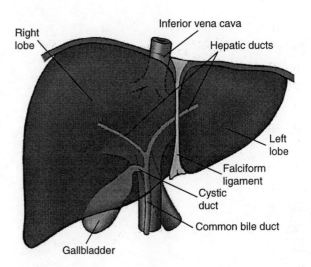

2. metabolism of carbohydrates, lipids, and fats; produces and secretes bile; filters foreign substances from the blood; detoxifies drugs, toxins, and hormones; stores glycogen, certain vitamins, minerals

3. inferior vena cava

4. glucose

5. jaundice, ascites, portal hypertension, hepatic encephalopathy, clotting disorders, nutritional deficiencies

6. fatty acids

7. amino acids

8. icterus

9. bile

10. sodium; fluid

11. D

12. A

13. C

14. B

	Value	Incr./Decr.
15. Urine urobilinogen	1–4 mg/24 hrs	I
16. Total serum protein	6.6–7.9 g/dL	D
17. Serum albumin	3.3–5.5 g/dL	D
18. Blood ammonia	15–49 mg/dL	I
19. Total cholesterol	< 200 mg/dL	D
20. Prothrombin time	9.5–11.8 sec	I
21. Alpha–fetoprotein	< 30 ng/mL	I
22. AST	10–30 U/L	I

23. C

24. B

25. B

26. C

27. D

28. A

29. A

30. B

31. A

32. C

33. B

34. D

35. C

36. A

37. C

38. C

39. A

40. D

41. B

42. D

43. B

44. D

45. C

46. B

47. B

48. A

49. C

50. B

51. A

52. Patient outcome: Patient's abdominal girth decreases daily.

Interventions: Strict intake and output daily. Monitor fluid restrictions. Administer diuretics. Weigh daily. Measure abdominal girth daily.

53. Patient outcome: Patient experiences no injury.

Interventions: Monitor level of orientation q4h. Restrict intake of protein. Monitor daily lab results. Keep side rail up at all times.

54. Nursing diagnosis: Alteration in nutrition related to anorexia and poor dietary intake secondary to alcohol use.

Patient outcome: Patient has a steady weight gain with no evidence of fluid retention. Patient takes in a balanced daily diet.

Interventions: Provide small feedings with consideration of food preferences. Provide Meals on Wheels or assistance with shopping and meal planning. Instruct patient to take antiemetic prior to meals if indicated. Teach patient basic dietary information. Provide referral to Alcoholics Anonymous for support system.

55. A

56. C

57. B

58. A

59. A

60. C

61. B

62. B

63. C

64. D

65. D

CHAPTER 26

Nursing Care of Patients with Hepatic Disorders

1. necrosis
2. parenteral
3. chronic
4. jaundice
5. passive
6. liver transplantation
7. necrosis
8. alcohol
9. sclerotherapy
10. final
11. true
12. false
13. true
14. true
15. true
16. false
17. true
18. false
19. false
20. true
21. A
22. B
23. A
24. D
25. B
26. C
27. B
28. D
29. A
30. A
31. B
32. C
33. C
34. C
35. C
36. D
37. B
38. B
39. C
40. A
41. D
42. C
43. A
44. D
45. D
46. A
47. C
48. B
49. B
50. A
51. B
52. C
53. D
54. B
55. A
56. D
57. A
58. Patient outcome: Patient verbalizes understanding of cause of viral hepatitis and ways to prevent transmission.

    Interventions: Explain mode of transmission to patient/family (fecal/oral route). Explain importance of hand washing. Institute enteric precautions. Teach patient to refrain from drugs, alcohol. Identify close contacts who may have been exposed.
59. Patient outcome: Patient experiences no injury.

    Interventions: Monitor orientation, speech, asterixis. Restrict protein intake. Monitor potassium intake. Administer neomycin, lactulose as ordered. Protect patient from injury.
60. Nursing diagnosis: Knowledge deficit related to postsurgical management and possible complications.

    Patient outcome: Patient can describe goals of medical management and ways to identify and treat complications.

    Interventions: Review signs of acute rejection: fever, jaundice, pain, elevated AST, LDH. Instruct patient on rationale for medication administration and the side effects of therapy (risk of infection, fluid and electrolyte problems with steroids, many for each drug). Discuss coping strategies.
61. D
62. A
63. C
64. A
65. C

66. C
67. C
68. B
69. A
70. B
71. B
72. D
73. A

CHAPTER 27

Knowledge Base for Patients with Endocrine Dysfunction

1.

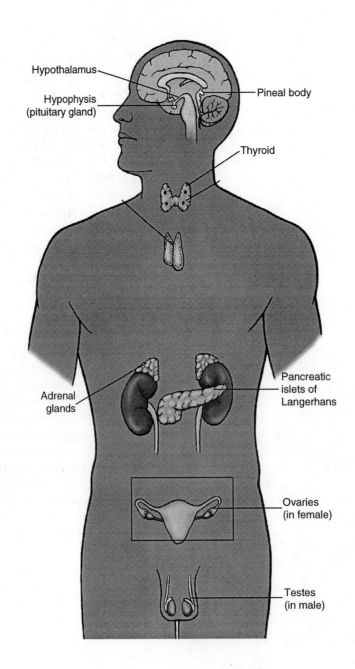

2. target organ

3. negative feedback control

4. hypophysis

5. islets of Langerhans

6. endocrine, nervous

7. stimulated

8. pituitary

9. cortisol

10. medulla

	Gland	Hormone
11.	Thymus	Thymine, thymosin
12.	Pineal	Melatonin
13.	Hypothalamus	ADH, oxytocin
14.	Pituitary	STH, GH, ACTH, LH, TSH, FSH
15.	Thyroid	T4, T3
16.	Adrenals	Glucocorticoids, miner-alocorticoids, sex hor-mones
17.	Pancreatic islets	Insulin, glucagon

18. I

19. F

20. D

21. H

22. J

23. A

24. G

25. C,D

26. E

27. B

28. true

29. false

30. true

31. true

32. false

33. A

34. C

35. D

36. B

37. B

38. A

39. A

40. A

41. A

42. B

43. A

44. A

45. E

46. C

CHAPTER 28

Nursing Care of Patients with Diabetes Mellitus

1. hyperglycemia

2. increase, decrease, increase

3. glucose

4. liver

5. blood glucose

6. renal threshold

7. U-100

8. mimic

9. hyperglycemia, dehydration

10. dawn

11. true

12. true

13. true

14. false

15. false

16. true

17. true

18. false

19. false

20. false

21. true

22. D

23. A

24. C

25. B

26. D

27. B

28. B

29. C

30. A

31. C

32. A

33. A

34. B

35. B

36. C

37. C
38. B
39. A
40. all
41. B
42. B
43. B
44. A
45. A
46. C
47. C
48. B
49. A
50. C
51. C
52. D
53. Patient outcome: Patient verbalizes a basic understanding of the pathophysiology of diabetes mellitus. Patient demonstrates willingness to learn about disease and to participate in self-care activities.

    Interventions: Explain the pathophysiology of diabetes at patient's level of understanding. Reinforce diet teaching. Demonstrate how to adjust diet for changes in activity level. Explain reason for insulin and how to administer. Teach patient how to test blood glucose. Teach signs of hypo- and hyperglycemia.

54. Nursing diagnosis: Altered tissue perfusion related to degenerative vascular changes of diabetes

    Patient outcome: Patient will maintain adequate systemic tissue perfusion as evidenced by BP WNL for patient, palpable peripheral pulses, skin warm, color pink, quick capillary refill, maintenance of skin integrity.

    Interventions: Assess for changes in vital signs. Assess for pain. Promote circulation through activity, including leg exercises. Keep patient warm. Teach patient to avoid smoking. Teach principles of self-care to prevent long-term problems. Teach patient about medications that promote vasodilation.

55. A
56. A,B,C

57. B
58. A
59. A,B
60. B
61. C
62. B
63. C
64. A
65. B
66. A

CHAPTER 29

Nursing Care of Patients with Other Endocrine Disorders

1. pituitary
2. autoimmune
3. glucocorticoid
4. pheochromocytomas
5. iodine, protein
6. thyroid stimulating hormone
7. calcitonin
8. Hashimoto's thyroiditis
9. regulate serum calcium and phosphate levels
10. rise
11. A
12. C
13. B
14. A
15. B
16. B
17. true
18. true
19. false
20. true
21. true
22. false
23. true
24. true
25. true
26. true
27. A
28. B
29. B
30. B

31. C
32. D
33. C
34. A
35. B
36. B
37. A
38. C
39. D
40. C
41. D
42. D
43. A
44. B
45. D
46. A
47. D
48. C
49. B
50. C
51. A
52. A
53. B
54. C
55. B
56. D
57. D
58. B
59. C
60. A
61. E
62. A
63. A
64. all
65. D
66. D
67. C
68. all
69. C
70. A
71. A
72. B
73. C
74. A
75. D

76. A
77. C
78. Patient outcome: Patient remains alert and oriented.

   Interventions: Elevate head of bed 30–45 degrees. Provide rest periods (decrease external stimuli). Administer oxygen as ordered. Assess neurologic status every two hours. Instruct patient not to cough, sneeze, or hyperflex the head. Administer antiemetic to avoid vomiting. Monitor for early signs of increased ICP.

79. Patient outcome: Patient demonstrates adequate extracellular fluid volume.

   Interventions: Administer intravenous hydrocortisone and isotonic dextrose and saline as prescribed. Monitor vital signs, neuro status, and urine output frequently. Administer antiemetics as needed.

80. Patient outcome: Patient identifies activities that will reduce risk of infection after discharge.

   Interventions: Discuss ways that the patient can contract an infection. Discuss the effect of excess cortisol on the immune system. Stress proper hand washing. Teach how signs and symptoms can be masked. If infection is suspected, have patient monitor temperature closely and notify physician. Take antibiotics as prescribed.

81. Patient outcome: Patient verbalizes understanding of the effects of disease and the need to follow prescribed treatment.

   Interventions: Offer explanation of disease and its treatment in easily understood terms. Encourage patient to ask questions and verbalize concerns. Teach patient name, dose, and side effects of medications. Teach patient to take medication in AM. Teach patient to take pulse and notify physician if > 100. Instruct patient to wear Medic-Alert.

82. Patient outcome: Patient maintains adequate tissue perfusion as evidenced by normal temperature, vital signs WNL, adequate urine output, normal neurologic status.

   Interventions: Monitor vital signs, pulse pressure, capillary refill, neurologic status, and urine output as indicated by condition. Monitor for signs of thyroid crisis and institute any needed interventions.

83. D
84. B

85. B

86. C

87. A,B,C,F

88. B

89. C

90. A

91. D

92. D

93. C

94. B

95. D

96. B,C,D

97. C

98. A

99. B

100. B, C, D

101. D

CHAPTER 30

Knowledge Base for Patients with Urinary Dysfunction

1.

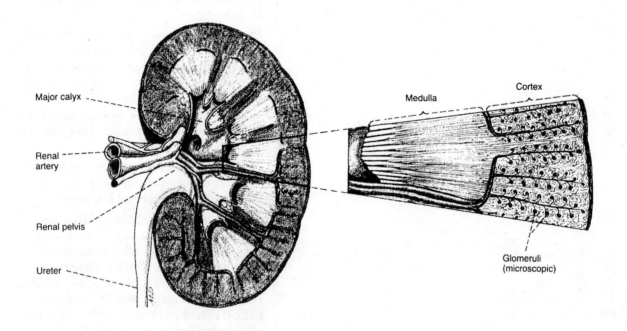

2.   parenchyma

3.   nephron

4.   1.   Excretion of metabolic waste products

     2.   Regulation of fluid and electrolyte balance

     3.   Maintenance of acid-base balance

     4.   Assist with calcium metabolism

     5.   Assist with blood pressure maintenance

     6.   Regulate red blood cell production

5.   1.   Permeability of the glomerular capillary walls

     2.   Blood pressure

     3.   Effective filtration process

6.   creatinine

7.   Renin-angiotensin-aldosterone

8.   Filtration, reabsorption, and secretion

9.   Appropriate bladder sensations during filling, closed bladder outlet during rest, absence of involuntary bladder contractions, strong and well-maintained bladder contractions, absence of any obstruction

10. symptom

11. nosocomial infection

12. maintain aseptic technique, maintain a closed drainage system, keep drainage bag below level of bladder, change catheter only if contaminated, empty every eight hours, assess patient on a routine basis,

13. D

14. A

15. B

16. C

17. E

18. G

19. E

20. C

21. A

22. F

23. D

24. B

25. B

26. B

27. D

28. A

29. A

30. B

31. C

32. A

33. A

34. B

35. C

36. B

37. B

38. D

39. B

40. C

41. C

42. C

43. C

44. B

45. D

46. A

47. B

48. C

49. A

50. C

51. A

52. B

53. A

54. C

55. B

56. B

57. A

58. C

59. B

60. true

61. false

62. true

63. false

64. false

65. Nursing diagnosis: Total incontinence related to loss of muscle tone and chronic disease

Patient outcomes: Client will have decrease in episodes of incontinence. Client will demonstrate a bladder regimen. Client will maintain intact skin. Client will verbalize feeling of self-worth.

Interventions: Establish a bladder training program. Set up a schedule for toileting. Teach bladder exercises. Teach ways to keep skin dry and intact.

66. Patient outcome: Patient voids adequate amounts within reasonable intervals. Patient has no visible bladder distention.

    Interventions: Determine normal elimination patterns. Assess for signs of retention. Monitor intake and output. Instruct patient to void when urge is felt. Provide privacy. Encourage adequate intake.

67. Patient outcome: Patient will reestablish normal pattern of urination within 24 hours.

    Interventions: Increase fluid consumption. Encourage ambulation. Encourage patient to empty bladder every 2–3 hours.

68. A
69. B
70. C
71. A
72. A
73. A
74. B
75. C
76. A

CHAPTER 31

Nursing Care of Patients with Urinary Disorders

1. infections and inflammations
2. uremia
3. antibiotics
4. obstruction
5. stricture
6. blunt or penetrating
7. F
8. B
9. E
10. A
11. C
12. G
13. D
14. D
15. C
16. D
17. D
18. B
19. A
20. A

21. B
22. C
23. C
24. B
25. A
26. C
27. B
28. B
29. C
30. C
31. E
32. D
33. D
34. D
35. B
36. B
37. C
38. A
39. C
40. B
41. B
42. B
43. D
44. D
45. B
46. D
47. A
48. A
49. A
50. C
51. B
52. B
53. C
54. C
55. C
56. B
57. B
58. A
59. A
60. C
61. A
62. D
63. C
64. B

65. Patient outcome: Patient reports relief of symptoms. Patient resumes normal voiding pattern.

    Interventions: Administer antimicrobial medications as ordered. Increase oral intake up to 3000 mL per day. Encourage voiding at regular intervals.

66. Patient outcome: Patient will have decreased manifestations of chronic renal failure.

    Interventions: Monitor fluid and electrolyte status. Maintain fluid restriction. Administer medication as ordered. Promote comfort. Provide extensive education. Provide psychological support.

67. Nursing diagnosis: Alteration in fluid and electrolyte status related to the procedure

    Patient outcome: Patient will achieve stabilization of fluid and electrolyte status.

    Interventions: Monitor blood pressure before and during procedure. Weigh patient before and after procedure. Maintain aseptic technique. Monitor for any signs of infection. Monitor intake and output.

68. A
69. B
70. A
71. A
72. D
73. B
74. C
75. A
76. A
77. D
78. D
79. A
80. A
81. B
82. D
83. C
84. A
85. B

CHAPTER 32

Knowledge Base for Patients with Immune Dysfunction

1. 1. defense
    2. surveillance
    3. homeostasis

2. thymus and bone marrow
3. thymus gland, cellular
4. bone marrow, antibodies
5. IgG
6. IgM
7. foreign substances
8. 1. Blood vessels in area dilate to become more permeable to chemical mediators. More blood and lymph go to injured area. Monocytes also phagocytize any harmful agent.
    2. Phagocytosis and exudate formation occur.
    3. Repair and regeneration of injured tissue occurs.
9. donor
10. antigens
11. C
12. D
13. A
14. B
15. physical barrier = N
16. interferon = N
17. inflammation = N
18. antigen = S
19. phagocytosis = N
20. B
21. A
22. D
23. C
24. false
25. true
26. false
27. true
28. true
29. true
30. true
31. D
32. A
33. B
34. A
35. B
36. A
37. B
38. B

39. C

40. A,B,C,D

41. C

42. D

43. C

44. B

45. A

46. B

47. D

48. A

49. C

50. C

51. Patient outcome: Patient states why test is being done. Patient states where test is being done. Patient understands sensations associated with procedure.

Interventions: Explain procedure, including reasons for test, sensations felt, equipment used, length of procedure, and expected outcome.

52. Nursing diagnosis: Knowledge deficit

Patient outcome: Patient will understand the essentials of self-care after bone marrow transplantation.

Interventions: Provide information on need for frequent rest periods. Gradually increase activity. Take medications as prescribed. Watch for any sign of bleeding and report promptly. Avoid contact sports until platelet count is normal. Avoid medications that impair clotting. Monitor for any signs of infection. Be meticulous in hygienic practices. Do frequent mouth care. Avoid crowds until WBC is normal. Monitor for signs of graft versus host disease. Follow up with physician, monitor lab results carefully.

53. C

54. B

55. A

56. C

57. B

58. D

59. D

60. D

61. D

62. B

CHAPTER 33

Nursing Care of Patients with HIV/AIDS and Other Immune Disorders

1. produce an adequate response to an antigen

2. primary or congenital

3. human immunodeficiency virus (HIV)

4. Kaposi's sarcoma

5. *Pneumocystic carinii*

6. mononucleosis-like illness, persistent generalized lymphadenopathy, AIDS-related complex, AIDS, AIDS-related dementia

7. an acute infection such as the flu; asymptomatic period lasting 2 months to 15 years; transitional or symptomatic disease period; period marked by development of opportunistic infections or malignancies

8. anaphylaxis

9. antihistamines

10. desensitization

11. anergy

12. autoimmunity

13. antinuclear antibodies (ANA)

14. true

15. true

16. false

17. false

18. true

19. true

20. true

21. true

22. true

23. false

24. true

25. false

26. A

27. D

28. C

29. D

30. A

31. D

32. B

33. C

34. E

35. D

36. A

37. B

38. D

39. B

40. B

41. C

42. A

43. C

44. E

45. C

46. D

47. D

48. B

49. A

50. all

51. A

52. B

53. C

54. C

55. C

56. B

57. A,B,E

58. Patient outcome: Patient can explain what AIDS is, how it is spread, symptoms that require attention, medical treatment options.

Interventions: Explain what causes the disease and method of transmission. Instruct the patient in self care. Explain medications. Instruct patient on when to seek medical attention.

59. Patient outcome: Patient will express or exhibit signs of increased comfort.

Interventions: Administer analgesic and anti-inflammatory drugs, maintain bed rest during flare-up, support joints, maintain joint mobility through active and passive ROM, keep skin lesions clean and dry

60. Patient outcome: Patient expresses feelings and concerns. Patient can set priorities for activities. Patient schedules periods of activity and rest.

Interventions: Help patient adapt to fatigue state. Encourage patient to express feelings, fears, and concerns. Guide the patient to modify activities. Stress consistency. Explain ways to conserve energy.

61. A

62. C

63. B

64. D

65. A

66. A

67. B

68. C

69. B

70. B

71. E

72. A

73. B

74. D

CHAPTER 34

Nursing Care of Patients with Oncologic Disorders

1. change in bowel or bladder habits, a sore that does not heal, unusual bleeding or discharge, thickening or lump in breast or elsewhere, indigestion or difficulty swallowing, obvious change in wart or mole, nagging cough or hoarseness

2. cigarette smoking, exposure to airborne carcinogens, family history

3. early sexual activity, multiple sexual partners, genital herpes

4. oncogenesis

5. staging

6. person with low self-esteem who sees him- or herself as a victim, lacks resiliency, and has narrow range of personal relationships

7. tumor markers

8. diagnosis, remove

9. hypogeusia

10. cytotoxic

11. increase

12. Genetic—individuals with specific genetic characteristics may have an increased risk of certain cancers

13. Environment—chemicals in the environment have been shown to contribute to certain oncologic disorders

14. Tobacco—single most preventable cause of disease and death; documented relationship between smoking and cancer

15. Diet—being studied, may be responsible for up to ⅓ of oncologic disorders.

16. Immunologic—when immune system fails, tumors can grow and spread

17. Psychosocial factors—there is a strong relationship between stress and illness, as well as outcome. Cancer often occurs following a major loss and depression.

18. Aging—defective repair of DNA and the decreased effectiveness of the immune system

19. D
20. A
21. E
22. C
23. B
24. F
25. A
26. B
27. B, C
28. A
29. C
30. B
31. D
32. B
33. C
34. A
35. D
36. C
37. B
38. A
39. A
40. A, D
41. D
42. D
43. D
44. C
45. D
46. A
47. C
48. C
49. A
50. A
51. B
52. E
53. A
54. B
55. A
56. C
57. C

58. B
59. A,B,E,F
60. B
61. A
62. B
63. B
64. C
65. Patient outcome: Patient will state an understanding of the treatment protocol associated with cancer.

Interventions: Review the type of cancer and associated risk factors. Encourage patient to ask questions. Explain any diagnostic tests and treatment being planned.

66. Patient outcome: Patient describes expected effects of radiation.

Interventions: Reinforce purposes and type of treatment. Instruct patient in self-care and comfort measures.

67. Anxiety and fear: Help patient talk about feelings; use of therapeutic communication is essential. Give patient information in clear simple terms. Help patient identify steps to reduce anxiety. Teach guided relaxation. Teach problem-solving techniques.

68. Sexuality: Differentiate between psychologic conflicts and results of medications. Explore the significant other's reaction to the treatment. Discuss alternative techniques to satisfy the patient's needs. Make referrals to counseling.

69. Helplessness: Discuss ways to enable the patient to make decisions and actively participate in planning for the future. Involve the patient in decision making. Explore support groups. Explore and encourage spiritual support.

70. Side effects of chemotherapy: nausea and vomiting; mucositis, stomatitis, esophagitis; diarrhea, constipation; skin rashes, alopecia.

71. Interventions: use relaxation therapy for stomatitis, good diet, adequate fluid intake, good oral hygiene

72. Radiation Therapy: Skin—erythema, dry desquamation, moist desquamation; mouth—mucositis, stomatitis; head—cerebral edema, alopecia; chest—esophagitis, pneumonitis, pulmonary fibrosis

73. Interventions: Skin—wear loose clothing to limit effects; dry desquamation—use water-soluble lubricant; mouth—may use liquid or high-protein diet; good oral hygiene

74. A

75. D

76. A

77. D

78. A

79. A

80. A

81. B

82. D

83. A

84. C

85. A

86. B

87. D

88. B

CHAPTER 35

Knowledge Base for Patients with Integumentary Dysfunction

1.

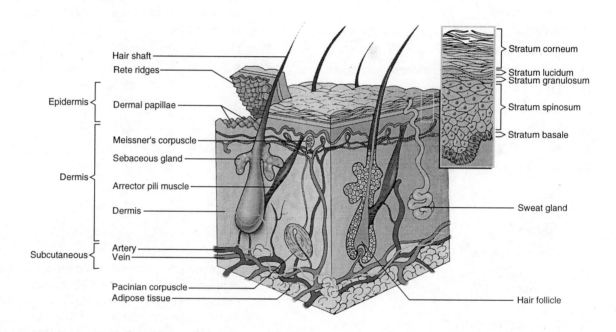

2. E
3. F
4. F
5. B
6. C
7. D
8. C
9. G
10. papule
11. staphylococcal
12. acne
13. hive, urticaria
14. eczema, impetigo
15. skin atrophy
16. itching
17. keratolytic
18. skin color, turgor, temperature, sensation
19. D
20. A
21. E
22. B
23. F
24. C
25. papule
26. pustule
27. cyst
28. ulcer
29. macule
30. true
31. true
32. true
33. true
34. true
35. false
36. true
37. true
38. B
39. A
40. C
41. D
42. A
43. B
44. A
45. D
46. C

47. A
48. B
49. B
50. C
51. B
52. C
53. C
54. C
55. A
56. Patient outcome: Spreading erythema around the graft is absent. Purulent drainage is absent. Foul odor from graft site is absent.

Interventions: Use aseptic technique. Change dressing as per order. Instruct patient on proper technique. Provide going-home instructions.
57. D
58. B
59. C
60. A
61. C
62. D
63. A
64. B
65. B
66. A
67. C
68. Wear pressure garments as directed over the recipient site. Elevate the upper arm to prevent swelling. Wear warm clothing, avoid exposure to sunlight or heat. Massage graft and donor site with lanolin to soften the skin, decrease itching, and increase circulation.

CHAPTER 36

Nursing Care of Patients with Integumentary Disorders

1. H
2. F
3. A
4. D
5. I
6. C
7. E
8. G
9. B
10. external

11. staphylococci or streptococci

12. dermatophyte (tinea) or nondermatophyte (yeast)

13. human papilloma virus

14. cutaneous

15. external

16. unrelieved pressure, shear

17. sun

18. true

19. false

20. false

21. true

22. true

23. true

24. true

25. false

26. B

27. C

28. B

29. C

30. E

31. B

32. C

33. B

34. C

35. A

36. C

37. A

38. C

39. C

40. B

41. C

42. A

43. C

44. C

45. C

46. Patient outcome: Skin lesions clear.

Interventions: Instruct patient to apply warm, moist compresses for 20 minutes t.i.d. Apply astringent compresses to promote crusting. Instruct in self-administration of antibiotics.

47. Patient outcome: Patient verbalizes anxiety. Patient discusses fear of malignancy. Patient states anxiety is reduced.

Interventions: Support patient during diagnostic and surgical procedures. Answer questions and correct misconceptions. Encourage patient to verbalize fears and concerns.

48. Patient outcome: Patient describes care of the wound. Wound heals without excessive scarring or infection.

Interventions: Instruct patient in care of wound. Instruct patient in specific type of solution and dressing to be used. Instruct patient to avoid activity that might disrupt the suture line.

49. A

50. B

51. C

52. B

53. A

54. C

55. C

56. B

57. C

58. A

59. C

60. A

61. A

62. D

63. C

64. A

65. A

66. A

67. D

CHAPTER 37

Nursing Care of Patients with Burns

1. What time did the injury occur? Was the victim in an enclosed space? How did the accident occur? Did the patient lose consciousness? Does the patient have any chronic illnesses?

2. Depth of the burn, size of the burn, part of the body burned, medical history, any other injuries

3. it is a quick and easy method to estimate the size of the burn

4. bloodstream into body tissues

5. 10, 50

6. thinner, deeper

7. respiratory

8. 3

9. debrided

10. hydrotherapy

11. comfort, scarring, graft adherence, and tissue growth

12. B

13. A

14. C

15. A

16. C

17. B

18. C

19. B

20. A

21. C

22. false

23. false

24. true

25. true

26. true

27. false

28. false

29. true

30. B

31. C

32. B

33. A

34. B

35. A

36. B

37. C

38. C

39. C

40. B

41. C

42. B

43. D

44. C

45. A

46. C

47. B

48. B

49. D

50. A

51. C

52. D

53. C

54. B

55. A

56. B

57. B

58. D

59. D

60. Patient outcome: Patient is alert, oriented, and able to follow commands. Patient has normal skin color. Patient's respirations are clear, unlabored, and >12 < 20.

    Interventions: Encourage deep breathing, administer high-flow oxygen as ordered. Observe for changes in level of consciousness. Monitor arterial blood gases. Monitor respiratory status and breath sounds to detect changes in condition.

61. Patient outcome: Patient is alert and oriented. Patient maintains adequate hydration.

    Interventions: Establish intravenous access. Administer and document fluid replacement. Insert Foley catheter and monitor output. Monitor vital signs. Monitor daily weights. Monitor lab results.

62. Patient outcome: Patient expresses relief from analgesics. Pain decreases in intensity as wounds heal.

    Interventions: Assess level of pain. Administer narcotic analgesics as needed. Monitor response to medication. Explain cause of pain and feelings of patient. Keep patient informed of need to do procedures. Explore use of other techniques to reduce anxiety and enhance pain relief.

63. C

64. C

65. A

66. C

67. C

68. A

69. B

70. B

71. C

72. B

73. A

74. A

75. C

76. A

77. all but C

78. C

79. C

80. A

81. all

82. A

CHAPTER 38

Knowledge Base for Men with Reproductive Dysfunction

1.

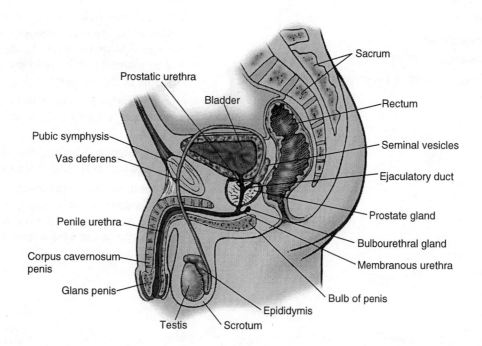

2. A
3. D
4. E
5. B
6. F
7. C
8. organ for copulation (sexual intercourse), urination
9. covers, protects, regulates the temperature of the testes
10. reproductive
11. epididymis and vas deferens
12. urine and semen
13. retention
14. prostate gland
15. sterilization
16. aspermia (to determine if sperm are being produced)
17. pain
18. 75%
19. false
20. true
21. true
22. false
23. true
24. true
25. false
26. false
27. false
28. true
29. B
30. D
31. A
32. B
33. C
34. C
35. B
36. all
37. C
38. B
39. C
40. D
41. B
42. B
43. C

44. A, C, D, E
45. C
46. B
47. A
48. C
49. A
50. A
51. B
52. B
53. C
54. Patient outcome: Patient expresses thoughts and concerns. Patient states that anxiety is decreased.

    Interventions: Acknowledge that his anxiety is normal. Encourage expression of his feelings. Assure the patient that his privacy will be maintained. Explain the normal outcome of this surgery.
55. Nursing diagnosis: Potential urinary retention related to obstruction of drainage catheter

    Patient outcome: Urinary drainage tubes remain patent and output is adequate.

    Interventions: Maintain the flow of the normal saline irrigant. Empty the urinary drainage bag frequently. Keep the tube in a straight line, avoid kinks. Irrigate the catheter as ordered.
56. B
57. C
58. B
59. A
60. C
61. B

CHAPTER 39

Nursing Care of Men with Reproductive Disorders

1. D
2. E
3. B
4. C
5. A
6. G
7. F
8. circumcision
9. manual reduction

10. cryptorchidism; varicocele

11. infection, hydrocele

12. medications, chronic diseases, disorders of the reproductive tract

13. testicular

14. aging; testicular

15. second

16. true

17. true

18. true

19. true

20. true

21. true

22. true

23. true

24. true

25. true

26. D

27. B

28. A

29. C

30. B

31. C

32. A

33. D

34. A

35. B

36. D

37. B

38. C

39. B

40. A

41. B

42. D

43. A

44. B

45. B

46. C

47. C

48. D

49. D

50. A

51. C

52. D

53. C

54. D

55. B

56. C

57. A

58. C

59. E

60. Explain the cause of epididymitis. Stress the need to take entire course of antibiotics. Maintain daily fluid intake of 2000 cc. Empty bladder frequently. Use ice packs as ordered. Elevate scrotum if swelling is present. Have him monitor temperature and take antipyretic as needed.

61. Nursing diagnosis: Pain (penile) related to constricted, retracted foreskin

    Patient outcome: Patient states relief of pain is obtained.

    Interventions: Administer a narcotic analgesic prior to reduction. Instruct the patient to elevate the penis after treatment. Apply cool compresses for edema and discomfort.

62. Patient outcome: Patient identifies alternative ways of dealing with sexual expression.

    Interventions: Encourage patient to express his concerns. Provide privacy for visits between patient and partner. Encourage alternative methods of sexual expression. Refer patient to a sex therapist or counselor if needed.

63. A

64. B

65. C

66. A

67. D

68. D

69. B

70. A

71. A

72. B

73. B

74. B

75. B

CHAPTER 40

Knowledge Base for Women with Reproductive Dysfunction

1.

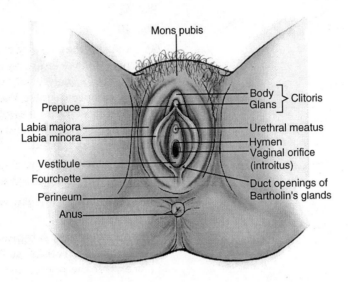

2.

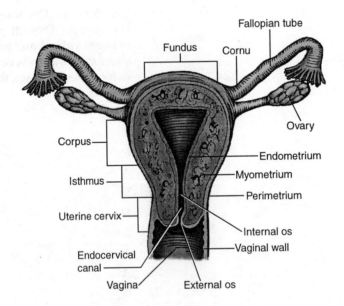

3. vagina
4. uterus
5. ligaments
6. fallopian tubes
7. ovaries
8. perimenopause
9. illness, fatigue, stress, anxiety, environmental change
10. hot flashes, insomnia, weakness, dizzy spells, palpitations, nervousness, headaches, weight gain
11. C
12. A
13. B
14. D
15. false
16. true
17. true
18. true
19. true
20. true
21. true
22. true
23. false
24. true
25. C
26. E
27. G
28. F
29. A
30. D
31. B
32. true
33. true
34. true
35. true
36. false
37. false
38. C
39. D
40. B
41. F
42. B
43. A

44. E
45. B
46. D
47. A
48. A
49. D
50. A
51. D
52. B
53. C
54. C
55. A
56. D
57. A
58. Patient outcome: Patient defines menopause. Patient can describe effects of menopause on lifestyle. Patient can describe the health practices relevant to the menopausal woman.

    Interventions: Explain what menopause is, discuss symptoms and treatment options. Instruct patient in related health-care practices. Provide information to prevent misconceptions. Provide information about hormone replacement therapy.
59. Patient outcome: Patient expresses feelings of anxiety.

    Interventions: Provide patient with needed information. Encourage patient to express feelings. Provide privacy for communication. Explore coping strategies.
60. A
61. C
62. B
63. C
64. A, B
65. B
66. C
67. C, D
68. A
69. C
70. C
71. C
72. B
73. C

CHAPTER 41

Nursing Care of Women with Reproductive Disorders

1.   C
2.   B
3.   D
4.   E
5.   B
6.   G
7.   F
8.   leukorrhea
9.   fever; vomiting; diarrhea; muscle aches; shock; impaired cardiopulmonary, hepatic, and renal function
10. menstruation
11. GI symptoms, breast swelling, tenderness, pain, neurologic sensitivities, tachycardia, back pain, joint pain, emotional symptoms (Table 41-2)
12. dysmenorrhea
13. childbirth
14. bladder or rectum
15. cervix
16. false
17. true
18. true
19. false
20. true
21. true
22. false
23. false
24. false
25. true
26. B
27. D
28. A
29. C
30. A
31. B
32. E
33. D
34. A
35. A
36. C
37. B
38. A

39. C
40. D
41. C
42. B
43. B
44. C
45. C
46. A
47. A,B,C,E
48. A,C,E,F
49. B
50. C
51. C
52. A
53. D
54. B
55. A
56. B
57. C
58. C
59. A
60. C
61. B
62. B
63. A
64. E
65. C
66. E
67. A
68. B
69. A
70. Patient outcome: Patient identifies the disease as real and identifies ways to cope with it.

     Interventions: Affirm that the disease is real and other women suffer from it. Explain the role of stress and PMS. Explore family support and coping strategies.
71. Rest/activity: adequate rest, naps, with periods of exercise

     Diet: high in protein, complex CHO, green vegetables

     Fluid: limit

     Anxiety: avoid tobacco, coffee, caffeine

72. Suture line remains intact.

    Interventions: Use a low-Fowler's or side-lying position. Place a pillow to support back and between the knees. Have the patient use a trapeze bar to move in bed. Use bed cradle. Prevent constipation to prevent pressure on the suture line.

73. Patient demonstrates interest in appearance.

    Interventions: Allow patient to express feelings. Discuss the meaning of the surgery to the patient. Discuss coping strategies. Elicit family support.

74. Patient describes radiation procedures that will be observed by staff and visitors.

    Interventions: Patient will be on bed rest with catheter and low-residue diet. Explain limited contact by staff and visitors. Explain that nausea, vaginal cramps, and discharge are normal.

75. C
76. B
77. C
78. C
79. A
80. A
81. B
82. C
83. A
84. A
85. A
86. B
87. C

CHAPTER 42

Nursing Care of Patients with Breast Disorders

1. glandular, fibrous, fat
2. fibrous
3. prolactin, growth
4. involution
5. upright then supine
6. family history of breast cancer; early menarche; delayed pregnancy; environmental factors; estrogen therapy
7. monthly
8. *Staphylococcus aureus*
9. fibroadenomas
10. estrogen
11. mammoplasty
12. C
13. A
14. D
15. B
16. E
17. true
18. false
19. false
20. false
21. false
22. true
23. true
24. true
25. true
26. B
27. A
28. B
29. D
30. B
31. C
32. C
33. C
34. B
35. D
36. B
37. B
38. A
39. C
40. D
41. C
42. A
43. D
44. A
45. Patient outcome: Patient states reason for surgery, pre- and postoperative activities.

    Interventions: Review all information on procedure with patient. Clarify the postoperative appearance. Demonstrate breathing exercises. Demonstrate arm exercises. Explain all postoperative equipment.

46. A
47. B
48. C
49. B
50. B

51. B
52. D
53. C
54. A
55. C
56. B

CHAPTER 43

Nursing Care of Patients with Sexually Transmitted Diseases

1. C
2. D
3. A
4. B
5. B, F
6. B
7. C
8. G
9. D
10. A
11. E
12. vulvovaginal itching
13. acidotic
14. penicillin G
15. skin-to-skin
16. topical application of podophyllin or cryosurgery
17. itching
18. application of Kwell
19. exposure to heat, stress, sexual intercourse
20. Chlamydia
21. true
22. false
23. true
24. true
25. true
26. false
27. false
28. false
29. false
30. true
31. true
32. true
33. all
34. B, C, E

35. A
36. B
37. C
38. C
39. A
40. D
41. D
42. B
43. B
44. A
45. C
46. D
47. C
48. B
49. A
50. C
51. D
52. C
53. A
54. B
55. C
56. B
57. A
58. B
59. D
60. B
61. C
62. D
63. D
64. Patient outcome: Patient describes changes in lifestyle that may prevent a recurrence.

    Interventions: Identify strategies for self-management to help patient feel in control of this disease. Review the factors that may precipitate outbreaks. Discuss with the patient the need to inform prospective partners about the disease.
65. Patient outcome: Participants can state cause and mode of transmission of STDs. Participants can state methods to prevent transmission to others.

    Interventions: Assess participants' learning needs and current level of understanding. Correct any misconceptions about the disease. Provide both written and verbal material to provide information and as a way of reinforcement later. Conduct a question-and-answer period.

66. Patient outcome: Patient lists potential long-term effects of untreated syphilis. Patient can state recommended treatment regimen.

    Interventions: Explain treatment plan and rationale in detail. Review all medications, dosage, and side effects. Discuss effects of untreated syphilis. Provide a resource to call if further questions occur. Caution patient to avoid sex until he or she is free from transmitting the disease.

67. Nursing diagnosis: Knowledge deficit related to ways to prevent recurrence of infection.

    Patient outcome: Patient identifies factors that may predispose her to infection. Patient describes methods for preventing recurrence of infection

    Interventions: Review the cause, symptoms, and treatment of infection. Review factors that promote growth of Candida. Review use of medications that may predispose to the development of Candida.

68. Patient outcome: Patient reports that using recommended measures reduces discomfort.

    Interventions: Review medications and treatment plan. Make sure patient uses all medication as ordered, not to stop when symptoms abate. Recommend cool compresses, sitz baths. Recommend use of cotton undergarments.

69. B

70. A

71. C

72. C

73. B

74. A

75. B

76. C

CHAPTER 44

Knowledge Base for Patients with Eye Dysfunctions

1.

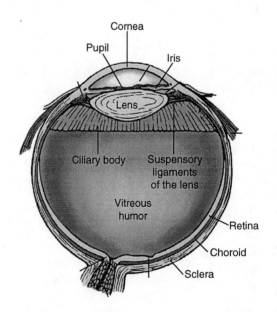

2. lacrimal

3. iris

4. choroid

5. retina

6. aqueous humor

7. lens

8. Light rays stimulate the retina and initiate the nervous impulses that travel to the optic nerve. They pass through the right or left optic tract to the geniculate nucleus of the thalamus where the neurons conduct the impulse to the right and left occipital lobe.

9. "Pupils equal, round, reactive to light and accommodation."

10. III, IV, VI

11. mydriatics, dilation

12. miotics, constriction

13. lower, aqueous humor

14. osmosis

15. keratoplasty

16. enucleation

17. B

18. D

19. A

20. C

21. F

22. E

23. F

24. E

25. D

26. B

27. C

28. A

29. A

30. C

31. B

32. D

33. true

34. false

35. true

36. false

37. true

38. true

39. true

40. A

41. B

42. C

43. A

44. A

45. C

46. B

47. B

48. B

49. D

50. A

51. B

52. C

53. B

54. A

55. Patient outcome: Patient will be able to describe the procedure and expected outcome.

    Interventions: Review the surgical procedure, describe the preoperative preparations (NPO, hair shampoo, draping during procedure, etc.), review the postoperative care, explain that improvement in vision may not be immediate

56. B

57. A

58. C

59. A

60. C

61. A,D,E

CHAPTER 45

Nursing Care of Patients with Eye Disorders

1. A

2. F

3. D

4. C

5. E

6. B

7. allergens, irritants
8. hyperemia
9. focusing
10. cornea
11. lens
12. glaucoma
13. A
14. C
15. D
16. B
17. E
18. F
19. true
20. true
21. false
22. false
23. true
24. D
25. D
26. B
27. C
28. A
29. E
30. B
31. B
32. D
33. A, B, D, E
34. B
35. D
36. A
37. A
38. C
39. B

40. D
41. B
42. C
43. C
44. D
45. A
46. C
47. A
48. Patient outcome: Patient reports improved visual acuity.

    Interventions: Use strict aseptic technique. Administer ophthalmic drops or ointments. Remove any drainage from eye, irrigate if needed. Follow universal precautions. Assess current visual acuity. Adjust the environment to facilitate independence.

49. Patient outcome: Patient's eye heals without evidence of trauma. Patient avoids injury.

    Interventions: Explain to patient how patching one eye changes depth perception. Use adaptive devices when necessary. Orient patient to surroundings. Keep call light within reach. Remove all environment hazards.

50. B
51. A
52. B,D
53. B
54. D
55. C
56. D
57. B
58. B
59. C

CHAPTER 46

Knowledge Base for Patients with Ear Dysfunction

1.

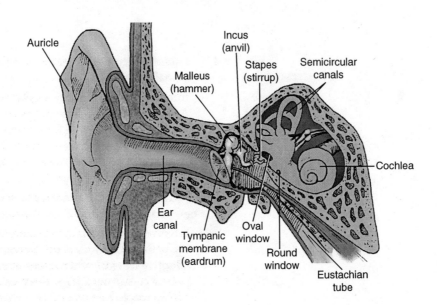

2.   A

3.   C

4.   D

5.   E

6.   B

7.   auricle (pinna) and the auditory meatus (ear canal)

8.   Air waves from the environment enter the external auditory canal and set the tympanic membrane in motion. The vibrations pass to the bony ossicle, through the oval window to the perilymph. Receptor cells in the cochlea are stimulated, which then send electric impulses to the brain.

9.   cochlea

10. Hertz (Hz)

11. decibels (db)

12. otoscope

13. B

14. C

15. A

16. D

17. A

18. E

19. C

20. B

21. F

22. true

23. true

24. false

25. true

26. true

27. false

28. true

29. D
30. all
31. A
32. B
33. A
34. B
35. D
36. B
37. C
38. C
39. A
40. B
41. A
42. D
43. B
44. A
45. D
46. B
47. Patient outcome: Patient reports no vertigo, dizziness, or unsteadiness and takes medications as ordered.

   Interventions: Administer medications as ordered. Explain purpose of medications. Explain that symptoms are not uncommon after surgery. Keep environment dim and quiet. Instruct patient to avoid sudden movements.
48. B
49. C
50. D
51. C
52. B
53. A
54. B
55. C
56. B
57. A ,D, E, F
58. D

CHAPTER 47

Nursing Care of Patients with Ear Disorders

1. B
2. A
3. D
4. H

5. G
6. F
7. E
8. C
9. C
10. D
11. B
12. A
13. pain
14. hole or tear
15. stapes
16. unknown
17. 90%
18. true
19. true
20. false
21. true
22. true
23. true
24. true
25. true
26. A
27. C
28. B
29. D
30. C
31. A
32. B
33. D
34. C
35. D
36. C
37. D
38. C
39. C
40. C
41. Patient outcome: Patient demonstrates ways to help open the eustachian tube and permit air to enter the middle ear.

   Interventions: Teach patient how to perform Valsalva maneuver, how to blow nose to open tubes, and to take decongestants as ordered.

42. Nursing diagnosis: Pain related to tissue disruption in the ear.

Patient outcome: Patient takes analgesic as prescribed, states relief of pain.

Interventions: Explain disease process and expected outcomes. Explain administration of analgesic. Explain other comfort measures.

43. Patient outcome: Patient expresses confidence in his ability to cope.

Interventions: Allow patient opportunities to express concerns, encourage independent problem-solving, and assist patient in identifying support systems.

44. Patient outcome: Patient instructs others on ways to increase effective communication.

Interventions: Provide quiet, calm environment. Face patient when speaking, speak slowly and clearly. Use normal conversational tone. Use gestures or written communication as needed.

45. C
46. A
47. B
48. C
49. A
50. C
51. A
52. B
53. D
54. D